Fundamentals of Chemotherapy

Fundamentals of Chemotherapy

William B. Pratt, M.D.

New York
Oxford University Press
London 1973 Toronto

Preface

Antibiotics and antimetabolites have played an important role as tools for the investigation of basic biochemical processes in the cell, and the use of these drugs by researchers has significantly expanded our knowledge of their mechanisms of action. In many cases, we are now able to explain the mechanisms by which a drug exerts its therapeutic effects at a depth of biochemical detail that extends to the direct interaction between the drug and its receptor. In some cases, the mechanisms of other clinically important drug effects such as toxicities, hypersensitivity phenomena, side effects, and idiosyncratic responses can be explained at a similar level of biological detail. In this discussion of the drugs used for the treatment of bacterial, fungal, and viral infections, parasitic infestations, and neoplastic disease, the emphasis is on the mechanisms of their effects.

The student's first exposure to the subject of chemotherapy was once largely a rote experience, which included the memorization of infecting organisms, drugs of choice, and long lists of undesirable toxicities, side effects, and drug interactions. In this text, I have tried to present chemotherapy as a logical application of the student's basic biological knowledge to the clinical management of infectious disease and cancer. The book is meant primarily for medical students and graduate students taking pharmacology courses. It is also meant for physicians, particularly those with a special interest in infectious disease, who would like to have available a brief and up-to-date reference on chemotherapy.

The book's chapters have been organized by grouping drugs according to their biochemical site of action. Thus, for example, the penicillins, the cephalosporins, vancomycin, ristocetin, cycloserine, and bacitracin, all inhibitors of cell wall synthesis, are considered together. But there are some instances when this organization cannot be utilized, as, for example, in the chemotherapy of parasitic infestations, because so little is known about the mechanism of action of many of the drugs. In most cases, the biochemical process affected by a drug is briefly described in the early part of the chapter, concurrently with the mechanism of the drug's action. References are listed at the end of each chapter.

The phenomena of drug resistance and drug interaction are given considerable space in this book. All known resistance mechanisms and drug interactions associated with each agent are not included; instead, I have chosen examples that illustrate fundamental principles in some detail. If he reaches the end of the book, the reader will have been exposed to most of the known basic mechanisms of resistance and to the numerous different ways that interactions between chemotherapeutic drugs take place. In addition, he will have encountered discussions of such general problems as multiple drug resistance, the use of resistant variants to determine mechanisms of drug action, and the large-scale emergence of resistant strains.

The amount of drug that should be administered to a patient is determined by a number of factors including his weight and age, his clinical state (for example, the presence of compromised renal or hepatic function, inability to take an oral preparation), and the etiology, anatomical location, and severity of the specific condition for which he is being treated. As this book is not a therapeutic guide, specific recommendations for drug dosage are not included. In special cases where unique properties of a drug (for example, extensive tissue binding, slow metabolism, unusual distribution, initial extreme reactions) determine an unusual dosage or regimen, specific recommendations for therapy are made. But this is only done when I have felt that fundamental concepts would be reinforced by showing how they are translated into an appropriate therapeutic regimen.

I am very grateful for the help and stimulation of my colleagues in the Department of Pharmacology at Stanford University and of the medical and graduate students in my classes. They have made this book possible. I am deeply indebted to Dr. Lewis Aronow, who read and provided a valuable commentary on the entire manuscript, and whose untiring patience was sincerely appreciated. I am also indebted to Dr. Avram Goldstein for his helpful criticism of major portions of the text. Moreover, I owe a great deal to both Dr. Aronow and Dr. Goldstein for their excellent teaching over a period of seven years. This book draws heavily on the concepts presented in their superb text, *Principles of Pharmacology* (A. Goldstein, L. Aronow, and S. M. Kalman, New York: Harper and Row, 1968). Many people have been kind enough to review parts of the manuscript dealing with specialized subjects, and I would like to thank Drs. John Frenster, Jean Grey, Dale Kaiser, Tag Mansour, and Leslie Wilson for their generous assistance. I would also like to thank Mrs. Diana Sickler for her efficient typing of the manuscript and my wife Dr. Diana Pratt for her labors in reading the proof.

New Haven, Connecticut   W. B. P.
October 1972

Acknowledgments

I would like to thank the authors, journals, and publishers for their permission to reprint the following figures and tables in this text:

Figs. 1-1, 1-2: D. D. Woods: "the biochemical mode of action of the sulfonamides," *J. Gen. Microbiol.* 29:687 (1962). Cambridge University Press

Fig. 2-1: C. L. Wisseman *et al., J. Bacteriol.* 67:662 (1954). American Society for Microbiology

Fig. 2-3: S. Pestka, *Proc. Natl. Acad. Sci.* 64:709 (1969). National Academy of Sciences

Fig. 2-4: H. K. Das *et al., Mol. Pharmacol.* 2:158 (1966). Academic Press, Inc.

Fig. 2-5: C. F. Weiss *et al., New Eng. J. Med.* 262:787 (1960). The Massachusetts Medical Society

Fig. 2-6: W. R. Best, *J.A.M.A.* 201:99 (1967). The American Medical Association

Figs. 5-4, 5-6, 5-7: J. L. Strominger *et al., Fed. Proc.* 26:9 (1967). Federation of American Societies for Experimental Biology

Fig. 5-5: M. Matsuhashi *et al., J. Biol. Chem.* 242:3191 (1967). American Society of Biological Chemists

Fig. 5-8: D. J. Tipper and J. L. Strominger, *Proc. Natl. Acad. Sci.* 54:1133 (1965). National Academy of Sciences

Fig. 5-10: B. B. Levine, *J. Exptl. Med.* 112:1131 (1960). The Rockefeller University Press

Fig. 5-11: B. B. Levine and Z. Ovary, *J. Exptl. Med.* 114:875 (1961). The Rockefeller University Press

Fig. 5-12: B. C. Brown *et al., J.A.M.A.* 189:599 (1964). The American Medical Association

Fig. 6-1: S. C. Kinsky *et al., Biochim. Biophys. Acta* 152:174 (1968). Elsevier Publishing Co.

Fig. 7-1: L. T. Coggeshall, in *Textbook of Medicine,* ed. by P. B. Beeson and W. McDermott. W. B. Saunders Co., 1963

Fig. 7-3: H. Polet and C. F. Barr, *Am. J. Trop. Med. Hyg.* 17:672 (1968). American Society of Tropical Medicine and Hygiene

Fig. 7-4: S. N. Cohen and K. L. Yielding, *Proc. Natl. Acad. Sci.* 54:522 (1965). National Academy of Sciences

Fig. 7-5: S. N. Cohen and K. L. Yielding, *J. Biol. Chem.* 240:3123 (1965). American Society of Biological Chemists

Fig. 7-6: S. N. Cohen and K. L. Yielding, *J. Biol. Chem.* 240:3123 (1965). American Society of Biological Chemists

Fig. 7-8: E. Beutler, *J. Lab. Clin. Med.* 49:84 (1957). The C.V. Mosby Co.

Fig. 7-12: I. M. Rollo, *Brit. J. Pharmacol.* 10:208 (1955). The Macmillan Co.

Fig. 8-3: A. P. Grollman, *J. Biol. Chem.* 243:4089 (1968). American Society of Biological Chemists

Fig. 8-5: T. E. Mansour and E. Bueding, *Brit. J. Pharmacol.* 9:459 (1954). The Macmillan Co.

Fig. 8-6: S. Norton and E. J. deBeer, *Am. J. Trop. Med. Hyg.* 6:898 (1957). American Society of Tropical Medicine and Hygiene

Fig. 9-2: C. E. Hoffmann et al., *J. Bacteriol* 90:623 (1965). American Society for Microbiology

Fig. 10-4: K. W. Kohn et al., *J. Mol. Biol.* 19:266 (1966). Academic Press, Inc.

Fig. 10-5: P. D. Lawley and P. Brookes, *Nature* 206:480 (1965). The Macmillan Co.

Fig. 10-11: H. M. Sobell et al., *Cold Spring Harbor Symp.* Vol 36. The Cold Spring Harbor Laboratory of Quantitative Biology

Fig. 10-12: H. M. Sobell and S. C. Jain, *J. Mol. Biol.* in press. Academic Press, Inc.

Table 1-1: B. Wolf and R. D. Hotchkiss, *Biochemistry* 2:145 (1963). American Chemical Society

Table 1-2: L. Weinstein, in *The Pharmacological Basis of Therapeutics*, ed. by L. S. Goodman and A. Gilman. The Macmillan Co., 1965, p. 117q.

Table 1-3: T. Watanabe, *Bacteriol. Rev.* 27:87 (1963). American Society for Microbiology

Table 2-1: D. Vazquez, *Nature* 203:257 (1964). The Macmillan Co.

Table 2-2: A. G. So and E. W. Davie, *Biochemistry* 2:132 (1963). American Chemical Society

Table 2-3: A. A. Ynis and G. R. Bloomberg, *Progress in Hematology* 4:138 (1964). Grune and Stratton, Inc.

Table 3-1: J. E. Davies, *Proc. Natl. Acad. Sci.* 51:659 (1964). National Academy of Sciences

Tables 3-2 and 3-3: M. Ozaki et al., *Nature* 222:333 (1969). The Macmillan Co.

Table 3-4: J. Daviet et al., *Mol. Pharmacol.* 1:93 (1965). Academic Press, Inc.

Tables 3-5, 4-3, 5-4, 6-3: *The Medical Letter* 13:39 (1971).

Table 3-6: J. C. Gingell and P. M. Waterworth, *Brit. Med. J.* 2:19 (1968).

Table 4-1: I. Suzuka et al., *Proc. Natl. Acad. Sci.* 55:1483 (1966). National Academy of Sciences

Table 4-2: S. Sarkar and R. E. Thach, *Proc. Natl. Acad. Sci.* 60:1481 (1968). National Academy of Sciences

Table 5-1: S. G. Nathenson and J. L. Strominger, *J. Pharmacol. Exp. Therap.* 131:1 (1961). The Williams & Wilkins Co.

Table 5-2: J. S. Anderson et al., *Proc. Natl. Acad. Sci.* 53:881 (1965). National Academy of Sciences

Table 5-3: G. Siewert and J. L. Strominger, *Proc. Natl. Acad. Sci.* 57:767 (1967). National Academy of Sciences

Table 5-5: *The Medical Letter* Vol. 14, No. 2, Issue 340 (1972).

Table 5-6: R. P. Novick, *Biochem. J.* 83:229 (1962). The Biochemical Society

Table 5-7: F. F. Barrett et al., *New Eng. J. Med.* 279:441 (1968). The Massachusetts Medical Society

Table 6-1: S. C. Kinsky, *Proc. Natl. Acad. Sci.* 48:1049 (1962). National Academy of Sciences

Table 6-2: D. S. Feingold, *Biochem. Biophys. Res. Commun.* 19:261 (1965). Academic Press, Inc.

Tables 6-3, 8-1, 8-5, 10-2, 10-3: *Medical Letter Reference Handbook* (1971). Drug and Therapeutic Information, Inc.

Table 8-4: E. Bueding and T. E. Mansour, *Brit. J. Pharmacol.* 12:159 (1957). The Macmillan Co.

Table III-1: M. R. Hilleman, *Science* 164:506 (1969). American Association for the Advancement of Science

Table 9-1: S. E. Luria and J. E. Darnell, *General Virology* (2nd ed.). John Wiley & Sons

Table 9-2: E. DeClercq and T. Merigan, *Ann. Rev. Med.* 21:17 (1970). Annual Reviews, Inc.

Table 9-3: A. W. Galbraith et al., *Lancet* 2:1026 (1969).

Contents

Part I
Drugs Employed in the Treatment of Bacterial and Fungal Infection

Introduction

In the chemotherapy of infectious disease, the goal is to assist the body in ridding itself of the infecting organism. This is done most effectively by exploiting differences between the biochemistry of the infecting agent and the host. The differential effect is known as "selective toxicity." It enables the physician to inhibit the growth of (or kill) the bacterium, fungus, virus, or parasite without seriously impairing the normal biochemical functions of the patient.

The use of a chemotherapeutic agent in the treatment of an infection allows the normal host defense mechanisms to gain control in their battle to eliminate the infecting agent. Most infections do not require therapy; they are taken care of by a person's defense mechanisms, and he may never become conscious of them. Infections are combatted in an orchestrated manner by a number of host mechanisms, such as antibody production, phagocytosis, interferon production, fibrosis, and gastrointestinal rejection reactions (e.g. vomiting and diarrhea). Sometimes, however, the host's ability to respond to infection is diminished. In a patient with diabetes, neoplastic disease, or any debilitating condition, these normal defense processes may be seriously weakened, and the therapeutic problem may become very complicated. Similarly, when a patient is being treated with immunosuppressive drugs, normal resistance to infection is depressed, and almost total reliance must be placed on the chemotherapeutic effect unaided by immunological responses.

The drugs used to treat bacterial infection may be divided into two groups. Some (e.g. the sulfonamides, chloramphenicol, erythromycin) are bacteriostatic; they inhibit bacterial cell replication, but, if the drug is withdrawn, bacterial growth can resume. Some (e.g. the penicillins) are bactericidal; they cause cell death and lysis. These effects are illustrated in Figure I-1. Treatment with a bacteriostatic agent stops bacterial growth, thereby allowing the host defenses to catch up in their battle. Treatment with a bactericidal agent superimposes the killing effect of the drug on the effects of host defenses. In a suppurative lesion, necrosis of

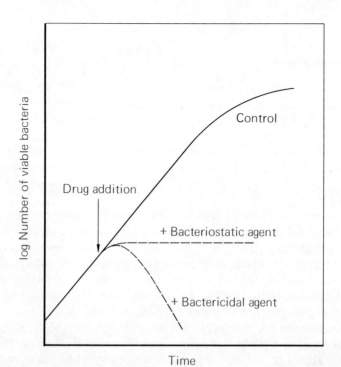

Figure I-1 Bacteriostatic and bactericidal effects of antibiotics. A suspension of bacteria in the log phase of growth is divided into three parts. A bacteriostatic drug such as chloramphenicol is added to one culture and a bactericidal agent such as penicillin to another; the third is a control. At various times, samples are taken from each culture, diluted, and plated on agar with new growth medium. The number of colonies obtained is a measure of the number of viable cells per culture. *BUT IN HOST CURVES CLOSER*

phagocytes interferes with the host's ability to kill bacteria. There is thus a poor response to bacteriostatic agents, and a bactericidal drug should be chosen. The same is true if there is severe depression of host immunological defense mechanisms.

NB

1. PUS
2. immune response

4

Chapter 1

The Antimetabolites
The Sulfonamides
The Sulfones
PAS

Discovery and Structure of the Sulfonamides

Sulfonamide-containing compounds were synthesized early in this century by German chemists for use as dyes. Their therapeutic potential was not exploited until 1935, when Domagk demonstrated that one of these dyes, prontosil, was effective in treating mice infected with streptococci. Later it was found that prontosil is metabolized in the tissues to para-aminobenzenesulfonamide, the chemotherapeutically active part of the molecule. Subsequently, thousands of compounds were synthesized, and many were introduced for the treatment of infection.

The sulfonamides are structural analogs of para-aminobenzoic acid (PABA). They differ from each other according to various substitutions on the sulfonamide group. The most active of the many sulfonamide compounds synthesized are those with a pK_a of about 6.5.

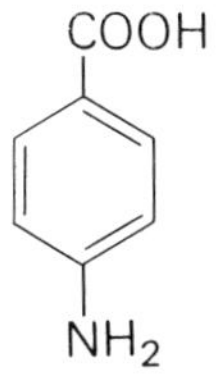

COOH

NH_2

para-Aminobenzoic acid

SO_2NHR

NH

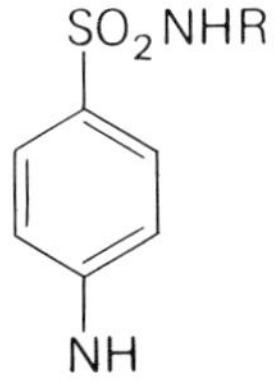

Sulfonamides

Mechanism of Action

The Sulfonamides

The sulfonamides are bacteriostatic agents. When they are added to a culture of bacteria, there is a delay period of several cell replications before there is inhibition of growth (Figure 1-1). These drugs arrest cell growth by inhibiting the synthesis of folic acid by the bacterium. During the delay period, before cell growth is arrested, the bacterium is exhausting its stores of folic acid.

Folic acid is required for growth by both bacterial and mammalian cells. Because animal cells are unable to synthesize folate, this compound must be supplied in the diet. Folic acid is taken into mammalian cells by an active transport mechanism. It does not enter most bacterial cells; these bacteria therefore must syn-

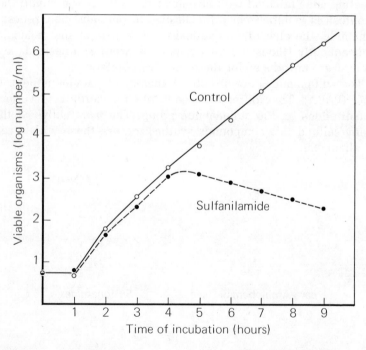

Figure 1-1 Early growth of hemolytic streptococci in blood broth without (o-o) and with (●--●) $10^{-5}M$ sulfanilamide. (From Woods.[1])

thesize the compound intracellularly. This difference between the biochemistry of the bacterial and mammalian cell is the basis of the selective toxicity of the sulfonamides, para-aminosalicylic acid, and the sulfones.

A reduced form of folic acid functions as a coenzyme, which transports one-carbon units from one molecule to another. Such one-carbon transfer reactions are essential for the synthesis of thymidine, all of the purines, and several amino acids. Thymidine is necessary for DNA synthesis, and the purines are necessary for all nucleic acid synthesis in the cell. When folate synthesis is inhibited, cell growth is arrested due to the cell's inability to synthesize these essential macromolecular precursors.

Folic acid consists of a pteridine unit, PABA, and glutamate. It was postulated some time ago that the sulfonamides, being structural analogs of PABA, might compete for the incorporation of this subunit into the folate molecule. Also, it was demonstrated

pteridine moiety   PABA

Folic acid

that the effect of sulfonamides in bacteria capable of taking up folic acid could be reversed in a non-competitive manner by adding to the culture the products of the inhibited reaction sequence such as folic acid or leucovorin, a reduced and methylated form of folic acid. If the mechanism of growth inhibition by the sulfonamides is competition for PABA, then increasing the level of PABA in the culture medium should reverse the action of sulfonamide in a competitive manner. Figure 1-2 shows these effects in cultures of *Clostridium tetanomorphum*. Folic acid can enter these

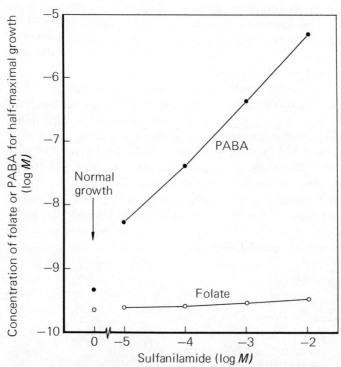

Figure 1-2 The requirement of *Clostridium tetanomorphum* for para-amino-benzoic acid or folic acid for growth in the presence of varying concentrations of sulfanilamide. Para-aminobenzoic acid (●-●); folic acid (o-o). From Woods.[1]

cells, and, in the presence of folic acid sufficient to maintain normal growth, the cell is not affected by any concentration of sulfonamide. In the presence of increasing concentrations of sulfanilamide, however, higher and higher concentrations of PABA are required to maintain growth.

The development of a cell-free system from bacteria that can form folate compounds from pteridines, PABA, and glutamic acid has permitted us to take a closer look at the mechanism of sulfonamide action. Sulfonamides inhibit the incorporation of PABA into dihydropteroic acid in such a system, but inhibition is not solely competitive.[2] If sulfathiazole and PABA are added to the *in vitro* system simultaneously, then competition can be demonstrated. If the enzyme system is first preincubated with sulfathiazole, then PABA cannot completely reverse the inhibitory effect of the drug. The enzyme system incorporates sulfonamide into a sulfonamide-containing analog of folic acid, and it is postulated that this product might itself be an inhibitor of the enzyme system. Therefore, the sulfonamides inhibit folic acid synthesis in two ways; the more important is competitive inhibition of PABA utilization. The enzyme that directs the incorporation of PABA and the pteridine moiety into dihydropteroic acid (dihydropteroate synthetase) has been purified 50-fold,[3] and definitive studies of the mechanism of sulfonamide action at the receptor level can now be carried out.

The inhibition of cell growth by sulfonamides may be reversed by adding the end products of one-carbon transfer reactions (thymidine, purines, methionine, and serine) to the growth medium. This reversal is of some clinical significance; in purulent infections the pus may contain a considerable amount of these substances as a result of cell breakdown. This may substantially decrease the efficacy of the sulfonamides in the treatment of these infections.[4]

PAS and the Sulfones

Para-aminosalicylic acid (PAS) and the sulfones are also structural analogs of PABA, and their bacteriostatic action is antagonized by PABA[5,6]; also PAS, like the sulfonamides, is joined to a pteroic acid moiety by the bacterial enzyme systems to produce PAS-containing folate analogs.[7]

para-Aminosalicylic acid

Diaminodiphenylsulfone
(dapsone)

There is a great deal of difference between the spectrum of antibacterial action of PAS and that of the sulfonamides. PAS is an effective bacteriostatic drug in *Mycobacterium tuberculosis*, but most organisms are not very sensitive to this compound. Sulfonamides are ineffective against *M. tuberculosis*, but they inhibit a number of organisms that are quite insensitive to PAS. There may be considerable variation in bacteria with regard to their relative permeability to these agents, but this cannot entirely explain the different sensitivities seen. As both the sulfonamides and PAS inhibit growth by competing for PABA, it seems entirely possible that the enzyme responsible for incorporating PABA into the folate molecule may vary considerably from one type of bacterium to another. Thus the PABA substrate site in *M. tuberculosis* may preferentially accept PAS over the sulfonamides. In other organisms this same site may have another configuration allowing a good fit for PABA and the sulfonamides but not for PAS. This possibility is suggested by work carried out with mutant strains of pneumococci which demonstrated varying degrees of resistance to the sulfonamides.[8] Cell-free extracts of the resistant cells, which incorporated PABA into folic acid, were found to require higher concentrations of sulfanilamide for inhibition of folate production than the wild type.[9] As shown in Table 1-1, the concentration of PAS required for inhibition of *in vitro* folate synthesis was higher in one strain than the wild type; but in the other resistant strain the enzyme was ten times more sensitive to PAS. Other experiments demonstrated that one of the altered

Table 1-1 **Relative effect of sulfanilamide and PAS in inhibiting folic acid synthesis in cell-free extracts of *Pneumococci***
Cell-free extracts were prepared from two sulfanilamide-resistant strains of *Pneumococci* and a wild type. The concentration of sulfanilamide or PAS required to reduce folic acid synthesis in each incubation to a fixed quantity was compared to that required for inhibition of the enzyme system from the wild type to the same level. (Data from Wolf and Hotchkiss.[9])

Strain	Sulfanilamide	PAS
Wild type	1	1
Fa	4	7.5
Fd	7	0.1

enzymes (Fd) was heat sensitive and had an affinity for PABA that differed from that of the wild-type enzyme. A model system is available, therefore, which allows us to test whether some of the great differences in sensitivity of different bacteria to growth inhibition by various members of three groups of drugs (the sulfonamides, PAS, and the sulfones) that act in a similar manner at the same receptor site may be explained by genetically determined variations in the structure of the receptor site.

Therapeutic Indications

The role of the sulfonamides in the chemotherapy of bacterial infection has diminished continually as newer, more effective antibiotics have been introduced. Sulfonamides are still useful in the treatment of acute urinary tract infections. In rheumatic patients who are hypersensitive to the penicillins, the sulfonamides may be used for prophylaxis against infection with Group A hemolytic streptococci. Although the penicillins are drugs of choice for meningococcal and Hemophilus infections, sulfonamides are useful alternatives. The combination of a sulfonamide and streptomycin is the treatment of choice for Nocardia infection. The sulfonamides are also useful in the treatment of melioidosis. In the past they were widely used in the treatment of acute bacillary dysentery, but the sulfonamides have now been supplanted by ampicillin and other antibiotics. The non-absorbable sulfonamides are employed to sterilize the bowel prior to colonic surgery (see Chapter 3). Lymphogranuloma venereum and trachoma both respond well to sulfonamides, but the tetracyclines are drugs of choice for these infections. The sulfonamides and sulfones are useful in the treatment of chloroquine-resistant Plasmodium falciparum infection—a role discussed in Chapter 7. Another sulfonamide-sensitive parasite is Toxoplasma gondii. Combined therapy with pyrimethamine and triple sulfonamides is the treatment of choice for toxoplasmosis.

The sulfones are the drugs of choice for the treatment of leprosy. These drugs are effective against a number of gram-positive and gram-negative bacteria, but because of their toxicity and the greater effectiveness of the antibiotics they are not used for treating bacterial infection other than that caused by *Mycobacterium leprae.*

PAS is used in the treatment of tuberculosis, and this application will be discussed later in the chapter.

Pharmacology of the Sulfonamides, PAS, and the Sulfones

all 3
P.101

Absorption and distribution. Most of the sulfonamides, PAS, and the sulfones are absorbed well from the gastrointestinal tract, and they are routinely given orally. The sulfonamides should not be topically administered, as this results in a fairly high incidence of allergic sensitization. There are exceptions to this rule, however. Sulfacetamide can be applied topically to the conjunctiva. Also, mafenide, a sulfonamide derivative, is employed for the topical treatment of burn infections. It is not known whether there is cross sensitivity between mafenide and other sulfonamides. Silver sulfadiazine is a new drug that will probably be of great value for the topical treatment of burns in the near future. The sulfonamides and sulfones are distributed throughout the tissues, and they enter the cerebrospinal fluid. PAS is distributed throughout the tissues and readily enters caseous tissue.[10]

NB

The sulfonamides belong to a large group of drugs that compete with bilirubin for plasma protein binding sites. Thus in the presence of sulfonamides less bilirubin is bound, and more of this compound circulates in the free form. The free bilirubin can pass the blood-brain barrier, and high concentrations in the brain of the newborn can cause kernicterus. If possible, therefore, another drug should be used for treating the newborn infant. As sulfonamides pass through the placenta and are excreted in the milk, they should not be administered during pregnancy approaching term or during nursing.

NB

Metabolism. The sulfonamides are metabolized extensively—primarily by acetylation. Isoniazid, one of the drugs used in combination with PAS for the treatment of tuberculosis, is extensively acetylated by the same mechanism as PAS. There is an interesting drug interaction between isoniazid and PAS at the level of the metabolizing enzymes. PAS inhibits the acetylation of isoniazid *in vitro*.[11] This *in vivo* effect results in higher blood levels of isoniazid in man.[12]

As there is a close structural similarity between PAS and salicylates such as aspirin, one might predict that PAS would have some analgesic or antipyretic effect and that drug interaction would occur when both agents are used simultaneously. This is not the case, however. PAS does not have an analgesic or antipyretic effect, and although it has been reported that very high concentrations of salicylic acid will antagonize the bacteriostatic effect of PAS *in vitro*[5], this is not of any clinical importance.

Excretion. The excretion of the sulfonamides is primarily renal. The sulfonamides are filtered and exhibit varying degrees of tubular reabsorption. In acid urine some sulfonamides are quite insoluble and will precipitate out in crystalline aggregates. This can easily lead to obstruction of the urinary tract. All patients who are receiving these drugs should have their urine sediment routinely examined for sulfonamide crystals. This problem of sulfonamide insolubility has been approached in three ways:

(1) The sulfonamides are more soluble in an alkaline urine (see Table 1-2), so bicarbonate or lactate can be administered. It is also necessary to maintain good urine output by a high fluid intake.

(2) Sulfonamide analogs with higher urine solubility have been synthesized to overcome this problem. Sulfisoxazole (gantrisin) is such a compound.

(3) Moderate doses of three different sulfonamides are administered simultaneously. The presence of one sulfonamide does

Table 1-2 **Solubility of sulfonamides in acidic and alkaline urine**
(Data from Weinstein.[13])

Drug	Urine pH	Urine solubility at 37°C (mg/100 ml)
Sulfadiazine	5.5	18
	7.5	200
Sulfamerazine	5.5	35
	7.5	160
Sulfisoxazole	5.5	150
	7.5	14,500

not decrease the solubility of another in the same aqueous solution. Thus, triple sulfonamides produce a higher total sulfonamide concentration than a single sulfonamide without causing crystalluria.

Toxicity and hypersensitivity. The sulfonamides are associated with such hypersensitivity phenomena as rashes, photosensitivity, drug fever, and, rarely, acute hemolytic anemia and Stevens-Johnson syndrome. Patients taking sulfonamides often experience some nausea and vomiting.

Three classes of drugs were developed by exploiting the side effects of the sulfonamides. It was observed that patients given sulfanilamide tended to develop metabolic acidosis with an alkaline urine. The finding that this was caused by the inhibition of carbonic anhydrase by sulfanilamide led to the development of acetazolamide and other diuretics of the carbonic anhydrase-inhibitor class. The observation that sulfonamide treatment caused hypoglycemia in some patients led to the development of the sulfonylurea group of oral antidiabetic agents. Finally, the observation that rats treated with sulfaguanidine developed goiters resulted in the development of the thiouracil group of antithyroid drugs. The interesting story of how side effects of the sulfonamides were exploited in the development of new drugs is related in detail by Goldstein *et al.*[14]

Long-term therapy with drugs capable of greatly reducing the bacterial population of the bowel (e.g. the sulfonamides, the aminoglycosides, the tetracyclines) may lead to a deficiency of vitamin K. Vitamin K is synthesized by microorganisms in the gut, and particularly if the dietary supply of the vitamin is inadequate, depletion of the gut flora can result in a deficiency of vitamin K and consequently of prothrombin and factors VII, IX, and X. This should be considered in patients who exhibit any bleeding tendency while taking these drugs. The condition will respond readily to small doses of vitamin K.

The sulfonamide preparations. Sulfadiazine, sulfamerazine, and sulfamethazine are rapid-acting sulfonamides with poor urine solubility. They are well absorbed in the gastrointestinal tract and are excreted rapidly. These drugs are often used in combination in triple sulfonamide therapy. Sulfisoxazole is also fast acting and in addition has a high urine solubility.

Sulfamethoxypyridazine, sulfadimethioxine, and the newer drug sulfameter were developed as long-acting drugs. They are long acting because they are excreted slowly. These drugs should certainly never be given in initial therapy, as the maintenance of high drug levels over a period of time is a distinct drawback if allergic reactions develop. Since the long action is not really of any great therapeutic advantage, there is probably no reason to employ these drugs.

Succinylsulfathiazole and phthalylsulfathiazole are nonabsorbable sulfonamides which are excreted almost entirely in the feces. In the past they have been used extensively for sterilizing the bowel prior to colonic surgery; they are usually used in combination with an antibiotic or an antifungal agent. Kanamycin and neomycin are now taking the place of the sulfonamides for prophylactic reduction of bowel flora (see Chapter 3).

Side effects of PAS and the sulfones. The most frequent side effect of PAS is irritation of the gastrointestinal tract. Liver damage and decreased iodine uptake with enlargement of the thyroid gland are also occasionally observed.

The sulfones are toxic and can cause a variety of drug reactions.[15] They often produce a non-hemolytic anemia and on occasion an acute hemolytic anemia. During the treatment of leprosy there may sometimes be an acute exacerbation of skin lesions with erythema, edema and flaking, acute neuritis, and fever.[16] These exacerbations can be serious, and permanent paralysis of the muscles supplied by the involved nerves may result. When this reaction occurs, sulfone therapy should be discontinued immediately and corticosteroid therapy instituted. The development of erythema nodosum is a common problem. If a patient has erythema nodosum associated with untreated leprosy, sulfone therapy should not be started until the reaction has regressed. At high dose levels liver damage is sometimes seen. Patients with leprosy who are treated for years with these drugs, must be kept under constant clinical supervision because of the anemia and other side effects that can develop.

Infectious, Multiple Drug Resistance

The Mechanism

At the end of World War II, the sulfonamides were introduced into Japan for the treatment of bacillary dysentery. As a result, the incidence of the disease decreased by about 80 per cent within two years.[17] After 1949, however, the incidence of dysentery rose above the level observed at the end of the war. This increased incidence of infection occurred despite the extensive use of sulfonamides; most of the *Shigella* strains isolated from cases at this time were found to be resistant to the drug. After 1952, newer antibiotics, such as streptomycin, chloramphenicol, and the tetracyclines, were employed for the treatment of the sulfonamide-resistant shigellae. With the advent of these newer drugs the number of dysentery patients fell somewhat, but within only four years it became clear that their therapeutic usefulness was also diminishing rapidly. After 1952 Japanese workers isolated one strain of *Shigella* from each dysentery epidemic and tested it for resistance to streptomycin, chloramphenicol, and the tetracyclines (see Table 1-3). By 1958 a number of the strains being recovered were simultaneously resistant to two or three of these antibiotics. Many of the strains listed in the table were resistant to sulfonamides as well.

In epidemiological studies *Shigella* strains isolated from some

Table 1-3   Antibiotic resistance in shigellae isolated from epidemics of bacillary dysentery in Japan

One strain of *Shigella* was isolated from each epidemic of bacillary dysentery occuring in Japan from 1953 to 1969 and tested for resistance to streptomycin (Sm), tetracycline (Tc), and chloramphenicol (Cm). (Data from Watanabe.[17])

| Year | Number of strains tested | Number of strains resistant to: | | | | | | |
		Sm	Tc	Cm	Sm, Cm	Sm, Tc	Cm, Tc	Sm, Cm, Tc
1953	4900	5	2	0	0	0	0	0
1956	4399	8	4	0	0	0	1	0
1958	6563	18	20	0	7	2	0	193
1960	3396	29	36	0	61	9	7	308

patients were completely sensitive while serologically identical strains isolated from other patients in the same epidemic were resistant to a number of drugs. Stool cultures from a single patient were sometimes found to contain both sensitive and multiple drug-resistant strains of the same serological type. Finally, it was observed that the administration of chloramphenicol alone to patients infected with sensitive *Shigella* could result in the appearance of organisms that were resistant to many drugs. These findings were tied together when one of the Japanese investigators postulated that multiple drug resistance might be transferred from multiple drug-resistant *Escherichia coli* to shigellae in the patient's intestinal tract. It was demonstrated that multiple drug-resistant *E. coli* could be cultured *in vitro* with sensitive *Shigella* and that the multiple resistance could then be transferred to the shigellae without the simultaneous transfer of a number of genetic markers that are a part of the genome of *E. coli*.[18]

We now understand many aspects of the transfer of multiple drug resistance.[19] The transfer of resistance requires cell to cell contact. Information for resistance is contained in extra-chromosomal pieces of DNA (although they can be integrated into the chromosome) that replicate autonomously and faster than the rest of the bacterial DNA. The plasmid or episome containing the information for multiple drug resistance is called an R-factor. In addition to the portion of DNA containing the information for drug resistance (the R-determinant) the R-factor includes a portion, called the RTF segment, that controls the transmission of the plasmid during bacterial conjugation. These two components may exist independently as closed circular DNA's or together as a complete R-factor.[20] These relationships are illustrated in Figure 1-3.

The Clinical and Epidemiological Problem

Infectious, multiple drug resistance has been transferred to such human pathogens as the agents of cholera, plague, and typhoid fever. Although clinical problems so far have been confined to multiple drug resistance in the common acute gastrointestinal infections, it is sobering to think of this phenom-

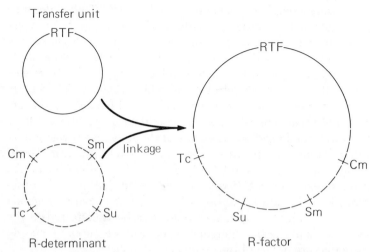

Figure 1-3 Diagram of an R-factor that contains information for determining resistance to tetracycline (Tc), sulfonamide (Su), streptomycin (Sm), and chloramphenicol (Cm). Genetic determinants for antibiotic resistance (R-determinants) can exist independently of the transfer factor or in combination with it.[19] The transfer unit contains the genetic information that directs the transfer of the whole plasmid during bacterial conjugation.

enon becoming prevalent in large-scale cholera or typhoid epidemics.

Multiple drug-resistance transfer has become increasingly widespread in the domestic livestock population. For about twenty years, it has been the practice to add antibiotics to the feed of livestock being fattened in feeder pens. The economic advantage of this practice has been clearly demonstrated. Antibiotics kill the microorganisms that commonly infect livestock living under crowded conditions and that depress the animals' rate of growth. But the prolonged use of antibiotics in animal feed results in the development of drug resistance in certain gram-negative organisms. In many cases the resistance is of the multiple drug type and is transferable.[21] As bacteria can be transferred from animals to man, many people feel that the drug resistance developing in the animal population could reduce the effectiveness of drug therapy in man. The prophylactic use of antibiotics in entire herds favors the spread of the very organisms they are intended to control. The use of antibiotics in animals has reached the point where the economic benefits of the practice and the potential risk to antibiotic therapy in humans must be carefully assessed. It may prove necessary to severely restrict this practice in the future.

The Chemotherapy of Tuberculosis

The treatment of tuberculosis is a special problem within the field of chemotherapy of bacterial infection. The disease requires a long course of treatment with multiple drugs. Many of the drugs find their only clinical application in the treatment of tuberculosis, and most of the effective drugs are quite toxic. The tubercle bacilli multiply in poorly vascularized caseous lesions that do not always receive high levels of the drugs. In addition, tubercle bacilli readily develop resistance to the drugs that are most effective against them.

The rapid emergence of drug resistance first prompted investigators to employ a combination of drugs in the therapy of tuberculosis. It was reasoned simply that the chance of resistance arising to two drugs is very much less than to a single drug. For example, if a bacterial strain produced a mutation for resistance to drug A at a rate of once in every 10^5 cell divisions and to drug B once in every 10^4 cell divisions, then simultaneous resistance to both drugs would be expected to occur with a frequency of once in every 10^9 cell divisions. The simultaneous use of two or more chemotherapeutic agents is the cornerstone of antituberculosis therapy.

The major drugs employed against tuberculosis are PAS, isoniazid, streptomycin, and ethambutol. Rifampin, a drug new to the U.S. market, may soon be included. If these drugs do not produce a good therapeutic response, then the less common and generally more toxic drugs must be employed. These include cycloserine, viomycin, pyrazinamide, kanamycin, capreomycin, and ethionamide. The mechanism of action and pharmacology of PAS have already been discussed. Both streptomycin and kanamycin are used for purposes other than the treatment of tuberculosis and are considered in detail in Chapter 3. Cycloserine, an inhibitor of bacterial cell wall synthesis, is discussed in Chapter 5.

Isoniazid. Isonicotinic acid hydrazide (INH) is the most useful of the antituberculosis agents. Despite many studies, which have been reviewed by Youatt,[22] the mechanism of action of this compound is unknown. One of the early metabolic responses to isoniazid is apparently an inhibition of carbohydrate metabolism. The drug produces an accumulation of phosphorylated hexoses in *Mycobacterium*, which may indicate inhibition of glycolysis.[23] Isoniazid is very specific for mycobacteria, having no activity against gram-positive or gram-negative bacteria, protozoa, or viruses. It is bactericidal.

Isoniazid is well absorbed from the intestine and is metabolized by acetylation, as is PAS. The rate of acetylation is subject to genetic variation.[24] When blood levels of isoniazid are recorded for a series of patients, two groups are found: patients who acetylate the drug rapidly and patients who do not. Patients in the first group may require larger doses to achieve appropriate serum

Isoniazid

$CONHNH_2$

levels. Peripheral neuritis is the principal toxic effect of isoniazid. This can be prevented by simultaneous administration of pyridoxine. Isoniazid can also cause hepatic dysfunction, and patients receiving the drug should be monitored for signs of liver toxicity. Preventive treatment for tuberculosis should be deferred in individuals with acute hepatic disease.

Ethambutol. This is the newest of the major antituberculosis drugs. Its mechanism of action is not known. A short time after the addition of ethambutol to a culture of mycobacteria, there is a decrease in the total cellular RNA. The effect of the drug in inhibiting growth is reversed by magnesium ion.[25] Ethambutol is given orally, and the greater part is excreted, unchanged, by the kidney. The chief side effect is a retrobulbar neuritis, with a loss of visual acuity and disburbances in color discrimination. Patients receiving this drug should be checked for these symptoms once a month.

$$\underset{\displaystyle \text{Ethambutol}}{H-\underset{\underset{C_2H_5}{|}}{\overset{\overset{CH_2OH}{|}}{C}}-NH-CH_2-CH_2-HN-\underset{\underset{C_2H_5}{|}}{\overset{\overset{CH_2OH}{|}}{C}}-H}$$

The use of the major drugs. A combination of two or three of the major drugs is used for initial intensive therapy of both pulmonary and extra-pulmonary tuberculosis. Virtually all the therapeutic regimens include isoniazid. This drug is very effective and has a relatively high therapeutic ratio. In two-drug regimens isoniazid is usually combined with PAS. In patients who cannot tolerate PAS (usually because of gastrointestinal distress) a combination of isoniazid and ethambutol is very effective. Many studies demonstrate that initial therapy should be carried out with a three-drug regimen, which usually includes isoniazid, PAS, and streptomycin[26] or isoniazid, ethambutol, and streptomycin. Streptomycin is very effective, but it has drawbacks: it must be given by deep intramuscular injection, which is often quite painful, and it can cause severe disturbances of balance and hearing (see Chapter 3). In the treatment of pulmonary tuberculosis, as soon as the sputum becomes negative streptomycin is usually stopped, and therapy continues with the two oral drugs. The minimum duration of treatment is about two years.

A special case of antibiotic prophylaxis is associated with tuberculosis. Because the risk of developing serious tuberculous disease (e.g. miliary tuberculosis or tuberculous meningitis) is especially severe in children, all children under the age of four who have a positive tuberculin test should receive prophylactic treatment. All tuberculin-positive people who are contacts of active cases and all people found to have recently changed from tuberculin negative to positive should receive chemoprophylaxis. The drug of choice for prophylaxis is isoniazid. It should be given for one year.

The use of the alternative drugs. In patients who have relapsed or who do not respond to initial intensive treatment with the major drugs, alternative drugs may be employed. The therapeutic margin of safety of many of these drugs is quite small, and great care must be exercised in their use.

Cycloserine. This drug is given orally. It has a severe, central nervous system toxicity, which can result in psychoses, convulsions, and coma (see Chapter 5).

Viomycin. Viomycin is given by intramuscular injection. It does not pass well into the cerebrospinal fluid. Its side effects include renal damage and vertigo and tinnitus.

Pyrazinamide. This drug is given orally. It causes liver damage and should be discontinued when disturbance of hepatic function is observed. Pyrazinamide also causes uric acid retention.

Ethionamide. Ethionamide is given orally, but it causes gastric irritation in many patients. Resistance to the drug emerges quite readily.

Kanamycin. This drug is a structural analog of streptomycin. Like streptomycin, it is given by intramuscular injection and can cause vertigo and deafness (see Chapter 3).

Capreomycin. Capreomycin is a mixture of several peptides isolated from Streptomyces capreolus. It is used in the retreatment of tuberculosis. The drug can cause loss of balance and hearing acuity; it has a mild renal toxicity.

Rifampin (rifampicin). Rifampin is one of a group of closely related antibiotics, called the rifamycins, which are produced by a strain of Streptomyces. Rifampin is available in the United States for the treatment of tuberculosis. There has been a great deal of experience with the use of this drug in Europe.

Our understanding of the mechanism of action of the rifamycins is fairly detailed. These drugs inhibit the synthesis of bacterial RNA[27] and bind to the RNA polymerase enzyme.[28] Experiments with rifampin have demonstrated that the initiation, not the continuation, of RNA synthesis is blocked by the drug.[29] It is clear that the effect on RNA polymerase is critical to the bactericidal effect of the drug, because the enzyme isolated from some resistant mutants does not bind the drug.[30] The polymerase enzyme is a very complex molecule with a number of subunits. It has been demonstrated by experiments in which polymerase was reconstituted from subunits prepared from rifampin-sensitive and rifampin-resistant enzymes that the core enzyme (β subunit), not the sigma factor, is affected by rifampin.[31] The mutant β subunit from resistant cells has demonstrably altered physical characteristics.[32] The selective toxicity of the rifamycins is explained by the fact that even high concentrations of rifampin do not affect the activity of human RNA polymerase[33] or the enzyme present in the nucleus of other eukaryotic cells.[34]

Rifampin is an effective drug for the oral treatment of tuberculosis. It has been used primarily in retreatment of tuberculosis after therapeutic failure with the major drugs. Rifampin has been so successful, however, that it is now being used for primary treatment. Two-drug primary therapy with rifampin and isoniazid, for example, was demonstrated in one study to be as effective as a three-drug regimen of isoniazid, streptomycin, and ethambutol.[35] In addition, there were fewer side effects. Resistance to rifampin does emerge, and it must, therefore, be used in combination with other drugs. It may turn out that rifampin is more toxic than present experience indicates. A few patients have experienced transient hearing loss, skin rashes, reversible increases in SGOT and alkaline phosphatase, reversible leukopenia, and, rarely, thrombocytopenia and purpura.[36] As rifampicin is eliminated mainly in the bile,[37] the risk of toxic effects is much higher in patients with liver disease; the dose should be lowered in these patients. At present, rifampicin seems to be quite safe compared to the other antituberculosis drugs. Its antituberculous activity is greater in animals than that of ethambutol.[38] Preliminary data suggest that rifampin may be as effective as isoniazid.[39] It is very effective in killing Mycobacterium leprae in experimental systems, and preliminary clinical studies indicate that the drug may be effective in treating leprosy.[40]

In closing this section it is worth noting that there seems to be a continuing decline of interest in research in antituberculosis therapy from a peak in the 1940s. With the advances that made chemotherapy the basis for treatment of tuberculosis, researchers' interest in the field naturally waned. Nonetheless, ideal agents for the treatment of tuberculosis have not yet been found, and we are still at a fairly primitive stage of development in this area. It would be very unfortunate if the interest in and funds for this research continue to decline.

References

1. D. D. Woods: The biochemical mode of action of the sulfonamides. *J. Gen. Microbiol.* 29:687 (1962).

2. G. M. Brown: The biosynthesis of folic acid: inhibition by sulfonamides. *J. Biol. Chem.* 237:536 (1962).

3. D. P. Richey and G. M. Brown: The biosynthesis of folic acid: Purification and properties of the enzymes required for the formation of dihydropteroic acid. *J. Biol. Chem.* 244:1582 (1969).

4. D. S. Feingold: Antimicrobial chemotherapeutic agents; the nature of their action and selective toxicity. *New Eng. J. Med.* 269:957 (1963).

5. H. Hurni: Über die quantitativen Verhältnisse bein Antagonisms zwischen p-Aminosalicylsaure (PAS) und p-Aminobenzoesaure (PABA). *Schweiz Z. Path. Bakt.* 12:282 (1949).

6. G. Brownlee, A. F. Green, and M. Woodbine: Sulfetrone; a chemotherapeutic agent for tuberculosis. *Brit. J. Pharmac. Chemother.* 3:15 (1948).

7. A Wacker, H. Kolm, and M. Ebert: Über den Stoffwechsel der p-Aminosalicylsaure und Salicylsaure bei *Enterococcus*. *Z. Naturforsch* 13b:147 (1958).

8. R. D. Hotchkiss and A. H. Evans: Fine structure of a genetically modified enzyme as revealed by relative affinities for modified substrate. *Fed. Proc.* 19:912 (1960).

9. B. Wolf and R. D. Hotchkiss: Genetically modified folic acid synthesizing enzymes of *Pneumococcus*. *Biochemistry* 2:145 (1963).

10. A. Heller, R. H. Ebert, D. Koch-Weser, and L. J. Roth: Studies with C^{14} labelled para-aminosalicylic acid and isoniazid. *Am. Rev. Tuberc.* 75:71 (1957).

11. W. J. Johnson: Biological acetylation of isoniazid. *Nature* 174:744 (1954).

12. W. Mandel, M. L. Cohn, W. F. Russell, and G. Middlebrook: Effect of para-aminosalicylic acid on serum isoniazid levels in man. *Proc. Soc. Exp. Biol. Med.* 91:409 (1956).

13. L. Weinstein: "Sulfonamides" in *The Pharmacological Basis of Therapeutics*, ed by L. S. Goodman and A. Gilman. New York; Macmillan, 1970, p. 1197.

14. A. Goldstein, L. Aronow and S. Kalman: Principles of Drug Action, New York: Harper and Row, 1968, pp. 783–791.
15. L. E. Millikan and E. R. Harrell: Drug reactions to the sulfones. Arch. Dermatol. 102:220 (1970).
16. J. R. Trautman: The management of leprosy and its complications. New Eng. J. Med. 273:756 (1965).
17. T. Watanabe: Infective heredity of multiple drug resistance in bacteria. Bacteriol. Rev. 27:87 (1963).
18. T. Akiba, K. Koyama, Y. Ishiki, S. Kimura, and J. Fukushima: On the mechanism of the development of multiple-drug-resistant clones of Shigella. Japan, J. Microb. 4:219 (1960).
19. T. Watanabe and T. Fukasawa: Episome-mediated transfer of drug resistance in Enterobacteriaceae, transfer of resistance factors by conjugation. J. Bacteriol. 81:669 (1961).
20. S. N. Cohen and C. A. Miller: Non-chromosomal antibiotic resistance in bacteria; molecular nature of R-factors isolated from Proteus mirabilis and Escherichia coli. J. Mol. Biol. 50:671 (1970).
21. E. S. Anderson: The ecology of transferable drug resistance in the enterobacteria. Ann. Rev. Microbiol. 22:131 (1968).
22. J. Youatt: A review of the action of isoniazid. Am. Rev. Resp. Dis. 99:729 (1969).
23. F. G. Winder, P. J. Brennan, and I. McDonnell: Effects of isoniazid on the composition of Mycobacteria, with particular reference to soluble carbohydrates and related substances. Biochem. J. 104:385 (1967).
24. D. A. P. Evans, K. A. Manley, and V. A. McKusick: Genetic control of isoniazid metabolism in man. Brit. Med. J. 2:485 (1960).
25. M. Forbes, E. A. Peets, and N. A. Kuck: Effect of ethambutol on Mycobacteria. Ann N.Y. Acad. Sci. 135:726 (1966).
26. W. Fox: Changing concepts in the chemotherapy of pulmonary tuberculosis. Am. Rev. Resp. Dis. 97:767 (1968).
27. G. Lancini, R. Pallanza, and L. G. Silvestri: Relationships between bactericidal effect and inhibition of ribonucleic acid nucleotidyltransferase by rifampicin in Escherichia coli K-12. J. Bacteriol. 97:761 (1969).
28. W. Wehrli, F. Knüsel, K. Schmid, and M. Staehelin: Interaction of rifamycin with bacterial RNA polymerase. Proc. Natl. Acad. Sci. 61:667 (1968).
29. A. Sippel and G. Hartman: Mode of action of rifamycin on the RNA polymerase reaction. Biochim Biophys. Acta 157:218 (1968).
30. E. di Mauro, L. Snyder, P. Marino, A. Lamberti, A. Coppo, and G. P. Tocchini-Valentini: Rifampicin sensitivity of the components of DNA-dependent RNA polymerase. Nature 222:533 (1969).
31. A. Heil and W. Zillig: Reconstitution of bacterial DNA-dependent RNA-polymerase from isolated subunits as a tool for the elucidation of the role of the subunits in transcription. FEBS Letters 11:165 (1970).

32. D. Rabussay and W. Zillig: A rifampicin resistant RNA-polymerase from *E. coli* altered in the β-subunit. *FEBS Letters* 5:104 (1969).

33. H. P. Voigt, R. Kaufmann, and H. Matthei: Solubilized DNA-dependent RNA polymerase from human placenta; a magnesium-dependent enzyme. *FEBS Letters* 10:257 (1970).

34. W. Wehrli, J. Nüesch, F. Knüsel and M. Staehelin: Action of rifamycins on RNA polymerase. *Biochim. Biophys. Acta* 157:215 (1968).

35. R. Newman, B. Doster, F. J. Murray, and S. Ferebee: Rifampin in initial treatment of pulmonary tuberculosis. *Am. Rev. Resp. Dis.* 103:461 (1971).

36. Rifampin and other drugs for treatment of tuberculosis. *Med. Letter* 13:73 (1971).

37. S. Furesz, R. Scotti, R. Pallanza, and E. Mapelli: Rifampicin: A new rifamycin III: Absorption, distribution, and elimination in man. *Arzneim.-Forsch.* 17:536 (1967).

38. F. Grumbach: Experimental *in vivo* studies of new antituberculosis drugs; capreomycin, ethambutol, rifampicin. *Tubercle* 50 Suppl: 12 (1969).

39. G. Canetti, M. le Lirzin, G. Porven, N. Rist, and F. Grumbach: Some comparative aspects of rifampicin and isoniazid. *Tubercle* 49:367 (1968).

40. R. J. W. Rees, J. M. H. Pearson and M. F. R. Waters: Experimental and clinical studies on rifampicin in treatment of leprosy. *Brit. Med. J.* 1:89 (1970).

Chapter 2
The Inhibitors
of Protein Synthesis I
Chloramphenicol
Erythromycin
Oleandomycin
Carbomycin
Lincomycin
Clindamycin

Introduction

Chemotherapeutic drugs have been discovered in a number of ways. Only rarely has their discovery been the result of logical design of a compound intended to interfere with a particular biochemical reaction in a predictable way. On occasion, drugs have been discovered by following up a chance observation in the laboratory. More often drugs used in the treatment of infectious disease have been discovered in search programs that screen chemicals and extracts of plants and fungi for antibacterial properties. These procedures, which are exceedingly repetitive, have yielded the bulk of the useful antibiotics. Chloramphenicol, erythromycin, streptomycin, and the tetracyclines were all isolated from soil actinomycetes discovered in large screening programs. Literally thousands of antibacterial compounds have been found in such screening programs, but the majority are not marketed either because they are too toxic to the patient or offer no advantages over antibiotics already in use.

The antibiotics chloramphenicol, erythromycin, oleandomycin, lincomycin, and clindamycin all inhibit bacterial protein synthesis, and they all bind to the 50 S subunit of the bacterial ribosome. These drugs are not all structural analogs of each other, and a knowledge of their structures does not afford any particular insight into their mechanisms of action at our current level of understanding. Structurally, the macrolide antibiotics (e.g., erythromycin, carbomycin, triacetyloleandomycin, and spiramycin) consist of a large lactone ring to which sugars are attached.

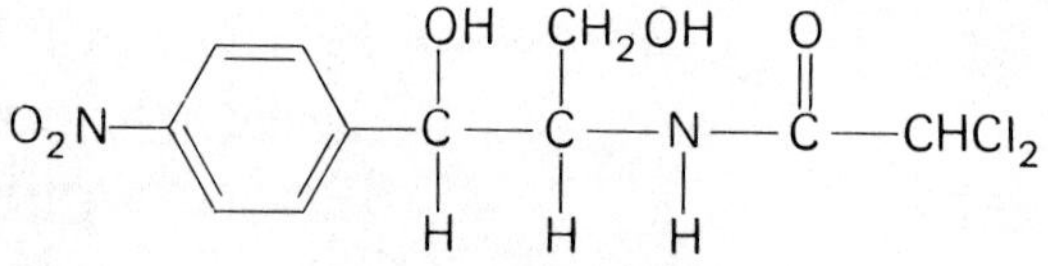

Chloramphenicol

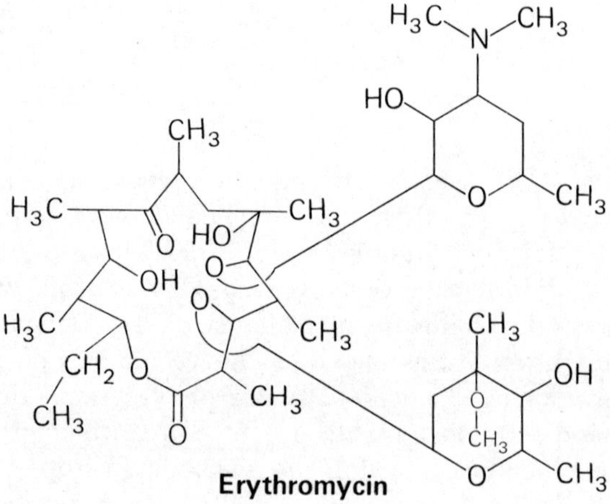

Erythromycin

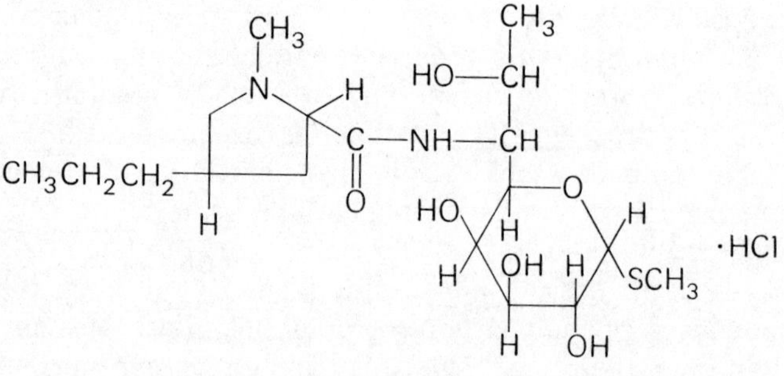

Lincomycin

Mechanism of Action

The Receptor

The extensive literature dealing with the mechanisms of action of chloramphenicol, erythromycin, and related drugs has been reviewed in detail by Weisblum and Davies.[1] The following discussion will focus on the mechansim of action of chloramphenicol as a representative member of this group, though this is not to imply that all the antibiotics that bind to the 50 S ribosomal subunit have the same mechanism of action at the molecular level.

It was demonstrated very early that exposure of bacteria to chloramphenicol caused an immediate cessation of protein synthesis with no immediate effect on the synthesis of nucleic acids (Figure 2-1).[2] There is a correlation between the ability of an

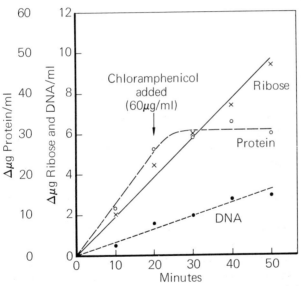

Figure 2-1 Chloramphenicol inhibition of protein synthesis in *Escherichia coli.* Chloramphenicol was added to *E. coli* in the logarithmic phase of growth, and portions of the culture were sampled at various time intervals and assayed for total cell protein and nucleic acid. The values represent the average of triplicate analyses expressed as increments in micrograms per milliliter over the initial concentration. (Reprinted from Wisseman *et al.*[2])

Table 2-1 Relationship between sensitivity to growth inhibition by chloramphenicol and the ability of isolated ribosomes to bind the radioactive-labeled drug

Here ^{14}C-labeled chloramphenicol was added to ribosome suspensions prepared from various sources, and the amount of drug bound was assayed by centrifuging the samples and determining the radioactivity in the ribosomal pellet. The results are expressed as picograms of chloramphenicol bound per milligram of ribosomes. (Data compiled from Vazquez[3])

Type of organism	Source of ribosomes	Response to chloramphenicol	Type of ribosome	In vitro binding to ribosomes
Bacteria	Staphylococcus aureus	Sensitive	70 S	18
	Bacillus megaterium	Sensitive	70 S	30
	Escherichia coli B	Sensitive	70 S	29
	Escherichia coli B 150	Resistant	70 S	30
Yeast	Saccharomyces fragilis	Resistant	80 S	
Protozoan	Strigomonas	Resistant	80 S	Less than 1
Mammal	Rat liver	—	80 S	

organism's ribosomes to bind chloramphenicol and the sensitivity of an organism to growth inhibition by the drug.[3] Table 2-1 shows that only 70 S ribosomes have the ability to bind the drug. The binding is readily reversible, and, if a chloramphenicol-treated culture is diluted with new growth medium, the culture will begin growing again. Chloramphenicol, erythromycin, clindamycin, and lincomycin are all bacteriostatic agents.

While the growth of E. coli B 150 is not inhibited by the drug, 70 S ribosomes from this strain are able to bind chloramphenicol just as well as are ribosomes from the drug-sensitive strain. It has been demonstrated that whole cells or spheroplasts of E. coli B 150 have a markedly reduced ability to take up the drug.[3] Thus it appears that these organisms may have become resistant to chloramphenicol by virtue of a mutation that altered the permeability of the bacterial membrane to the drug or altered a transport mechanism in the membrane responsible for drug uptake.

It is clear that interaction of chloramphenicol with the ribosome is responsible for the inhibition of protein synthesis by the drug. This inhibition of protein synthesis is maximal when one molecule of chloramphenicol is bound per ribosome.[4] The results presented in Table 2-2 show that chloramphenicol inhibits protein synthesis in a cell-free system only when 70 S ribosomes are present.[5] There is very little inhibition when protein synthesis is directed by a soluble fraction from *E. coli* and 80 S ribosomes prepared from yeast.

The 70 S ribosome is composed of two particles of different size, the 50 S and the 30 S ribosomal subunits. Each subunit is composed of ribosomal RNA and a number of different proteins. Chloramphenicol binds only to the 50 S subunit.[6] The binding of chloramphenicol to ribosomes is inhibited by lincomycin and such macrolide antibiotics as erythromycin, carbomycin, and oleandomycin.[7] It may be that the other drugs can compete for chloramphenicol binding because they are competing for the same receptor site and, therefore, may have a similar mechanism of action. It is just as likely, however, that the other drugs are interacting with the 50 S particle at another location and in

Table 2-2 Effect of chloramphenicol on ^{14}C-lysine incorporation with yeast and *E. coli* supernatant and ribosomes

Ribosomal and soluble (105,000 × g supernatant) fractions were prepared from *E. coli* and the yeast *S. fragilis.* The ribosomes and supernatant were incubated with ^{14}C-lysine and nonradioactive amino acids with or without chloramphenicol (2 μmoles/ml), and the amount of radioactivity incorporated into trichloroacetic acid-insoluble material was assayed. The results are expressed as counts per minute incorporated per incubation. (From So and Davie.[5])

			Amino acid incorporation		
Supernatant	Ribosomes	Chloramphenicol	Experiment 1	Experiment 2	Average inhibition (%)
Escherichia coli	Escherichia coli	—	5,625	3,905	95
		+	196	239	
Escherichia coli	Saccharomyces fragilis	—	4,804	10,369	14
		+	4,460	8,236	

some way are preventing the association of chloramphenicol with its receptor as a secondary phenomenon.

The use of antibiotic-resistant, mutant strains of bacteria is often a potent tool in elucidating the mechanism of action of a compound. For example, a strain of *E. coli* resistant to the drug erythromycin was isolated after exposure of a sensitive culture to the mutagen N-methyl-N-nitroso-N'-nitroguanidine. The 50 S ribosomal subunits from these resistant cells did not bind erythromycin.[8] To detect alterations in ribosomal proteins resulting from the mutation to erythromycin resistance, samples of 30 S or 50 S ribosomal protein obtained from ^{3}H-lysine-labeled sensitive cells and ^{14}C-lysine-labeled resistant cells were mixed and simultaneously chromatographed on a carboxymethyl-cellulose column. There were no differences in the 30 S proteins from the two strains. When the protein components of the 50 S subunits of the parent and resistant strain were compared, however, one of the 21 protein peaks in the resistant strain appeared in a different place. It would appear that this protein had undergone a mutation that altered its physical characteristics so that the protein was eluted elsewhere. This altered protein may well be the receptor for erythromycin. Similar experiments will help define the protein(s) receptor for chloramphenicol.

The Inhibition of Protein Synthesis

It is appropriate to review our current understanding of protein synthesis[9] before discussing inhibition of the process by drugs. The synthesis of proteins, which, for the purpose of this discussion, equals the process of messenger RNA (mRNA) translation, can be conveniently divided into three stages—initiation, elongation, and termination (Figure 2-2).

The first stage in protein synthesis is the formation of an initiation complex. In bacteria the first or N-terminal amino acid for all proteins is formyl-methionine. Formyl-methionine and its appropriate transfer RNA (tRNA) are first united under the direction of an aminoacyl-tRNA-synthetase to form aminoacyl-RNA. The mRNA becomes attached to the 30 S subunit, a process in which two proteins called initiation factors participate. The

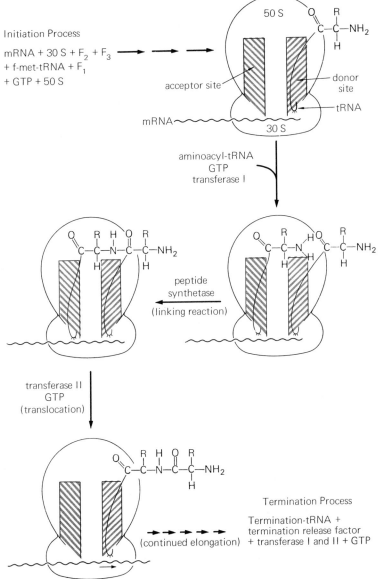

Figure 2-2 Protein synthesis in bacteria. This schematic presentation of this process is described in detail in the text. The linking reaction directed by peptide synthetase is the step that seems to be inhibited by chloramphenicol. The shapes representing the tRNA and the ribosome are, of course, highly schematic and are not intended to represent their actual form.

formyl-methionine-charged tRNA then combines with the mRNA-30 S-ribosomal complex. The anticodon triplet portion of the tRNA is juxtaposed to the start signal (AUG initiation codon) on the mRNA. This requires the participation of a third initiation factor. In the next step, the 50 S ribosomal subunit becomes bound to the mRNA-30 S-tRNA-amino acid complex in a reaction requiring GTP. The initiation complex is now complete.

Chain elongation commences with the insertion of a second aminoacyl-tRNA in the ribosomal acceptor site under the direction of an enzyme called transferase I. The first two tRNA's are now oriented appropriately with their anticodon ends opposite their respective code triplets on the mRNA and their attached amino acids adjacent to each other on the surface of the 50 S portion of the ribosome. The two amino acids then become linked by a peptide bond under the direction of a peptide synthetase enzyme. This enzyme is one of the more than 20 protein components of the 50 S ribosomal subunit. The carboxyl group of formyl-methionine is linked to the amino group of the second amino acid, and the dipeptide is now attached to the second tRNA. After the formation of the peptide bond, a translocation takes place. Under the direction of a transferase II (translocase) enzyme the tRNA for formyl-methionine is released from the donor site, the tRNA with the attached dipeptide moves from the acceptor to the donor site, and the 30 S subunit moves one codon along the mRNA. The acceptor site is then unoccupied and ready to receive the next aminoacyl-tRNA directed by the next code triplet on the mRNA. The process of elongation continues with the addition of single amino acid units until a termination code triplet (UAA, UGA, or UAG) in the mRNA signals that the protein chain is complete. A termination tRNA with the appropriate anticodon occupies the acceptor site under the direction of transferase I, and, with the participation of transferase II, GTP, and a termination release factor, the completed protein is released into the cell, and the ribosome becomes detached from the mRNA.

The mechanisms of action of chloramphenicol, erythromycin, and the other antibiotics affecting protein synthesis now can be at least partially explained. The probable site of action of chloramphenicol in the scheme of events presented in Figure 2-2 has been identified largely by the process of elimination—that is, as a result of many experiments which demonstrated where the drug was not working. It is clear that chloramphenicol does not preferentially inhibit the initiation of new protein chains or chain termination and detachment from ribosomes.[4] The binding of aminoacyl-tRNA[10] and the binding of mRNA[4] to the 30 S ribosome subunit is not affected by the drug.

In the presence of chloramphenicol, newly formed, pulse-labeled mRNA enters poly-ribosomes of all sizes without concomitant synthesis of protein.[11] It would then seem that in the presence of chloramphenicol, ribosomes attach to and move along mRNA (a process that requires translocation) without producing peptide bonds. The conclusion that chloramphenicol must inhibit peptide bond formation was also reached by an entirely different experimental approach.[12] The uncoupling of translocation and peptide bond formation is difficult to understand. It is postulated that binding of chloramphenicol to the ribosome causes a distortion in the ribosomal components and thus relaxes the requirement for the coupling of peptide bond formation and ribosome movement. In this case translocation would continue in an ordered manner by virtue of the correct orientation of the tRNA molecules in the acceptor and donor sites on the ribosome.

If we visualize the orientation of the amino acid-charged tRNA on the ribosome, the tRNA is attached to the 30 S portion in that region of the molecule containing the anticoden triplet. The region of the tRNA containing the attached amino acid must be correctly oriented on the surface of the 50 S portion of the ribosome for peptide bond formation to take place. This can be inferred from the fact that the enzyme directing the synthesis of the peptide bond (peptide synthetase) is a structurally integral part of the 50 S ribosome. If the binding of tRNA at the codon recognition site is undisturbed, then translocation might very well proceed in the presence of chloramphenicol. One would predict that a disturbance in the binding of the amino acid-containing end of the tRNA to the 50 S subunit would interfere with peptide bond formation.

This hypothesis has been tested in a more direct manner: tRNA charged with tritium-labeled phenylalanine was digested with T_1 ribonuclease. After this limited digestion, a ^{3}H-phenylalaninepentanucleotide was isolated. It was presumed that this radio-active amino acid-oligonucleotide represented the aminoacyl portion of an amino acid-charged tRNA. Several antibiotics were then tested for their effect on the ability of ribosomes to bind the radioactive phenylalanine-oligonucleotide (Figure 2-3).[13] Chlor-amphenicol and lincomycin markedly inhibited the binding at concentrations that inhibited protein synthesis in *in vivo* systems. If this system indeed mimics the association between the amino-acyl-terminal of the tRNA and the 50 S ribosomal subunit, then it should be a good tool for further defining the mechanism of action of chloramphenicol and the other antibiotics. Clearly, a precise definition of the inhibition of protein synthesis by antibiotics that bind to the 50 S ribosomal subunit depends upon a complete understanding of the process of mRNA translation at the molecular level.

Chloramphenicol Particles

Even though protein synthesis is inhibited almost immediately by chloramphenicol, RNA synthesis continues, and RNA accumu-lates in the cell. The RNA that accumulates in the cell appears

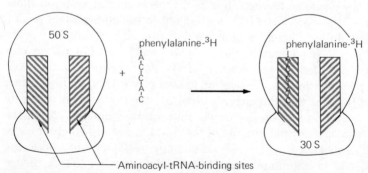

Figure 2-3 A schematic illustration of the binding of phenylalanyl-oligonucleo-tide to ribosomes. It has not been demonstrated that the binding of phenylalanyl-oligonucleotide to the ribosome replicates the specific binding of the amino acid-containing end of a complete aminoacyl-tRNA. The binding that does occur between the phenylalanyl-tRNA and the ribosome is inhibited by chloramphenicol but not by erythromycin. (Adapted from Pestka.[13])

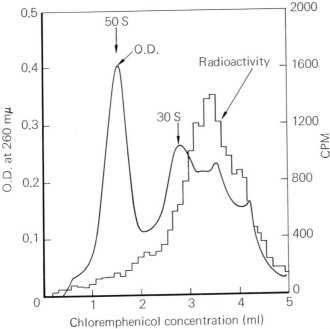

Figure 2-4 Chloramphenicol particles as seen by sucrose density gradient centrifugation. Chloramphenicol (10 μg/ml) was added to an exponentially growing culture of *E. coli*. After 1 minute, ^{14}C-uridine was added, and, after 45 minutes, the culture was harvested, lysed, and a high speed pellet was centrifuged on a (5–20%) sucrose gradient. The chloramphenicol particles are indicated by the radioactivity peak. (Adapted from Das *et al.* [4])

in the form of ribosome-like particles which are a combination of ribosomal RNA and protein. These units are called "chloramphenicol particles" (Figure 2-4), and for a long time they were considered to be defective, partially formed ribosomes. These bodies result from the chloramphenicol-mediated inhibition of protein synthesis, they appear well after protein synthesis is inhibited, and they are not associated with the mechanism of action of chloramphenicol as some older texts imply.

The concept that these particles represent partially synthesized ribosomes (that is, combinations of ribosomal RNA and ribosomal protein) is incorrect. There is good evidence that the sequence of events in the chloramphenicol-treated cell is as follows:[14] protein synthesis is inhibited; production of ribosomal precursor RNA continues; as apparently there is only a very small pool of free ribosomal protein in the cell[15], the ribosomal RNA combines randomly with soluble cell protein to produce the hybrid product the chloramphenicol particle. When cells are returned to a growth medium in the absence of chloramphenicol, the chloramphenicol particle RNA enters functioning ribosomes, while the protein previously associated with it does not.

Therapeutic Indications

When first introduced, chloramphenicol (Chloromycetin) was used to treat a variety of infections. Because serious side reactions (most notably, fatal marrow aplasia) were recognized, this drug is now the treatment of choice only for acute typhoid fever caused by *Salmonella typhosa*. Otherwise chloramphenicol should be used only under strict guidelines (outlined later in this chapter) in the in-hospital treatment of severe infections when the drug of choice cannot be used and sensitivity testing demonstrates that chloramphenicol is the best alternative. Chloramphenicol is a broad-spectrum drug. It inhibits the growth of both gram-positive and gram-negative organisms as well as rickettsia and filterable, disease-producing agents (such as the agents responsible for psittacosis, lymphogranuloma venerum, and inclusion conjunctivitis).

Erythromycin is a drug of choice for the treatment of Eaton agent infections *(Mycoplasma pneumoniae)*. Its main role in antibacterial therapy is as an alternative to penicillin when sensitivity testing indicates that an organism is readily inhibited by the drug. If a patient is allergic to the pencillins, erythromycin is a preferred alternative for the treatment of streptococcal or pneumococcal infection.

Lincomycin does not have the broad spectrum of activity of erythromycin. It is a useful alternative in the treatment of a number of infections due to gram-positive cocci. Clindamycin (7-chlorolincomycin) is similar to lincomycin in antibacterial spectrum and activity.[16] In addition to being active against many strains of staphylococci (including many penicillinase producers), streptococci (but not enterococci), and pneumococci, clindamycin and lincomycin are also effective against many isolates of bacteroides. Clindamycin has a better oral absorption, is somewhat more potent *in vitro*, and causes fewer cases of diarrhea than lincomycin.

The status of a drug in the treatment of infectious disease varies continually with the introduction of new drugs, the development of large resistant populations, and the discovery of toxicities and hypersensitivity phenomena. One of the best ways for the medical student and the practicing physician to keep himself informed of the relative efficacy of drugs for the treatment of specific infections is to read *The Medical Letter*. This biweekly review of therapeutics publishes listings of the consensus recommendations of a number of experts in infectious disease therapy regarding the choice of antimicrobial drugs. The recommendations are updated every two years as the therapeutic situation changes.

Pharmacology of Chloramphenicol and Erythromycin

Absorption. Chloramphenicol is well absorbed from the gastrointestinal tract. Erythromycin base is destroyed by gastric juice and should be taken when the stomach is empty. Many of the erythromycin preparations have acid-resistant coatings or are in a salt form for greater acid resistance. Peak serum levels are attained with both drugs in approximately two hours.

Metabolism and excretion. Erythromycin is concentrated in the liver, and large amounts of the unaltered, biologically active form of the drug are excreted in the bile. Chloramphenicol is extensively metabolized to the glucuronide. A small amount of the drug is excreted unchanged.

Toxicity. Chloramphenicol was used for a time by some pediatricians for prophylaxis as well as therapy in nursery infections. With premature and newborn infants this sometimes led to a series of events starting with abdominal distention, progressing with a pallid cyanosis, and ending sometimes in death from cardiovascular and respiratory collapse a few hours after onset of the symp-

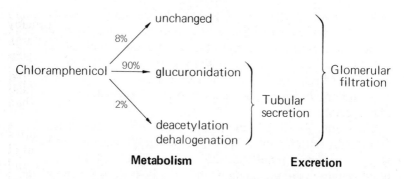

toms.[17] This toxic reaction to chloramphenicol has been called the "gray syndrome." It develops because the liver of a newborn infant is unable to conjugate chloramphenicol to the glucuronide. In addition to an inability to metabolize the drug, infants have depressed rates of glomerular filtration and tubular secretion. As a result, prolonged high levels of the unaltered drug build up in the newborn (Figure 2-5) even though the dose of the drug, after adjustment for body weight and surface area, would be suitable in an older baby. Termination of therapy upon early development of symptoms often reverses the process.

It would seem at first glance that the use of chloramphenicol in the adult patient with compromised renal function would be especially hazardous. It is not, however, because the drug is extensively metabolized by the liver to the glucuronide, and the glucuronide is not toxic. Even though higher levels build up in the patient who excretes it in reduced amounts, they are not of great consequence providing there is normal liver function.

Erythromycin has a good therapeutic index. Treatment is sometimes accompanied by mild gastrointestinal upset, but hypersensitivity reactions are uncommon. Some preparations of erythromycin and oleandomycin can cause a cholestatic hepatitis.[18] The basic forms of the drugs cannot cause hepatitis, and this phenomenon seems to be associated with the lauryl sulfate salt of the drug. Lincomycin taken orally produces diarrhea in a reasonably high percentage of patients. On occasion the diarrhea can be quite severe. This is a relatively new drug, but it seems to elicit only occasional allergic reactions according to information presently available.

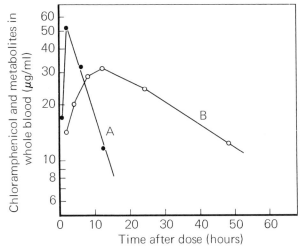

Figure 2-5 Mean whole-blood levels of free chloramphenicol and its metabolites in newborn infants and older children after oral administration of chloramphenicol palmitate in single doses of 50 mg/kg body weight. A, age one to eleven years (mean of thirteen subjects); B, age one to two days (mean of five subjects). (From Weiss *et al.* [17])

Effects of Chloramphenicol on the Hematopoietic System

Chloramphenicol affects the hematopoeitic system in two ways. One is a toxic phenomenon manifested by bone-marrow depression, and the other is an allergic or idiosyncratic response manifested by aplastic anemia.

Toxic bone-marrow depression. Chloramphenicol can cause a reversible, dose-related depression of bone-marrow function which presents as an anemia, sometimes with leukopenia or thrombocytopenia.[19] This occurs at a fairly high frequency. For example, in one well-controlled study, bone-marrow depression developed in 2 of 20 patients given 2 gm and in 18 of 21 receiving 6 gm of the drug daily.[20] As a reference figure, approximately 3 to 4 gm of the drug per day is administered routinely to adults in the treatment of typhoid fever or rickettsial diseases.

The mechanism of this toxic effect is not completely elucidated. It is clear that chloramphenicol can inhibit protein synthesis in certain mammalian erythroid cells (for example, rabbit reticulo-cytes).[21] The inhibition of protein synthesis by chloramphenicol is different in bacterial and mammalian systems. Concentrations of approximately $10^{-3}M$ are required for inhibition in erythroid cells, whereas a concentration of approximately 10^{-5} M will inhibit bacterial protein synthesis. Both RNA and protein syn-thesis are inhibited to the same degree in reticulocytes.

Earlier in this chapter it was noted that chloramphenicol inhibits the protein synthesis directed by 70 S ribosomes. This would seem to be the basis for its selective toxicity, since, in cells higher on the evolutionary scale than bacteria, the bulk of protein synthesis takes place on 80 S ribosomes. Mitochondria, however, have ribosomes similar to the 70 S bacterial ribosome, and chloramphenicol has been shown to inhibit mitochondrial protein synthesis.[22] Ribosomes from chloroplasts are also sensitive to chloramphenicol.[23] The fact that these cytoplasmic organelles are sensitive to chloramphenicol has been used as an argument to support the hypothesis that they may have arisen from primitive infecting organisms which gradually became obligatory endosym-bionts.[24]

Chloramphenicol also decreases ATP content of reticulocytes at the concentration where cellular protein and RNA synthesis are inhibited.[21] It is possible that by virtue of its effect on mito-chondria chloramphenicol may interfere with the energy supply of the bone-marrow cells; this could explain the inhibition of both protein and RNA synthesis and the resulting toxic anemia.

Aplastic anemia. Another type of response of the blood-forming cells to chloramphenicol is the development of aplastic anemia. Only after three years of extensive use did it become evident that chloramphenicol was able to completely depress bone-marrow activity in some patients. It was in response to this three-year delay in recognition that the American Medical Association established the Registry on Blood Dyscrasias to collect data on such drug-associated reactions. Chloramphenicol has been implicated in more reports to the registry than any other single drug. This suppression of bone-marrow activity is different from the toxic phenomenon just discussed (Table 2-3). The response is characterized by pancytopenia with an aplastic marrow. It can

Table 2-3 Features of two types of blood dyscrasia resulting from treatment with chloramphenicol

There are two different responses of the hematopoietic system to chloramphenicol. Separation of the responses into the toxic effect (bone-marrow depression) and the aplastic response was first made by Yunis and Bloomberg.[19]

Feature	Toxic effect	Aplastic response
Appearance of bone-marrow spears	Normocellular	Hypoplastic or aplastic
Peripheral blood	Anemia (with or without leukopenia or thrombocytopenia)	Pancytopenia
Relation to dosage of drug given	Dose related	No dose relationship
Time of appearance	During therapy	Most often days to months after cessation of therapy
Most common presenting symptoms	Anemia	Purpura and/or hemorrhage
Prognosis	Recovery is usually complete on cessation of treatment	Fatal in many cases

occur during treatment, but it often appears long after treatment has ended. It is not related to the dose of the drug. The prognosis is very poor, with a high percentage of fatalities. Estimates of the frequency of marrow aplasia have ranged from 1 in 40,000 to 1 in 100,000 cases.

It is not clear whether the development of aplastic anemia represents an allergic response to the drug or a type of drug idiosyncrasy. The hypothesis of an allergic basis for the response is supported by observations that there is no dose relationship; aplastic anemia frequently occurs in people who have received the drug previously, and it usually occurs long after the patient's course of treatment has ended.[25] But many workers in the field seem to feel that the marrow response involves some sort of biochemical lesion. Although there have been no extensive genetic studies, two reports have been published in which both members of sets of identical twins being treated with chloramphenicol developed severe marrow depression.[26,27] One could also imagine rare individuals with altered routes of metabolism that result in the production of a toxic metabolite of chloramphenicol. One intriguing hypothesis is that the gut flora in individuals who have an aplastic response may degrade small amounts of chloramphenicol to a substance that affects the blood-forming cells adversely. One investigator has noted that there ". . . seems to be no recorded case in which marrow aplasia has followed administration of chloramphenicol by parenteral routes alone."[28] It has also been demonstrated that the gut flora in about 2 per cent of English children studied were able to degrade chloramphenicol to various degrees. A complete review of all cases of chloramphenicol-associated blood dyscrasias submitted to the Registry on Blood Dyscrasias has been published by Best.[25]

The Use of Chloramphenicol

Chloramphenicol was introduced to the American drug market in 1949 under a patent issued to Parke, Davis and Co. It was found to be a useful broad-spectrum antibiotic noted for its relative lack of adverse side effects. By 1950, however, it had become apparent that chloramphenicol produced aplastic anemia, a fatal side affect, in a few patients. A continuing argument regarding the proper use of this drug then developed. On one side were the drug firm and a number of physicians who felt the risk of aplastic anemia to be trivial when compared with the therapeutic usefulness of the antibiotic. On the other side were a steadily increasing number of authorities in the treatment of infectious disease, many hematologists, advisors in the Food and Drug Administration, and at least two congressional committees who held hearings on the drug (chaired by Senator Estes Kefauver in 1960 and by Senator Gaylord Nelson in 1968). The controversy has not been concerned with the right of the company to market the drug or the right of the physician to use it. Rather it has been concerned with the way the drug company advertised its product and the uninformed way many physicians employed the drug. Many critics felt that the company played down the problem of side effects in their advertisements to physicians. The story of the commercial side of the controversy has been reviewed in *Consumer Reports*.[29]

A number of factors contributed to the use of the drug: the increasing incidence of infection resistant to other antibiotics, failure to check on the antibiotic sensitivity of an organism, and, in some cases, patient pressure to change the therapeutic regimen.

A great part of the problem with the use of this drug centers upon the way practicing physicians are exposed to information about drugs. The indications given for therapy with chloramphenicol in those cases of chloramphenicol-associated blood dyscrasia reported to the Registry on Blood Dyscrasias from 1953 through 1964 demonstrate how ignorant many physicians were of the proper use of this antibiotic. As seen in Figure 2-6, the second most common indication for therapy was the treatment of the common cold, a virus infection against which the drug is totally useless. In other cases the drug was prescribed for minor infec-

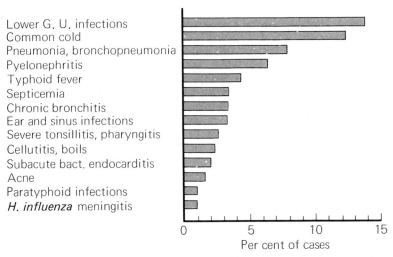

Figure 2-6 Some specific conditions for which chloramphenicol was given in instances of chloramphenicol-associated blood dyscrasia reported to the Registry on Blood Dyscrasias from 1953 through 1964. (From Best.[25])

tions where therapy with chloramphenicol is definitely not indicated. One would think that after repeated warnings the unwarranted use of chloramphenicol would plummet—but this has not been the case. Periodically (usually immediately after Senate committee hearings) a new level of awareness is temporarily achieved, and use of the drug drops, but there has always been a gradual rebound in sales.[29] As there is presumably no increase in the incidence of typhoid fever or severe infection for which other antibiotics cannot be used, one must assume that physicians are again using the drug indiscriminately. In a system where the principal exposure of many physicians to drug information is through the drug industry itself (e.g., the *Physicians' Desk Reference*[30] with its product descriptions prepared by manufacturers, the drug company detailmen and drug advertisements) there is simply not enough weight placed on unbiased reporting of the relative value of a drug in the best treatment of disease.

The use of chloramphenicol in some countries is much more lax than in the United States. In Mexico and in some countries in South America, chloramphenicol is sold over the counter. A correspondent writes in the *New England Journal of Medicine* that chloramphenicol is used by many people in South America as ". . . a daily self-medication for all ills and aches. . .".[31] In Japan the drug is marketed in combination with seven B-complex vitamins.[29] Actual restriction of chloramphenicol use by the physician is being discussed in the United States. Such a control might take the form of a regulation restricting the drug to in-hospital use.

What sort of guidelines should be used for this drug at the present time? The following set of criteria seem appropriate.

(1) *Chloramphenicol should be used only for the treatment of typhoid fever and as an alternative in severe infections where the drugs of choice cannot be used, and chloramphenicol is clearly the superior alternative. It should never be used for prophylaxis or for the treatment of mild or uncharacterized infections.*

(2) *Prolonged usage and repeat exposure should be avoided.*

(3) *Leukocyte counts with a differential should be taken daily,* and therapy should be discontinued when leukopenia occurs.

References

1. B. Weisblum and J. Davies: Antibiotic inhibitors of the bacterial ribosome. *Bact. Rev.* 32:493 (1968).
2. C. L. Wisseman, J. E. Smadel, F. E. Hahn, and H. E. Hopps: Mode of action of chloramphenicol. I. Action of chloramphenicol on assimilation of ammonia and on synthesis of proteins and nucleic acids in *Escherichia coli. J. Bacteriol.* 67:662 (1954).
3. D. Vazquez: Uptake and binding of chloramphenicol by sensitive and resistant organisms. *Nature* 203:257 (1964).
4. H. K. Das, A. Goldstein, and L. C. Kanner: Inhibition by chloramphenicol of the growth of nascent protein chains in *Escherichia coli. Mol. Pharmacol.* 2:158 (1966).
5. A. G. So and E. W. Davie: The incorporation of amino acids into protein in a cell-free system from yeast. *Biochemistry* 2:132 (1963).
6. D. Vazquez: The binding of chloramphenicol by ribosomes from *Bacillus megaterium. Biochem. Biophys. Res. Commun.* 15:464 (1964).
7. D. Vazquez: Binding of chloramphenicol to ribosomes; the effect of a number of antibiotics. *Biochim. Biophys. Acta* 114:277 (1966).
8. K. Tanaka, H. Teraoka, M. Tamaki, E. Otaka, and S. Osawa: Erythromycin-resistant mutant of *Escherichia coli* with altered ribosomal protein component. *Science* 162:576 (1968).
9. F. Lipmann: Polypeptide chain elongation in protein biosynthesis. *Science* 164:1024 (1969).
10. M. Cannon, R. Krug, and W. Gilbert: The binding of sRNA by *Escherichia coli* ribosomes. *J. Mol. Biol.* 7:360 (1963).
11. C. Gurgo, D. Aprion and D. Schlessinger: Polyribosome metabolism in *Escherichia coli* treated with chloramphenicol, neomycin, spectinomycin or tetracycline. *J. Mol. Biol.* 45:205 (1969).
12. G. R. Julian: ^{14}C-lysine peptides synthesized in an *in vitro Escherichia coli* system in the presence of chloramphenicol. *J. Mol. Biol.* 12:9 (1965).
13. S. Pestka: Studies on the formation of transfer ribonucleic acid-ribosome complexes. XI. Antibiotic effects on phenylalanyloligonucleotide binding to ribosomes. *Proc. Natl. Acad. Sci. U.S.* 64:709 (1969).
14. R. F. Schleif: Origin of chloramphenicol particle protein. *J. Mol. Biol.* 37:119 (1968).
15. R. F. Schleif: Control of production of ribosomal protein. *J. Mol. Biol.* 27:41 (1967).
16. B. R. Meyers, K. Kaplan, and L. Weinstein: Microbiological and pharmacological behavior of 7-chlorolincomycin. *Appl. Microbiol.* 17:653 (1969).
17. C. F. Weiss, A. J. Glazko, and J. K. Weston: Chloramphenicol in the newborn infant; a physiologic explanation of its toxicity when given in excessive doses. *New Eng. J. Med.* 262:787 (1960).

18. F. I. Gilbert: Cholestatic hepatitis caused by esters of erythromycin and oleandomycin. *J. Am. Med. Assoc.* 182:1048 (1962).

19. A. A. Yunis and G. R. Bloomberg: Chloramphenicol toxicity, clinical features and pathogenesis. *Progress in Hematology* 4:138 (1964).

20. J. L. Scott, S. M. Finegold, G. A. Belkin, and J. S. Lawrence: A controlled double-blind study of the hematologic toxicity of chloramphenicol. *New Eng. J. Med.* 272:1137 (1965).

21. W. Godchaux and E. Herbert: The effect of chloramphenicol in intact erythroid cells. *J. Mol. Biol.* 21:537 (1966).

22. L. W. Wheeldon and A. L. Lehninger: Energy-linked synthesis and decay of membrane proteins in isolated rat liver mitochondria. *Biochemistry* 5:3533 (1966).

23. J. M. Eisenstadt and G. Brawerman: The protein-synthesizing systems from the cytoplasm and the chloroplasts of *Euglena gracilis. J. Mol. Biol.* 10:392 (1964).

24. D. B. Roodyn and D. Wilkie, *The Biogenesis of Mitochondria,* London: Methuen and Co. Ltd., 1968. An extensive discussion of the possible evolutionary origin of mitochondria and a review of the effects of chloramphenicol on mitochondrial protein synthesis.

25. W. R. Best: Chloramphenicol-associated blood dyscrasias. *J. Am. Med. Assoc.* 201:99 (1967). Copyright 1967, American Medical Association

26. D. J. Fernbach and J. J. Trentin: "Isologous bone marrow transplantation in an identical twin with aplastic anemia" in *Proceedings of the Eighth International Congress on Hematology,* Vol. 1 Tokyo: Pan-Pacific Press, (1962). p. 150.

27. T. Nagao and A. M. Mauer: Concordance for drug-induced aplastic anemia in identical twins. *New Eng. J. Med.* 281:7 (1969).

28. R. Holt: The bacterial degredation of chloramphenicol. *Lancet* 1:1259 (1967).

29. *Consumer Reports,* October 1970, p. 616.

30. *Physicians' Desk Reference* (Pub.) Medical Economics Inc. (1970).

31. S. Aladjem: Chloramphenicol in South America. *New Eng. J. Med.* 281:1369 (1969).

Chapter 3
The Inhibitors
of Protein Synthesis II
Streptomycin
Neomycin
Kanamycin
Paromomycin
Gentamicin

Introduction

The drugs streptomycin, neomycin, kanamycin, and paromomycin are all structurally related aminoglycoside antibiotics. They affect protein synthesis in the bacterial cell similarly, but there is no definitive evidence to indicate that they all occupy the same receptor site and have precisely the same mechanism of action. They are polycationic compounds composed of amino sugars connected by glycosidic linkages. They are all derived from different species of *Streptomyces*. Gentamicin is a useful new drug (approved for the United States market in 1969) structurally related to the aminoglycosides.

Streptomycin

Mechanism of Action

Inhibition of Protein Synthesis

Most of the work on the mechanism of action of the aminoglycoside antibiotics has been carried out with streptomycin; it has been reviewed by Brock[1] and by Weisblum and Davies.[2] When growing bacteria are exposed to streptomycin, there is a rapid inhibition of protein synthesis.[3] As described in the preceding chapter, the process of mRNA translation consists of many reactions, and the inhibition of any one of these reactions by an antibiotic would block protein synthesis. The best evidence available at present indicates that streptomycin blocks bacterial protein synthesis in intact cells at the stage of initiation.

In one experiment that lends support to this conclusion, streptomycin was added to a culture of growing E. coli in which stable RNA had been labeled with radioactive uracil, the cells were lysed at various times after the streptomycin was added, and the lysate was centrifuged on a sucrose gradient.[4] Over a period of several minutes the ^{14}C activity disappeared from the polysome region and appeared in the 70 S region of the sucrose gradient. The largest polysomes were the first to disappear, followed by the smaller units until essentially all of the radioactivity in the portion of the gradient occupied by the polyribosomes had been shifted to 70 S material. In the same experiment it was demonstrated by pulse labeling with tritiated uridine that streptomycin treatment prevented the newly synthesized RNA from entering both polysomes and 70 S monosomes. The disappearance of polysomes indicates that protein synthesis in progress when the streptomycin was added continues, but that new protein synthesis does not start, presumably due to an inability to initiate synthesis. If the rate of chain elongation were reduced by streptomycin without a change in the rate of initiation, one would expect polysomes to accumulate.

The 70 S units that accumulate are called "streptomycin monosomes," and they are incapable of protein synthesis. The accumulation of the 70 S monosomes takes place at the expense of 50 S and 30 S ribosomes as well as polyribosomes. These streptomycin monosomes consist of a complex of 30 S and 50 S ribosomal particles, mRNA, and streptomycin. The streptomycin is bound very tightly, and the 70 S units accumulate irreversibly in the cell. This accumulation of 70 S monosomes at the expense of both large and small ribosomal units is what one would expect if the effect of streptomycin were to "freeze" protein synthesis at the initiation complex stage. Thus the drug allows the initiation complex to form, but this streptomycin-bound complex is inactive. There is a good correlation between the accumulation of 70 S monosomes and the loss of cell viability after exposure to streptomycin. The effects of streptomycin on bacterial protein synthesis are schematically presented in Figure 3-1.

The conclusion that streptomycin affects initiation is supported by experiments with mutant bacteria.[5] In a temperature-sensitive mutant of E. coli protein synthesis in intact cells stops when the temperature is raised from 30 to 42° C. Analysis of the distribution of polyribosomes after the shift to a higher temperature suggests that initiation of protein synthesis is defective. This temperature-sensitive mutation maps at the streptomycin locus.

Although streptomycin had been found to block protein synthesis in intact bacteria rapidly, for some time it proved difficult to demonstrate a complete inhibition of protein synthesis in bacterial extracts. This was difficult because the subcellular protein synthesizing systems initially used to study the drug effect utilized a synthetic mRNA (such as poly U) to direct the incorporation of amino acids into protein. If, however, a natural mRNA was added to a cell-free protein synthesizing system from bacteria, complete blockage of protein formation could be demonstrated at an appropriate streptomycin concentration.[4] This difference in sensitivity between natural mRNA-directed and synthetic mRNA-directed protein synthesis to inhibition by streptomycin is important in the elucidation of the mechanism of action of the drug. As we have already seen, protein synthesis directed by natural mRNA requires formyl-methionine-tRNA for the formation of an initiation complex, which is necessary for translation to commence. Protein synthesis directed by poly U initiates artificially (presumably a structural change in the ribosome is brought about by magnesium ion); it does not require formyl-methionine-tRNA and does not mimic the natural process.

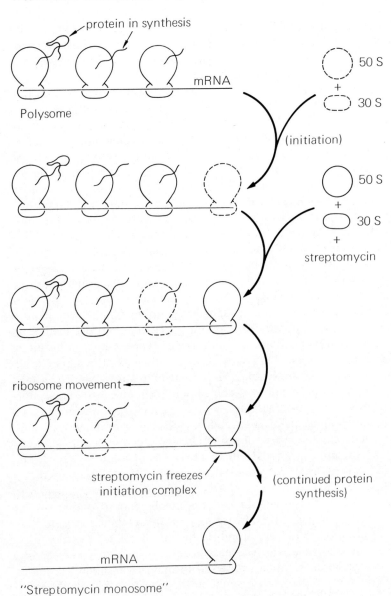

Given that protein synthesis requiring a normal initiation procedure is more sensitive to inhibition by streptomycin than synthesis directed by synthetic messenger, it can be predicted that protein synthesis directed by poly AUG (which contains the natural initiating codon AUG) would be very sensitive to the drug. This is indeed the case. Protein synthesis carried out at low magnesium concentrations with poly AUG is completely inhibited by streptomycin.[6] At higher concentrations of magnesium ion, where the variant mechanism of initiation is operative, the streptomycin effect is greatly reduced.

Streptomycin is a bactericidal drug. It is not yet clear why the drug is bactericidal.

The Receptor

The aminoglycoside antibiotics have a selective toxicity because they bind only to bacterial ribosomes. They differ from chloramphenicol and erythromycin in that they interact with the 30 S subunit of the ribosome. This site of interaction was first indicated by experiments that utilized ribosomes from streptomycin-sensitive and streptomycin-resistant cells to support poly U-directed protein synthesis.[7] The 70 S ribosome can be dissociated into its 50 S and 30 S subunits by lowering the Mg^{++} concentration; raising the Mg^{++} concentration permits reassociation. Accordingly, cell extracts of E. coli were made in buffer of low Mg^{++} concentration and centrifuged on a sucrose gradient to separate the heavier 50 S subunits from the 30 S particles. Cross-over experiments were then carried out by raising the magnesium ion concentration to produce hybrid 70 S ribosomes with one subunit from sensitive cells and one from resistant cells. These reassoci-

Figure 3-1 Streptomycin blocks bacterial protein synthesis at initiation. After intact bacteria are exposed to streptomycin, polysomes become rapidly depleted, and 70 S particles, the "streptomycin monosomes," build up.[4] Although the formation of the initiation complex is not affected, the complex formed in the presence of streptomycin cannot synthesize protein and remains fixed in position. Apparently ribosomes beyond the initiation stage are able to continue their movement and detachment so that a 70 S complex of mRNA and 50 S and 30 S units with bound streptomycin results. In effect, the initiation complex is "frozen."

Table 3-1   The effect of streptomycin on the incorporation of phenyl-alanine in a system utilizing hybrid ribosomes from sensitive and resistant cells

Ribosomes reconstituted from 30 S and 50 S subunits purified from streptomycin-sensitive and streptomycin-resistant *E. coli* were added to a phenylalanine incorporation system directed by poly U. Incubations were carried out with or without streptomycin (5 × 10^{-5}M), and the amount of radioactivity incorporated into the acid-insoluble form was assayed. The results are presented as the average per cent inhibition of incorporation by streptomycin for four experiments. (Data from Davies.[7])

Constitution of hybrid ribosomes:		Inhibition of phenylalanine incorporation by streptomycin (%)
30 S	50 S	
Sensitive	Sensitive	62
Sensitive	Resistant	60
Resistant	Resistant	6
Resistant	Sensitive	15

ated ribosomes were then incubated with poly U and streptomycin in an appropriate system for protein synthesis. The results of the experiment, summarized in Table 3-1, demonstrate that substantial inhibition of protein synthesis is achieved only when the 30 S subunit is derived from sensitive cells.

This type of experiment has been carried further by Nomura and his co-workers; they separated purified 30 S ribosomes into 16 S RNA and more than 20 different proteins, which could be fractionated by phosphocellulose column chromatography.[8] These proteins and the 16 S RNA were then reassociated into 30 S ribosomal subunits that support protein synthesis. Protein-synthesizing experiments utilizing such reconstituted ribosomes prepared with 30 S ribosomal protein purified from streptomycin-sensitive and streptomycin-resistant cells demonstrate that a single protein (designated P$_{10}$ in accordance with its migration on polyacrylamide gel electrophoresis) determines the streptomycin sensitivity of the reconstituted particles (Table 3-2).[9]

Clearly the P$_{10}$ protein is necessary not only for streptomycin sensitivity but also for streptomycin binding. This has been demonstrated by incubating reconstituted 30 S particles with radio-

Table 3-2 **Poly U-directed phenylalanine incorporation activity of reconstituted 30 S ribosomal particles and their sensitivity to streptomycin**

RNA prepared from 30 S ribosomes and 30 S ribosomal protein purified by phosphocellulose chromatography from streptomycin-sensitive and streptomycin-resistant *E. coli* were reconstituted into 30 S subunits. Two protein fractions were prepared: the protein P_{10}, which was essentially pure, and the protein mixture containing all the other 30 S subunit proteins except P_{10}. Particles were reconstituted in the combinations indicated and assayed for their activity in poly U-directed phenylalanine incorporation with or without streptomycin (5 $\times$ $10^{-5}M$) Values in cpm of phenylalanine incorporated per incubation; S, sensitive; r, resistant; Sm, streptomycin. (Data from Ozaki *et al.*[9])

Origin of proteins used for reconstituted 30 S subunits: All proteins but P_{10}	P_{10}	Incorporation activity (cpm):		Inhibition by streptomycin
		−Sm	+Sm	(%)
S	S	6354	4153	35
S	r	6209	5755	7
S	—	2926	3116	0
r	r	4214	4031	4
r	S	4236	2771	35

active dihydrostreptomycin and then separating the bound 30 S-streptomycin complex from the free drug by filtration.[9] The results presented in Table 3-3 show that there is significant binding of dihydrostreptomycin to ribosomes only when the P_{10} in the reconstituted ribosome is derived from sensitive cells. In dialysis experiments P_{10} alone (that is, not in combination with RNA as a reconstituted 30 S particle) does not bind the drug, while complete 30 S particles under the same conditions bind well. Therefore some structure involving both P_{10} and other components of the 30 S subunit of the ribosome is essential to the formation of the complete, functioning receptor site for the drug.

Streptomycin Distortion of the Fidelity of Translation

One result of the interaction of streptomycin (or other aminoglycoside antibiotics) with the ribosome is a higher frequency of

Table 3-3   **Binding of dihydrostreptomycin to reconstituted 30 S ribosomal particles**

30 S particles reconstituted from 16 S RNA and purified 30 S subunit protein from streptomycin-sensitive or streptomycin-resistant *E. coli* were incubated at 30°C with radioactive dihydrostreptomycin (3.4 $\mu g/ml$). After 20 minutes, the bound drug-30 S complex was separated from the free drug by filtration on cellulose acetate. The radioactive drug remaining on the filter was assayed in a scintillation counter; values in cpm of dihydrostreptomycin bound per 1.5 O.D.$_{260}$ units of 30 S particles; S, sensitive; r, resistant, (From Ozaki *et al.*[9])

Origin of proteins used for Reconstituted 30 S subunits :		Dihydrostreptomycin bound (cpm)
All proteins but P$_{10}$	P$_{10}$	
S	S	1198
S	r	65
S	—	83
r	r	31
r	S	691
Control 30 S (S)		943
Control 30 S (r)		35

incorrect codon-anticodon interaction. This effect on the fidelity of messenger translation can be seen *in vitro* as an increased incorporation of the "wrong" amino acid in protein synthesis directed by synthetic mRNA.[10] The effect can be also seen *in vivo* as "phenotypic suppression": that is, the drug masks the phenotypic expression of certain mutations.

An example of the misreading seen with streptomycin is presented in Table 3-4. Under rountine assay conditions poly U directs the incorporation of phenylalanine (codes UUU and UUC) much more readily than leucine, isoleucine, or serine, all of which have codons that differ from a phenylalanine codon by only one base. In the presence of streptomycin, neomycin, or gentamicin, however, the incorporation of isoleucine relative to phenylalanine increases several-fold.[10] This misreading effect of streptomycin has also been examined in a poly-U-directed protein-synthesizing system utilizing ribosomes with reconstituted 30 S particles, and the presence of protein P$_{10}$ from sensitive cells was found to be a

Table 3-4   Amino acid incorporation with poly U in the presence of aminoglycoside antibiotics
A subcellular protein-synthesizing system prepared from *E. coli* was incubated with poly U and a mixture of 20 amino acids; one amino acid was ^{14}C-labeled. Incubation was with or without aminoglycoside (4 μg/ml). Values represent the incorporation of the amino acid as per cent poly U-directed incorporation of phenylalanine in the absence of drug; Sm, streptomycin; Nm, neomycin; Gm, gentamicin. (Data from Davies *et al.*[10])

Amino acid incorporated	No drug	Relative incorporation: +Sm	+Nm	+Gm
Phenylalanine	100	60	40	55
Leucine	5	10	6	15
Isoleucine	8	30	37	55
Serine	4	20	48	100

prerequisite for extensive streptomycin-induced incorporation of "wrong" amino acids (Ile, Ser, and Tyr).[9]

The distortion of codon recognition in intact, growing bacteria should result in the frequent insertion of the "wrong" amino acid and a consequent alteration in (or loss of) activity of the protein. If distortion led to false UGA, UAA, or UAG (termination codons) recognition, then premature chain termination would result. In a number of current articles it is postulated that the growth inhibitory effect of streptomycin is due to the production of faulty protein in the bacterium exposed to the drug. Altered protein is certainly produced in the bacterium, but extensive misreading can be demonstrated in some mutant bacteria without the occurrence of cell death.[11] This argues against extensive misreading as the primary cause of cell death after streptomycin is administered.

Phenotypic Suppression and Streptomycin Dependence

That streptomycin induces misreading of the genetic code can be demonstrated in the intact bacterium by the ability of the drug to reverse the effect of certain mutations. For example, an *E. coli* mutant was isolated which required an arginine-containing medium for growth. In the presence of streptomycin, however, growth could proceed in the absence of arginine.[12] Thus, the drug was able to suppress the phenotypic expression of the mutation. It was found that when the mutant bacterium was grown without streptomycin, ornithine transcarbamylase activity was absent. This enzyme converts ornithine to citrulline, a reaction necessary for the synthesis of arginine by the bacterium. The mutant was shown to possess a defective structural gene that led to the production of an inactive enzyme, and thus no arginine could be produced. Exposure to streptomycin apparently introduced enough ambiguity into the reading process so that an amino acid acceptable for enzyme activity was occasionally inserted during translation. In this way the mutation became phenotypically corrected by streptomycin at the level of translation. Enough active enzyme molecules were then produced so that cells in the presence of streptomycin grew in an arginine-free medium. These mutants are called "conditionally streptomycin dependent," which means that another compound, such as an amino acid, can be substituted for streptomycin to support growth.

There is another form of streptomycin dependence in which streptomycin is needed for growth, and only this drug, or perhaps one of the other aminoglycosides, can support growth. Genetic analysis in E. coli has demonstrated that sensitivity to streptomycin, single-step resistance to high levels of the drug, and streptomycin dependence are determined by multiple alleles at a single genetic locus, the Sm locus.[13] The Sm locus seems to be the locus for the P_{10} protein. In these streptomycin-dependent mutants there is presumably a genetic impairment of ribosomal structure so that extensive misreading occurs in the absence of streptomycin. Under conditions of streptomycin deprivation there is a marked imbalance in the pattern of enzyme synthesis and a decline in the rate of total protein synthesis in these organisms.[14] The binding of streptomycin presumably restores the altered 30 S subunit to a more normal configuration. This in turn allows a higher frequency of correct codon recognition, and consequently enough functional protein is produced to permit growth.[15]

The phenomenon of mutation to antibiotic dependence is of bacteriological and genetic interest, but it is not of great importance in the clinical treatment of infection. Bacterial drug dependence has been found for chloramphenicol as well, but the case of streptomycin is the most fully understood.

Therapeutic Indications

The principal use of the aminoglycoside antibiotics is the treatment of infection by gram-negative bacilli. Kanamycin and gentamicin are often effective against. *S. aureus*, and they can be used as alternatives to penicillin in patients who are allergic to that drug and when sensitivity testing indicates that one or the other is the best alternative. A selected list of gram-negative infections in which the aminoglycoside antibiotics are therapeutically effective is presented in Table 3-5. The use of streptomycin in the chemotherapy of tuberculosis has been discussed in Chapter 1.

The value of gentamicin in treating a number of gram-negative infections has been well established over the past few years. Gentamicin is one of the three most effective antibiotics in treating infection due to *Pseudomonas aeruginosa*—the others are carbenicillin and the polymixins. It is also the drug of choice for treating infections due to *Aerobacter* and *Serratia*. There is wide

Table 3-5 **Infections in which an aminoglycoside antibiotic is the drug of choice**
The role of streptomycin in the treatment of infection with mycobacteria has been considered in the first chapter (according to recommendations from *The Medical Letter*[16]).

Infecting organism	Drug of choice
Escherichia coli sepsis	Kanamycin
hospital acquired	
Klebsiella pneumoniae	
community acquired	Kanamycin with or without Cephalothin
hospital acquired	Gentamicin
Aerobacter	Gentamicin
Serratia	Gentamicin
Proteus other than	Kanamycin
Proteus mirabilis	
Pseudomonas aeruginosa	Gentamicin and Carbenicillin
other than urinary tract	
infection	
Actinobacillus mallei (glanders)	Streptomycin and a tetracycline
Pasturella tularensis (tularemia)	Streptomycin
Pasturella pestis (bubonic plague)	Streptomycin
Nocardia	Streptomycin and a sulfonamide

variability in the sensitivity of *E. coli* to the penicillins and in the treatment of *E. coli* sepsis acquired in the hospital, where a high percentage of the strains are resistant to the penicillins, parenteral kanamycin is the treatment of choice. Kanamycin and gentamicin are the drugs of choice in treating infection due to *Klebsiella pneumoniae*. Both are employed as alternative drugs for a variety of infections due to gram-negative organisms. Streptomycin alone is very effective in the treatment of plague *(Pasturella pestis)* and tularemia *(Pasturella tularensis)*. It is used to treat glanders in combination with tetracycline and nocardiosis in combination with a sulfonamide.

Antibiotic Preparation of the Bowel for Colonic Surgery

There is a special case for the prophylactic use of antibiotics in bowel surgery. Before elective colon surgery, antibiotics are given to "sterilize the bowel" and thereby reduce the risk of postoperative complication due to infection with gram-negative enteric organisms. The goal of this bowel preparation is to eliminate bacteria from the intestine without achieving high blood levels of antibiotic or irritating the bowel mucosa. The antibiotic regimen is combined with a low residue diet and cleansing enemas for two to three days before surgery.

One of the dangers of this treatment is that it can disturb the balance of the normal bacterial flora, resulting in an overgrowth of pathogenic organisms. Because an increased incidence of postoperative diarrhea and staphylococcal and yeast infection has been reported, there is some controversy over the value of preoperative antibiotic preparation of the bowel. One report has indicated that there may be less wound complication and diarrhea in patients who do not receive antibiotics before open colon resection.[17] Some surgeons have abandoned the practice, but some studies suggest that it may not be harmful. Thieme and Fink.[18] for example, studied the use of neomycin or a poorly absorbed sulfa, or a combination of the two, for bowel preparation before colonic surgery. They found that the change in flora did not result in staphylococcal overgrowth leading to staphylococcal enterocolitis or staphylococcal wound infection. There is at present no clear resolution to the controversy. Since the colon is the largest reservoir of bacteria in the body, and the risk of infection after elective operations on the colon can be high, it seems clear that bowel antisepsis will continue to be a widely used procedure for some time. There is a growing body of surgeons, however, who place their reliance on careful surgical technique and thorough mechanical cleansing of the bowel.

Many drug combinations have been used for preoperative bowel preparation. These involve a non-absorbable sulfa, neomycin, or kanamycin, one of which is usually combined with a poorly absorbed broad-spectrum antibiotic or an antifungal agent, such as nystatin. When a single drug is used, kanamycin is probably preferable to neomycin or a non-absorbable sulfa.[19] A comparison of the efficacy of the various antibiotic preparations in suppressing colon bacteria and a discussion of the advantages and complications of intestinal antisepsis have been presented by Cohn.[20]

Pharmacology of the Aminoglycoside Antibiotics

Absorption, distribution, and elimination. All of the aminoglycosides are very poorly absorbed from the gastrointestinal tract, though they are absorbed well from intramuscular and subcutaneous injection sites. They are given orally for bowel antisepsis before intestinal surgery. Although they have a marked effect on the gastrointestinal flora after oral administration, there is little effect after parenteral administration. These drugs are excreted primarily in their unchanged form by the kidney, and very little of the parenterally administered drug reaches the intestine.

The aminoglycoside antibiotics are excreted almost entirely by the kidney, the predominant mechanism being glomerular filtration. If renal function is impaired, the blood levels of these drugs, which are all toxic to the eighth nerve, will rise rapidly with a consequent increased risk of toxic effects. In order to prevent a toxic reaction, it is important to adjust the dose of these drugs (as well as such other drugs heavily dependent upon the renal route for excretion as the tetracyclines, polymyxin B, and vancomycin) when there is impairment of renal function. This is done by lowering the maintenance dose, by increasing the interval between doses, or both. The reader should see the literature for precise recommendations on modifying the dosage of various antibiotics in the presence of compromised renal function.[21,22]

Gentamicin provides an example of how such an adjustment of therapy can be made. There is a direct correlation between the serum half-life of gentamicin and creatinine clearance. A creatinine clearance value is often not available when treatment must be begun, but an initial dosage schedule may be approximated from the blood urea levels (Table 3-6).[23]

Aminoglycoside concentrations much higher than peak blood levels can occur in the urine. As these drugs have a greater antibacterial effect in an alkaline environment, bicarbonate should be given when aminoglycosides are used to treat urinary tract infections. The effectiveness of gentamicin against S. aureus, for example, is 17 times greater in vitro at pH 8 than at pH 6.[24]

The aminoglycoside antibiotics pass with difficulty into the cerebrospinal fluid. These antibiotics (particularly gentamicin) are useful in treating meningitis due to susceptible gram-negative bacilli when less toxic alternatives are ineffective.[25,26] In such cases the drugs must be given by intrathecal injection combined with intramuscular therapy. Intrathecal injection, however, can produce severe central nervous system dysfunction.

Table 3-6 **Approximate dosage schedule for gentamicin in adult patients with impaired renal function**
Creatinine clearances and blood urea and serum gentamicin levels were measured in normal subjects and patients with impaired renal function. An approximate dosage schedule for gentamicin in an adult with impaired renal function weighing between 60 and 80 kg was derived by measuring the blood urea level and creatinine clearance; these schedules yield an average peak serum level of gentamicin of 7 μg/ml. (From Gingell and Waterworth.[23])

Blood urea (mg/100ml)	Creatinine clearance (G.F.R.) (ml/min)	Dose and frequency of administration
<35	>70	80 mg every 8 hours
50-100	30-50	80 mg every 12 hours
>200	5-10	80 mg every 48 hours
Twice weekly intermittent hemodialysis	<3	80 mg after dialysis

Hypersensitivity reactions. Aminoglycosides elicit the common allergic reactions. One type of hypersensitivity response, which can cause some confusion, is the development of allergic dermatitis after topical application. Neomycin, either alone or in combination with another antibiotic such as bacitracin, is often used in the topical treatment of superficial skin infections. Especially after long-term therapy, neomycin can produce contact dermatitis, which is, in many cases, clinically similar to the condition being treated.[27] When there is such a conversion from a complex of signs and symptoms of infectious origin to an allergic contact dermatitis, the patient benefits from withdrawal of therapy rather than continuation. It stands to reason that systemic administration of the other aminoglycoside antibiotics in the person who has been so sensitized may result in a hypersensitivity reaction.

Neuromuscular reactions. The aminoglycoside antibiotics act to block conduction at the neuromuscular synapse when the levels of drug are high enough.[28] This effect is additive to that of *d*-tubocurarine. If these antibiotics are placed directly on the peritoneal surface, respiratory arrest, which can be reversed with atropine and prostigmine, may result; the aminoglycosides, therefore, should not be applied directly to the peritoneum.

Toxicity. All the aminoglycoside antibiotics have a dose-related toxic effect on the function of the eighth cranial (auditory) nerve. A disturbance of labyrinthine function causes vertigo, past-pointing and a positive Romberg test, and impairment of cochlear function causes tinnitus and loss of hearing acuity. The target for the toxic effect of streptomycin appears to be the end organ, not the brain stem. There is a loss of sensory cells in the vestibulo-cochlear organs of the cat, which can be readily viewed histologically, and this correlates well with observed changes in function as a result of toxicity to streptomycin and dihydrostreptomycin.[29] Streptomycin and dihydrostreptomycin have different patterns of toxicity. Streptomycin is mainly toxic for the vestibular system, and dihydrostreptomycin and kanamycin for the auditory system. The dihydro-form is not often used for this reason. If streptomycin therapy is stopped soon after symptoms appear, both functions will return, although there is sometimes residual damage. If treatment is continued, permanent damage (including complete deafness) can result. Patients receiving these drugs should be given balance and audiometry tests before therapy is started and tests on a biweekly basis while therapy is in progress. The aminoglycosides are also nephrotoxic. Damage to the kidney can lead to increased levels of plasma creatinine and BUN. Renal damage is usually reversible.

Resistance to the Aminoglycosides

It was demonstrated some time ago that resistance to an antibiotic could develop either gradually in small steps or that resistance to a high level of the same drug could develop suddenly.[30] The former process is called a multi-step resistance pattern, and it results from the selection of several mutations, often in a number of different genes. Each mutation confers a small amount of resistance, and a cumulative effect builds up in the bacterial culture. The second type of resistance development, called the large-step pattern, is commonly seen with streptomycin. In this case a mutation in a single gene leads to a very high degree of resistance or to drug insensitivity. This is the type of mutation that was discussed earlier in the chapter: a mutation at the Sm locus which resulted in an alteration of the 30 S ribosomal subunit protein, P_{10}, making the mutant cells insensitive to streptomycin. The large-step pattern can be clinically significant, as a single mutational event can release an infecting organism from antibiotic control. In the multi-step pattern, which is more commonly seen, for example, with penicillin, the chance of developing highly resistant strains can be minimized by using doses of the drug sufficiently large to prevent survival of first-step resistant mutants.

The degree of cross resistance among the aminoglycoside antibiotics varies. Sometimes resistance to all the drugs develops. Sometimes one or another of the drugs may be useful when there is a high degree of resistance to the others. Gentamicin, for example, is effective in inhibiting the growth of staphylococci that are resistant to neomycin and kanamycin.[24] *Escherichia coli* strains have been isolated that carry resistance factors that direct the production of enzymes that modify the structure of the various aminoglycosides by phosphorylation or acetylation.[31] Some aminoglycosides are much better substrates than others for these enzymes. The altered drug may or may not retain antibiotic activity. It is easy to see how different patterns of cross resistance can develop depending upon the nature of the resistance mechanism.

Combined Therapy with Aminoglycosides and Other Antibiotics

When a combination of two antibiotics is used to treat an infection, it may have one of the following patterns of therapeutic effectiveness:

(1) The combination may be more effective than either of the drugs given alone. This response is called an additive effect, and it is often seen when streptomycin and penicillin are used together to treat endocarditis due to *Streptococcus viridans*.

(2) The combination may have a much greater effect than the sum of the two individual drug effects. This is called a synergistic response, and it is seen with certain mixtures of two bactericidal drugs. The combination of gentamicin and carbenicillin is synergistic *in vitro* for some strains of *Pseudomonas*.[32][33] Such a synergistic response has been reported in the clinical treatment of severe *Pseudomonas* infection.[34] Although these two antibiotics are used at the same time, they should never be mixed in the same solution because gentamicin loses activity in solution with carbenicillin.

(3) The combination may produce less of a response than one of the drugs alone. This is drug antagonism. Such antagonism occurs when streptomycin and chloramphenicol are combined,[35] but its basis in this case is not clear. Treatment with a bactericidal drug (streptomycin) in combination with a bacteriostatic drug (chloramphenicol) sometimes leads to a response that is less than that of the bactericidal drug alone. A common explanation of this observation is that many bactericidal agents will have a killing effect only on cells that are growing and actively synthesizing protein and that bacteriostatic drugs prevent such growth and thereby counter the effect of a bactericidal drug. This explanation is simplistic. It fits certain situations, the combination of penicillins with bacteriostatic agents, for example, but it does not fit others.

References

1. T. D. Brock: Streptomycin. *Symp. Soc. Gen. Microbiol.* 16:131 (1966).
2. B. Weisblum and J. Davies: Antibiotic inhibitors of the bacterial ribosome. *Bact. Rev.* 32:493 (1968).
3. D. T. Dubin, R. Hancock, and B. D. Davis: The sequence of some effects of streptomycin in *Escherichia coli. Biochim. Biophys. Acta* 74:476 (1963).
4. L. Luzzatto, D. Apirion, and D. Schlessinger: Polyribosome depletion and blockage of the ribosome cycle by streptomycin in *Escherichia coli. J. Mol. Biol.* 42:315 (1969).
5. S. Kang: A mutant of *Escherichia coli* with temperature-sensitive streptomycin protein. *Proc. Natl. Acad. Sci., U.S.* 65:544 (1970).
6. L. Luzzatto, D. Aprion and D. Schlessinger: Mechanism of action of streptomycin in *E. coli;* interruption of the ribosome cycle at the initiation of protein synthesis. *Proc. Natl. Acad. Sci., U.S.* 60:873 (1968).
7. J. E. Davies: Studies on the ribosomes of streptomycin-sensitive and resistant strains of *Escherichia coli. Proc. Natl. Acad. Sci., U.S.* 51:659 (1964).
8. P. Traub and M. Nomura: Structure and function of *Escherichia coli* ribosomes; VI. Mechanism of assembly of 30 S ribosomes studied *in vitro. J. Mol. Biol.* 40:391 (1969).
9. M. Ozaki, S. Mizuchima, and M. Nomura: Identification and functional characterization of the protein controlled by the streptomycin-resistant locus in *E. coli. Nature* 222:333 (1969).
10. J. Davies, L. Gorini, and B. D. Davis: Misreading of RNA codewords induced by aminoglycoside antibiotics. *Mol. Pharmacol.* 1:93 (1965).
11. L. Gorini and E. Kataja: Streptomycin-induced oversuppression in *E. coli. Proc. Natl. Acad. Sci., U.S.* 51:995 (1964).
12. L. Gorini and E. Kataja: Phenotypic repair by streptomycin of defective genotypes in *E. coli. Proc. Natl. Acad. Sci., U.S.* 51:487 (1964).
13. K. Hashimoto: Streptomycin resistance in *Escherichia coli* analyzed by transduction. *Genetics* 45:49 (1960).
14. C. R. Spotts: Physiological and biochemical studies on streptomycin dependence in *Escherichia coli. J. Gen. Microbiol.* 28:347 (1962).
15. C. R. Spotts and R. Y. Stanier: Mechanism of streptomycin action on bacteria; a unitary hypothesis. *Nature* 192:633 (1961).
16. Editorial: Antimicrobial drugs of choice. *Med. Letter* 13:39 (1971).
17. M. A. Polacek and P. Sanfelippo: Oral antibiotic bowel preparation and complications in colon surgery. *Arch. Surg.* 97:412 (1968).
18. E. T. Thieme and G. Fink: A study of the danger of antibiotic preparation of the bowel for surgery. *Surgery* 67:403 (1970).
19. I. Cohn: Intestinal antisepsis. *Dis. Colon and Rectum* 8:11 (1965).
20. I. Cohn: Intestinal antisepsis. *Surg. Gynec. Obstet.* 130:1006 (1970).
21. C. M. Kunin: A guide to use of antibiotics in patients with renal disease; A table of recommended doses and factors governing serum levels. *Ann. Int. Med.* 67:151 (1967).

22. B. L. Mirkin: Drug therapy in patients with impaired renal function. *Postgrad. Med.* 47:159 (1970).

23. J. C. Gingell and P. M. Waterworth: Dose of gentamicin in patients with normal renal function and renal impairment. *Brit. Med. J.* 2:19 (1968).

24. M. Barber and P. M. Waterworth: Activity of gentamicin against pseudomonas and hospital staphylococci. *Brit. Med. J.* 1:203 (1966).

25. R. L. Neuman and R. J. Holt: Intrathecal gentamicin in treatment of ventriculitis in children. *Brit. Med. J.* 2:539 (1967).

26. M. C. McHenry, D. F. Dohn, F. R. Tingwald, and T. L. Gavan: Meningitis due to *Escherichia coli. J.A.M.A.* 212:156 (1970).

27. E. Epstein: Allergy to dermatologic agents. *J.A.M.A.* 198:103 (1966).

28. O. Vital Brazil and A. P. Corrado: The curariform action of streptomycin. *J. Pharm. Exptl. Therap.* 120:452 (1957).

29. T. M. McGee and J. Olszewski: Streptomycin sulfate and dihydrostreptomycin toxicity. *Arch. Otolaryngol.* 75:295 (1962).

30. M. Demerec: Origin of bacterial resistance to antibiotics. *J. Bacteriol.* 56:63 (1948).

31. R. Benveniste and J. Davies: Enzymatic acetylation of aminoglycoside antibiotics by *Escherichia coli* carrying an R factor. *Biochemistry* 10:1787 (1971).

32. W. Brumfitt, A. Percival, and D. A. Leigh: Clinical and laboratory studies with carbenicillin; A new penicillin active against *Pseudomonas pyocyanea. Lancet* 1:1289 (1967).

33. M. Sonne and E. Jawetz: Combined action of carbenicillin and gentamicin on *Pseudomonas aeruginosa in vitro. Appl. Microbiol.* 17:893 (1969).

34. C. B. Smith, J. N. Wilfert, P. E. Dans, T. A. Kurrus, and M. Finland: *In vitro* activity of carbenicillin and results of treatment of infections due to *Pseudomonas* with carbenicillin singly and in combination with gentamicin. *J. Infect. Dis.* 122:S14 (1970).

35. P. Plotz and B. D. Davis: Absence of a chloramphenicol-insensitive phase of streptomycin action. *J. Bacteriol.* 83:802 (1962).

Chapter 4
The Inhibitors of Protein Synthesis III
The Tetracyclines

Introduction

The tetracycline antibiotics were isolated from various species of *Streptomyces* recovered by large-scale screening of soil samples. The first of these compounds chlortetracycline (Aureomycin) was introduced in 1948. The tetracyclines are all very closely related, structurally. The structure of chlortetracycline is presented as an

Chlortetracycline

example of the basic polycyclic unit of all these compounds. The antimicrobial properties of these drugs are essentially the same. When resistance arises to one of the compounds there is cross resistance with the others.

These drugs, which are stable in powder form, are not very stable in aqueous solution. The stability decreases with increasing pH. Many solutions of tetracycline prepared for intravenous administration also contain ascorbic acid to buffer the solution at a mildly acidic pH. The fact that the tetracyclines are more stable at an acidic pH causes problems when these drugs are being infused over several hours along with a drug that is unstable at an acidic pH. Penicillin G, methicillin, and cephalothin, for example, are unstable in acid solution. If tetracyclines are mixed with penicillin G in an intravenous solution, the penicillin is extensively inactivated after a few hours of standing at room temperature.[1] When administering any antibiotic intravenously, it is important to pick the appropriate vehicle solution carefully and to instruct the attending personnel to watch for evidence of decomposition and drug incompatibility, as indicated by changes in color or clarity of the solution or the formation of a precipitate. In the case of incompatibility between the tetracylines and penicillin G or methicillin, however, the second drug is slowly inactivated but no such obvious signs appear.

The tetracyclines form stable chelates with a number of metal ions such as calcium, magnesium, iron, and aluminum. The formation of an insoluble complex with any of these compounds decreases the absorption of the drug from the gastrointestinal tract. Therefore, tetracyclines should never be administered with milk, which contains calcium, or with antacids, such as Maalox, which contains magnesium and aluminum hydroxide or Amphojel, which is an aluminum hydroxide gel. Ferrous sulfate administered with a tetracycline markedly reduces the absorption of the antibiotic,[2] so even small doses of iron should be avoided during tetracycline therapy.

Mechanism of Action

At the blood concentrations achieved in antibacterial therapy, the tetracyclines are bacteriostatic. At much higher concentrations they are bactericidal. Various biochemical sites of action have been proposed for these drugs, based on reports of their inhibition of several bacterial enzyme systems, oxidative phosphorylation, glucose oxidation, and membrane transport.[3] One of the earliest studies demonstrated that protein synthesis is particularly sensitive to inhibition by the tetracyclines.[4] Studies with *in vitro* protein-synthesizing systems from resistant organisms have shown that tetracycline resistance can reside in altered ribosomal particles,[5] and this confirms that the inhibition of protein synthesis is responsible for the inhibition of growth by these drugs.

The receptor for tetracyclines has not been defined as precisely as that for streptomycin or erythromycin. The tetracyclines bind to both ribosomes and mRNA. It is clearly the binding of the drug to the ribosome that inhibits protein synthesis.[6] This binding is largely reversible, and the bulk of the bound tetracycline is associated with the 30 S ribosomal subunit.[7,8] A poly U-directed cell-free protein-synthesizing system from E. coli containing 30 S ribosomal subunits from tetracycline-resistant cells is much less sensitive to inhibition by tetracycline than the same system containing 30 S units from sensitive cells.[5] But it has not been demonstrated, as it has with streptomycin, that the 30 S particles from resistant cells bind the drug less well.

The basis for the selective toxicity of the tetracyclines is not entirely clear. It has been shown that a cell-free protein-synthesizing system from E. coli is more sensitive to inhibition by chlortetracycline than a cell-free system prepared from rat liver.[9] The rat-liver system was nevertheless appreciably inhibited by the drug.

In bacteria, tetracycline inhibits protein synthesis by blocking the binding of aminoacyl-tRNA to the mRNA-ribosome complex. As shown in Table 4-1, when tetracycline and phenylalanyl-tRNA are added simultaneously to a system containing 30 S subunits and poly U, binding of the radioactive phenylalanyl-tRNA to the 30 S subunits is markedly inhibited.[10] When the phenylalanyl-tRNA is added to the system twenty minutes before the tetracy-

Table 4-1 The effect of tetracycline on the binding of phenylalanyl-tRNA to the 30 S ribosomal subunit

Phenylalanyl-tRNA binding to ribosomes was measured by incubating ^{3}H-labeled phenylalanyl-tRNA with poly U and 30 S subunits at $24°C$ for 20 minutes. After incubation the samples were filtered and washed. The ribosome-bound radioactivity remained on the filter, while the unbound radioactive aminoacyl-tRNA passed through. The values in the table represent the total phenylalanyl-tRNA bound per 7 μg of 30 S subunit. (Data from Suzuka et al.[10])

| Conditions of prebinding | Binding of ^{3}H-phenylalanyl-tRNA: | |
	Tetracycline added with 30 S subunits	Tetracycline added 20 minutes after 30 S subunits
Control	781	851
Tetracycline $(4.5 \times 10^{-4} M)$	226	674

cline, inhibition of binding is much less. Thus, once the aminoacyl-tRNA is bound to the 30 S particles, tetracycline cannot dissociate it.

There are two binding sites for aminoacyl-tRNA on the mRNA-70 S-ribosome complex (see chapter 2). An aminoacyl-tRNA can bind to the first site, the acceptor site, when the 30 S subunit is present. It is only when the 50 S subunit is bound to the 30 S ribosome subunit that a second binding site (the donor site) is generated. This second binding site normally binds the tRNA to which the growing polypeptide is attached. It has been shown that tetracycline inhibits the binding of lysyl-tRNA to the ribosome but has no effect on the binding of polylysyl-tRNA.[11] This might indicate that the drug inhibits binding to the acceptor site but not to the donor site. A similar conclusion was reached by investigators who demonstrated that, although tetracycline inhibits virtually 100 per cent of the protein synthesis, it is only able to inhibit 50 per cent[12] of the binding of N-acetyl-phenylalanyl-tRNA. Protein synthesis then is halted at the same concentration of tetracycline that inhibits the binding of aminoacyl-tRNA to one-half of the tRNA binding sites on the ribosome.

The conclusion that tetracycline affects the binding to the acceptor site is supported by investigations using another antibiotic, puromycin, as an experimental tool. Puromycin is an analog of aminoacyl-tRNA.[13] It causes the separation of the growing peptide chain from the peptidyl-tRNA-messenger-ribosome complex with the formation of peptidylpuromycin.[14] Puromycin does not prevent the binding of aminoacyl-tRNA to the acceptor site nor does it effect the release of aminoacyl-tRNA from that site. It was reasoned that if tetracycline inhibits only the binding of amino-acyl-tRNA to the acceptor site, then the one-half of the aminoacyl-tRNA that remains bound in the presence of tetracycline should be occupying the peptidyl-tRNA (donor) site and should be released by puromycin. Correspondingly only one-half of the aminoacyl-tRNA bound in the absence of the drug should be sensitive to puromycin. In the experiment presented in Table 4-2 and Figure 4-1, only one-half of the aminoacyl-tRNA was bound in the presence of tetracycline, and all of this was released as phenylal-anyl-puromycin.[15] In the absence of tetracycline, twice as much

Table 4-2   The release by puromycin of radioactive phenylalanyl-tRNA prebound to ribosomes: with and without tetracycline
14C-labeled phenylalanyl-tRNA was bound to ribosomes with and without tetracycline. The phenylalanyl-tRNA was present in amounts sufficient to assure maximal binding. Puromycin was then added, the incubation was continued for one hour, and the amount of phenylalanyl-puromycin formed was extracted and assayed. Values represent the number of $\mu\mu$moles of phe-tRNA bound or phe-puromycin released per incubation. (From Sarkar and Thach.[15])

Conditions of prebinding	Phenylalanyl-tRNA prebound ribosomes	Phenylalanyl-puromycin synthesized and released	Prebound phenylalanine released by puromycin
	($\mu\mu$ moles)		(%)
Control	14.1	6.74	47.7
Tetracycline (6 $\times$ 10^{-4}M)	7.35	7.21	98.1

of the aminoacyl-tRNA was bound, and only one-half of it (presumably that portion occupying the donor site) was released as phenylalanyl-puromycin.

This use of one antibiotic to investigate the mechanism of action of another points up one important role that chemotherapeutic drugs have played outside the clinical field of infectious disease management. Many of these drugs are valuable investigative tools for the study of biological phenomena. Much of what we now know

Figure 4-1   The release by puromycin of phenylalanyl-tRNA bound to ribosomes with and without tetracycline. A. In the normal process of mRNA translation the tRNA with the attached peptide occupies the donor site (I). When puromycin is added, an aminoacyl-tRNA can still bind in the acceptor site; however, puromycin becomes linked by a peptide bridge to the carboxy terminal of the growing peptide (II), and this complex is released as peptidylpuromycin (III). B and C. The experiment as carried out with tetracycline by Sarkar and Thach.[15] When phenylalanyl-tRNA is bound to ribosomes in the presence of tetracycline (B), tetracycline blocks binding to the acceptor site but binding to the donor site is permitted. When the bound complex is exposed to puromycin all of the phenylalanine is released as phenylalanyl puromycin. In the absence of tetracycline (C), phenylalanyl-tRNA can bind to both the acceptor and donor sites; therefore, twice as much is bound. As puromycin can release only the phenylalanine occupying the donor site, one-half of the bound puromycin is released as phenylalanyl-puromycin. P, puromycin; T, tetracycline; phe, phenylalanine; aa, amino acid.

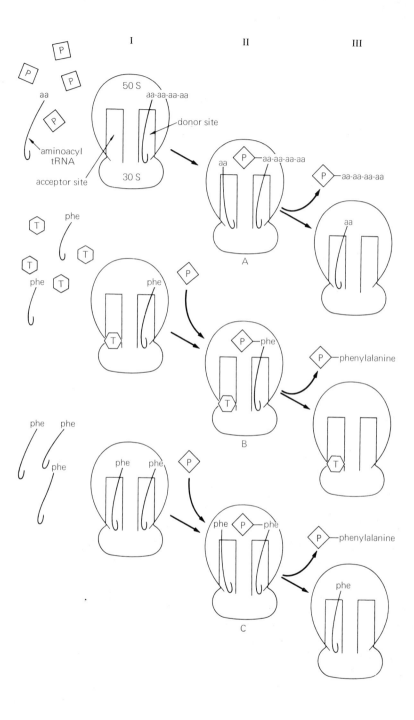

I   II   III

50 S
aa-aa-aa-aa
donor site

aa
aminoacyl
tRNA

acceptor site
30 S

A

phe

B

phe   phe

phe

phenylalanine

C

phenylalanine

about intermediary metabolism, protein and nucleic acid synthesis, and the sequence of the cell cycle was determined by using drugs that specifically block particular biochemical events. The investigative use of these drugs is most productive when the mechanism of action of the drug is precisely defined. If they are employed when only scant data regarding their mechanism of action are available, interpretation of experimental results is impossible.

Therapeutic Indications

The tetracyclines have a very broad spectrum of action. They inhibit the growth of many bacteria, actinomycetes, rickettsiae, mycoplasma, and agents of the psittacosis-lymphogranuloma venerum-trachoma group. The true viruses are not susceptible to the tetracyclines.

A list of those infections for which a tetracycline is a drug of choice is presented in Table 4-3. Tetracycline is the drug of choice for only a few bacterial infections. These include cholera, granuloma inguinale, chancroid, and gastrointestinal infection with *Bacteroides*. Tetracyclines are used in combination with streptomycin for the treatment of glanders and either alone or in combination with a sulfonamide or streptomycin for the treatment of melioidosis and brucellosis, respectively. They are not drugs of choice for infection with many enterobacteria because of the increasingly common resistance to tetracyclines of many strains of these organisms. Other than those few and relatively uncommon infections in which a tetracycline is a drug of choice, the use of these drugs in the treatment of bacterial infections depends upon the results of sensitivity testing and the ability of the patient to tolerate therapy with other antibiotics. They are often effective alternatives in the treatment of infection due to gram-positive bacilli (such as infection due to *Listeria*, tetanus, anthrax, and gas gangrene) and to a wide variety of gram-negative organisms. They are not useful alternatives to penicillin in the treatment of infection due to gram-positive cocci.

The tetracyclines are the best drugs for the treatment of rickettsial diseases such as Rocky Mountain spotted fever, Q fever, and typhus.

Table 4-3   A selected list of infections for which a tetracycline is the agent of choice in treatment
(According to recommendations from *The Medical Letter.* [16])

Infecting organism	Drug of choice
Gram-negative bacilli	
Bacteroides (gastrointestinal strains)	Tetracycline
Actinobacillus mallei (glanders)	Tetracycline with streptomycin
Pseudomonas pseudomallei (melioidosis)	Tetracycline alone or with a sulfonamide
Brucella (brucellosis)	Tetracycline alone or with streptomycin
Haemophilus ducreyi (chancroid)	Tetracycline
Calymmatobacterium granulomatis (granuloma inguinale)	Tetracycline
Vibrio cholerae (cholera)	Tetracycline
Spirochetes	
Borrelia recurrentis (relapsing fever)	Tetracycline
Rickettsia	
(Rocky Mountain spotted fever, typhus, Q fever)	Tetracycline
Filterable agents	
Mycoplasma pneumoniae (atypical pneumonia)	Tetracycline or erythromycin
Agent of psittacosis	Tetracycline
Lymphogranuloma venerum	Tetracycline
Chlamydia trachomatis (trachoma)	Tetracycline (topical)
Virus of inclusion conjunctitis	Tetracycline

Some infections are caused by organisms that are roughly classified as "filterable agents" and chlamydia ("large viruses"). The tetracyclines and erythromycin are equally effective in the treatment of infection with Mycoplasma pneumoniae (primary atypical pneumonia). The diseases resulting from infection with chlamydia include psittacosis, lymphogranuloma venerum, trachoma, and inclusion conjunctivitis. They all respond to the tetracyclines.

The spectrum of action of an antibiotic is roughly defined as broad or narrow depending upon the variety of disease agents susceptible to it. The tetracyclines and the chloramphenicol-erythromycin group have the broadest spectra of action and are the most useful in treating non-bacterial infections. If a tetracycline cannot be used, chloramphenicol is the preferred alternative for the treatment of rickettsial infections, psittacosis, and inclusion conjunctivitis. But of course the use of chloramphenicol is accompanied by the risk of producing aplastic anemia. The spectrum of action of the tetracyclines also encompasses certain fungal and parasitic diseases. They are useful alternatives for the treatment of actinomycosis and many *Nocardia* infections. In combination with other antiparasitic drugs, they are occasionally employed in the treatment of amebiasis.

Tetracycline Preparations

The tetracycline preparations vary according to extent of plasma binding, rate of absorption, and rate of excretion. These differences dictate different dosages and schedules of administration. Aside from these minor variations, the different tetracycline preparations do not vary significantly in clinical effectiveness. The antibacterial spectrum for all of the tetracyclines is the same. When resistance arises to one member of the group, it generally includes all the drugs. All preparations produce the same side effects, and most of these are dose related. The drugs are usually administered orally, but in severe infection they are given intravenously. They should never be administered intrathecally. When it is necessary to give a tetracycline to a patient with renal insufficiency, doxycycline should be used, as this compound depends less upon the renal route of excretion than the other tetracyclines. Because of its low renal clearance, doxycycline is probably not as useful as the other tetracyclines for the treatment of urinary tract infections.

Although the clinical effectiveness of the various tetracyclines at recommended doses and at recommended frequencies of administration is roughly the same,[17] there are nevertheless many generic and brand name preparations to choose from. A partial list of the preparations available is presented in Table 4-4. Tetracycline hydrochloride itself is available under a number of different brand names. This proliferation of different brand names for the same product injects a great deal of confusion into a physician's education. The tetracyclines are by no means a unique example,

Table 4-4 **Generic and brand names of some tetracycline preparations available in the United States**

Generic name	Brand name	Manufacturer
Tetracycline hydrochloride	Achromycin	Lederle
	Panmycin	Upjohn
	Tetracyn	Roerig
	Tetrachel	Rachelle
	Rexamycin	Rexall
	Kesso-Tetra	McKesson
Oxytetracycline	Terramycin	Pfizer
Chlortetracycline	Aureomycin	Lederle
Demethylchlortetracycline	Declomycin	Lederle
Methacycline	Rondomycin	Pfizer
Doxycycline	Vibramycin	Pfizer

but they serve to point out the problems involved in the dual drug-naming system existing today. The immediate problem for the medical student is that he first learns the generic name of the drug in the basic course in pharmacology. When he enters the clinical years, he is forced to completely overhaul his drug vocabulary in order to understand the clinician who, instead of referring to tetracycline hydrochloride, will talk about Achromycin, Panmycin, Tetrachel, or Tetracyn. All of these are brand names for the same compound, produced by different companies, and they indicate no clinically useful differences between the preparations.

The second problem resulting from this proliferation of names is that the practicing physician's awareness of new drug information can be considerably blunted. When a physician is informed of the advantages or disadvantages of a drug called by its brand name, he may not associate this information with other products that are identical. Chloramphenicol, for instance, is sold in the United States by three different companies under the names Chloromycetin, Amphicol, and Mychel, and it is sold abroad under 43 different trade names. This can of course make international communication between physicians difficult at times. It is clear that our redundant drug nomenclature system is not in the best interest of the physician or the patient.

Pharmacology of the Tetracyclines

Absorption and distribution. The tetracyclines are absorbed from the stomach and the upper gastrointestinal tract. As already mentioned, their absorption is impaired by milk, certain antacids, and iron compounds. They are distributed in a space larger than the body water, and they readily penetrate most body cavities. Their concentration in the cerebrospinal fluid is much lower than in the blood. They are concentrated in some tissues, particularly the liver, kidney, and spleen. The amount of drug bound to plasma protein varies from a low of 20 per cent with oxytetracyline to a high of 50 to 70 per cent with chlortetracycline.[18] This variation in the relative level of free drug has been taken into account in recommending therapeutic dosages. Tetracyclines remain bound to certain malignant tissues longer than to nonmalignant cells. This property has been used as an aid in the diagnosis of carcinoma of the stomach. Patients are given tetracycline, and 36 to 48 hours after the last dose exfoliated cells are recovered in gastric washings and examined for drug fluorescence. The reason for this longer binding to malignant cells is unknown.

The concentration of the tetracyclines in the liver, kidney, and spleen is a transient phenomenon lasting only a few hours. The tetracylines may be sequestered in bone for much longer periods. They become bound to newly forming bone but apparently not to bone that is already laid down.[19] Tetracycline is incorporated into calcifying tissue as a tetracycline-calcium orthophosphate complex. It is also incorporated into growing teeth and gives them a yellow or brownish color. The yellow color appears first and then is converted to brown, a process accelerated by exposure to light. The discoloration probably results from an oxidation product of tetracycline. The tetracyclines can cross the placenta, and their administration to pregnant women can discolor the deciduous teeth of the children they are carrying.[20] These drugs also appear in the milk of lactating patients. As would be expected, tetracycline taken by the mother during pregnancy does not affect the color of the child's permanent teeth.[21] Oxytetracycline binds calcium less readily than the other tetracyclines[22] and is less likely to produce a noticeable discoloration.[23] In children under eight years of age, the risk of discoloration of permanent teeth must be taken into account when the tetracyclines are being considered for long-term therapy.

Metabolism and excretion. The tetracyclines are eliminated in the urine and the feces; renal clearance is by glomerular filtration. The concentration of tetracyclines in the bile may be 10 to 20 times that in the serum. Some of the tetracycline released into the intestine in the bile is reabsorbed during passage through the rest of the gastrointestinal tract. Even if the drugs are given parenterally, they are found in the bowel; this is an important observation, since enteritis can result from superinfection of the bowel after parenteral as well as oral therapy. Some tetracyclines are excreted more slowly than others and have half-lives longer than the 9 hours observed for tetracycline hydrochloride: demethylchlortetracycline, 12 hours; methacycline, 15 hours; doxycycline, 20 hours.

Toxicity and side effects. The tetracyclines are irritative substances. Given intravenously, they can cause thrombophlebitis. Given orally, they cause epigastric burning, abdominal discomfort, nausea, and vomiting. If the irritation is severe, symptoms can sometimes be controlled, at the risk of some impairment of absorption, by having the patient take tetracyclines immediately after meals. The irritative effects on the mucosa of the bowel can cause diarrhea, which must be distinguished from enteritis due to superinfection with staphylococci.

Damage to the liver and kidneys may occur in tetracycline therapy, and serious liver damage occasionally occurs in pregnant women and in patients with renal disease. As with all antibiotics, expired or degraded tetracyclines should never be used. Both nephropathy[24] and Fanconi syndrome[25] have been reported after ingestion of outdated tetracyclines.

The tetracyclines cause occasional photosensitivity reactions, which disappear when the drug is withdrawn. These reactions occur most frequently with demethylchlortetracycline.

Superinfection

The normal microbial population of the gut, the respiratory tract, the skin, and the vagina is a complex community of both bacteria and fungi, some of which are potentially pathogenic. Growth of the potentially pathogenic organisms is normally suppressed by the more numerous nonpathogenic organisms. Such microbial antagonism can suppress the growth of bacteria and fungi in different ways. For example, two organisms may compete for essential nutrients. Some enteric bacilli produce proteins, called colicins, that kill sensitive bacteria in very specific ways.[26] These substances apparently act at the bacterial membrane and somehow elicit responses such as inhibition of macromolecular synthesis, degradation of DNA, or inhibition of oxidative phosphorylation. The nature of the cell response depends upon the colicin involved. In other cases resident bacteria may alter the chemical environment so that it is unfavorable for the growth of less desirable organisms. For example, the growth of lactobacilli in the adult vagina contributes to the maintenance of an acidic pH (4.0 to 4.5), which is probably not optimal for the growth of a number of potential pathogens.[27]

When the balance of the microbial population is altered by treatment with a broad-spectrum antibiotic, the usually dominant antibiotic-sensitive population is reduced, and superinfection with pathogenic organisms not sensitive to the drug can result. Two of the most common organisms involved in such superinfection are *Staphylococcus* and *Candida*. Superinfection with *Candida albicans* occurs in the oropharynx, vagina, and bowel; it can even occur as systemic infection. A number of tetracycline preparations contain both a tetracycline and nystatin, an antifungal agent included to suppress superinfection with *Candida*. This does not constitute rational prophylactic use of an antibiotic. The use of these two drugs in a fixed-ratio combination has not been demonstrated to reduce the incidence of intestinal superinfection with *Candida*. As stated in a drug efficacy study conducted by the National Academy of Sciences, "It is preferable . . . to prescribe antifungal drugs when clinically indicated, rather than to use them indiscriminately as 'prophylaxis' against an uncommon clinical entity seen during therapy with tetracyclines and other antibiotics."[28]

One of the most dangerous types of superinfection is overgrowth of *S. aureus* in the bowel, which can cause enterocolitis. Staphylococcal enteritis is a life-threatening condition, characterized by severe diarrhea, fever, and leukocytosis. It must be immediately considered when a patient receiving tetracyclines develops diarrhea. It can be differentiated from the milder diarrhea which results from the irritative effect of the drug on the mucosa of the colon by the presence of large numbers of gram-positive cocci in the stool and the growth of large numbers of coagulase-positive staphylococci on culture. Blood is often found in the liquid stool. When staphylococcal enteritis appears, tetracycline therapy must be stopped, fluid and electrolyte management begun, and oral treatment with large amounts of another antibiotic such as vancomycin initiated immediately. Although superinfection has been discussed here in regard to the tetracyclines, it can also occur during therapy with other antibiotics such as chloramphenicol, erythromycin, the aminoglycosides, and the penicillins.

References

1. S. Im and C. J. Latiolais: Physico-chemical incompatibilities of parenteral admixtures—penicillin and tetracyclines. Am. J. Hosp. Pharm. 23:333 (1966).

2. P. J. Neuvonen, G. Gothoni, R. Hackman, and K. Bjorksten: Interference of iron with the absorption of tetracyclines in man. Brit. Med. J. 4:532 (1970).

3. A. I. Laskin: Tetracyclines in D. Gotlieb and P. D. Shaw (ed.), Antibiotics, Vol. 1, New York: Springer-Verlag, 1967, pp. 331-359.

4. E. F. Gale and J. P. Folkes: The assimilation of amino acids by bacteria. Actions of antibiotics on nucleic acid and protein synthesis in Staphylococcus aureus. Biochem. J. 53:493 (1953).

5. G. R. Craven, R. Gavin, and T. Fanning: The transfer RNA binding site of the 30 S ribosome and the site of tetracycline inhibition. Symp. Quant. Biol. 34:129 (1969).

6. L. E. Day: Tetracycline inhibition of cell-free protein synthesis. II Effect of the binding of tetracycline to the components of the system. J. Bacteriol. 92:197 (1966).

7. R. H. Connamacher and H. G. Mandel: Binding of tetracycline to the 30 S ribosomes and to polyuridylic acid. Biochem. Biophys. Res. Commun. 20:98 (1965).

8. I. H. Maxwell: Studies of the binding of tetracycline to ribosomes in vitro. Mol. Pharmacol. 4:25 (1967).

9. T. J. Franklin: The inhibition of incorporation of leucine into protein of cell-free systems from rat liver and Escherichia coli by chlortetracycline. Biochem. J. 87:449 (1963).

10. I. Suzuka, H. Kaji, and A. Kaji: Binding of specific sRNA to 30 S ribosomal subunits; effect of 50 S ribosomal subunits. *Proc. Natl. Acad. Sci.* 55:1483 (1966).

11. M. E. Gottseman: Reaction of ribosome-bound peptidyl transfer ribonucleic acid with aminoacyl transfer ribonucleic acid or puromycin. *J. Biol. Chem.* 242:5564 (1967).

12. G. Suarez and D. Nathans: Inhibition of aminoacyl-tRNA binding to ribosomes by tetracycline. *Biochem. Biophys. Res. Commun.* 18:743 (1965).

13. M. Yarmolinsky and G. de la Haba: Inhibition by puromycin of amino acid incorporation into protein. *Proc. Natl. Acad. Sci.* 45:1721 (1959).

14. J. D. Smith, R. R. Traut, G. M. Blackburn, and R. E. Monroe: Action of puromycin in polyadenylic acid-directed polylysine synthesis. *J. Mol. Biol.* 13:617 (1965).

15. S. Sarkar and R. E. Thach: Inhibition of formylmethionyl-transfer RNA binding to ribosomes by tetracycline. *Proc. Natl. Acad. Sci.* 60:1481 (1968).

16. Editoral: Antimicrobial drugs of choice. *Med. Letter* 13:39 (1971).

17. Editorial: The choice and uses of tetracycline drugs. *Med. Letter* 11:62 (1969).

18. C. M. Kunin and M. Finland: Clinical pharmacology of the tetracycline antibiotics. *Clin. Pharm. Ther.* 2:51 (1961).

19. R. A. Milch, D. P. Rall, and J. E. Tobie: Bone localization of the tetracyclines. *J. Nat. Canc. Int.* 19:87 (1957).

20. A. C. Douglas: The deposition of tetracycline in human nails and teeth. A complication of long-term treatment. *Brit. J. Dis. Chest* 57:44 (1963).

21. J. R. Anthony: Effect on deciduous and permanent teeth of tetracycline deposition *in utero*. *Postgrad. Med.* 48:165 (1970).

22. M. Schach von Wittenau: Some pharmacokinetic aspects of doxycycline metabolism in man. *Chemotherapy* 13:41 (1968).

23. I. S. Wallman and H. B. Hilton: Teeth pigmented by tetracycline. *Lancet* 1:827 (1962).

24. F. Mavromatis: Tetracycline nephropathy. *J.A.M.A.* 193:91 (1965).

25. J. M. Gross: Fanconi syndrome (adult type) developing secondary to the ingestion of outdated tetracycline. *Ann. Int. Med.* 58:523 (1963).

26. M. Nomura: Mechanism of action of colicines. *Proc. Natl. Acad. Sci.* 52:1514 (1964).

27. B. D. Davis, R. Dulbecco, H. N. Eisen, H. S. Ginsberg, and W. B. Wood: *Microbiology*. New York: Harper and Row, 1969, p. 620.

28. Editorial: Candida infections. *Med. Letter* 12:29 (1970).

Chapter 5

The Inhibitors
of Cell Wall Synthesis
The Penicillins
The Cephalosporins
Vancomycin
Ristocetin
Bacitracin
Cycloserine

Discovery of the Penicillins

The discovery of penicillin is a now classic story of serendipity in scientific investigation. In 1928, Fleming noted that bacteria growing in culture in the vicinity of a contaminating mold were lysed.[1] He followed up this observation by culturing the mold in broth and demonstrating that filtrates of the broth were bactericidal *in vitro*. Almost a decade later, a group at Oxford led by H. W. Florey isolated a crude preparation of the bactericidal agent from cultures of *Penicillium notatum*. These investigators subsequently demonstrated the usefulness of this antibiotic in the treatment of bacterial infections in man. Although the basic unit of the penicillins has been synthesized, penicillin is produced commercially by isolation from cultures of mold that have been genetically altered to produce a very high yield.

In many cases, a detailed knowledge of the structure of an antibiotic is not particularly critical for developing an understanding of the current state of knowledge regarding its mechanism of action. For the penicillin group, however, a knowledge of the basic structure of the molecule is critical for understanding, at the molecular level, the basis of the mechanism of action, the development of bacterial cell resistance, and the mechanisms underlying the allergic response. The molecule, penicillin G. is composed of a thiazolidine ring attached to a four-membered (β-lactam) ring and a side chain attached in peptide linkage to the β-lactam ring. The four-membered ring is somewhat strained, and a number of important ring-opening reactions take place here. The cephalosporins, another group of compounds isolated from fungi, have the same mechanism of action as the penicillins and a similar structure with the characteristic β-lactam ring.

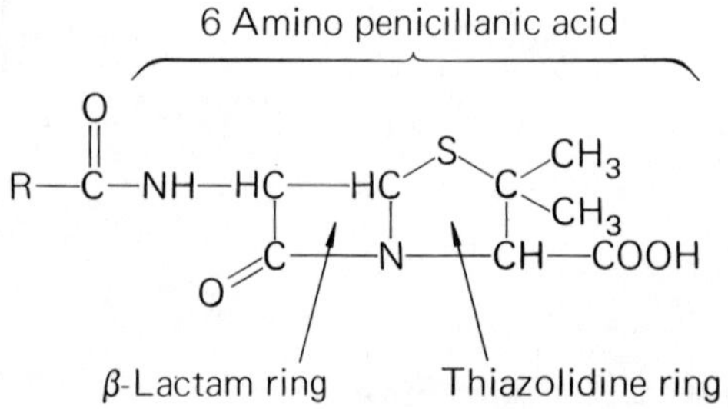

6 Amino penicillanic acid

β-Lactam ring   Thiazolidine ring

Penicillin G

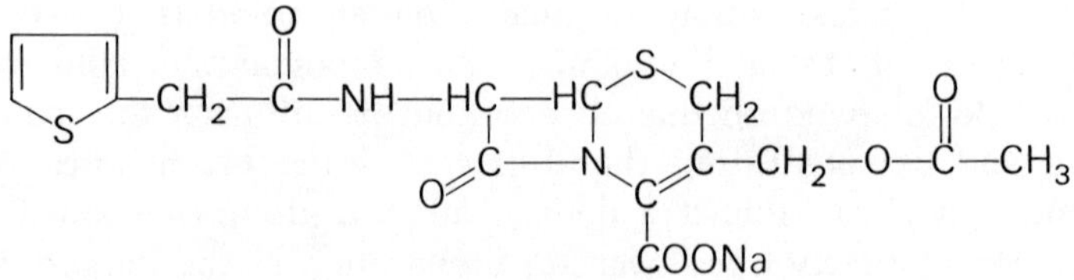

Cephalothin

Mechanism of Action

Site of Action

The cell wall of a bacterium forms a rather rigid skeleton on the outer surface of the cell membrane. The bacterial cell membrane in essence encases a volume hypertonic to the environment of the organism. Although the cell membrane is critical to the maintenance of the osmotic gradient between the organism and its environment, it is not strong enough in itself to keep the hypertonic sac from rupturing by osmotic shock. Thus the cell wall, which encases the cell membrane as a continuous, highly cross-linked molecule, prevents the cell membrane from rupturing. The penicillins inhibit the formation of cross-links between the units of the cell wall. As a result a strong cell wall network is not made, the cell membrane extrudes through the cell wall, and the cell ruptures by osmotic lysis and is, of course, no longer viable. Thus the penicillins are bactericidal agents.

When the bacterium is growing in a medium isotonic to the cytoplasm, exposure to penicillin, rather than rupturing the bacterium, can lead to the production of organisms that have no cell wall.[2] Such bacteria, encased solely in their cell membranes, are called protoplasts or spheroplasts. The site of synthesis of the cell wall and, therefore, the site of action of the penicillins, is oriented as a narrow girdle around the organism. If bacteria are exposed to penicillin the spheroplast emerges at the division furrow.[3] The sequence of events in bacterial cell growth and in the production of penicillin spheroplasts is presented schematically in Figure 5-1.

Early experiments demonstrated that exposure of S. aureus to penicillin resulted in a marked inhibition of radioactive precursor (leucine or phosphate) incorporation into the cell wall but not into bacterial protein or nucleic acid[4] (Table 5-1). It was clear that the process of cell wall biosynthesis would have to be explained in order to understand its inhibition by antibiotics. Our present knowledge of the biosynthesis of bacterial cell walls and the mechanisms of action of the various antibiotics inhibiting this process is largely the result of the research of Strominger and his co-workers.[5]

Table 5-1 Incorporation of isotopes into cell wall, cell protein, and nucleic acid in S. aureus
Penicillin was introduced into cultures of S. aureus, and the cultures were incubated for 20 minutes with radioactive leucine or phosphate. Incorporation as cpm/mg protein. (From Nathenson and Strominger,[4] Table 1.)

| Culture | Incorporation of ^{14}C-lysine into: | | Incorporation of ^{32}P-inorganic phosphate into: | |
	Cell wall	Cell protein and nucleic acid	Cell wall	Cell protein and nucleic acid
Control	34,800	5,100	155,000	11,600
Penicillin (100 µg/ml)	3,290	4,960	48,900	11,600

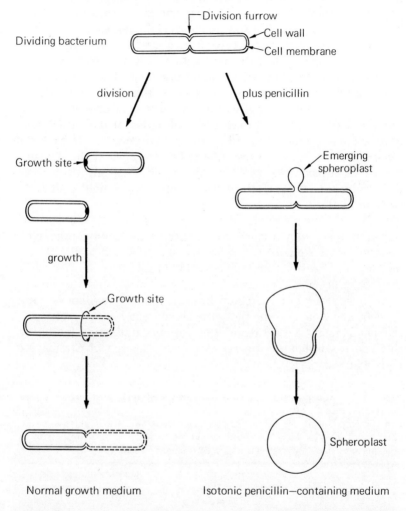

Figure 5-1 Normal cell growth and division compared to the formation of penicillin spheroplasts. Normal cell wall synthesis appears to take place at a growth site that encircles the cell. In the presence of penicillin, cross-linking of the cell wall units is inhibited, and the cell membrane then protrudes out of the structurally defective cell wall.

Inhibition of Cell Wall Synthesis

Synthesis of a bacterial cell wall can be divided into three stages according to where in the cell the reactions are taking place (Figure 5-2). The first series of reactions, resulting in the production of the basic cell wall building block (the UDP-acetyl-muramyl-pentapeptide), takes place inside the cell. Cycloserine, a second-choice antibiotic in the treatment of tuberculosis, inhibits one of the terminal reactions in this sequence. In the second stage of cell wall synthesis the precursor unit is carried from inside the cell membrane outside. During this process a number of modifications occur in the chemical structure of the basic repeating unit of the cell wall, and the units are linked covalently to the pre-existing cell wall. The antibiotics vancomycin, ristocetin, and bacitracin act during this second stage. The third stage of the process is a single reaction that takes place outside the cell membrane and results in the cross-linking of linear molecules to form the highly cross-linked, tough outer envelope of the cell. This cross-linking reaction is inhibited by the penicillins and cephalosporins.

Stage I—Precursor Formation

The sequence of reactions comprising the first stage of cell wall synthesis in *S. aureus* is presented in Figure 5-3. In the first reaction UTP is bound covalently to N-acetylglucosamine-1-P to form UDP-N-acetylglucosamine. Subsequent reactions add a three-carbon unit from phosphoenolpyruvate and three amino acids to form a UDP-acetylmuramyltripeptide. In the final reaction of this stage- a D-alanyl-D-alanine dipeptide is joined to the UDP-acetylmuramyltripeptide to produce the UDP-acetylmuramyl-pentapeptide, which is then available to participate in the second stage of cell wall synthesis. Exposure of bacteria to the antibiotics that inhibit stages II and III of cell wall synthesis will result in an accumulation of the pentapeptide in the cell.

Exposure of organisms to cyloserine prevents the formation of the pentapeptide. D-Cycloserine is a structural analog of D-alanine. The antibiotic is a competitive inhibitor of both alanine

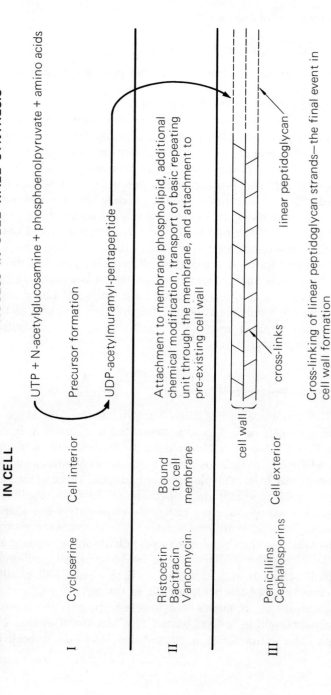

Figure 5-2 The three stages of bacterial cell wall biosynthesis and the antibiotics that inhibit this process at each stage.

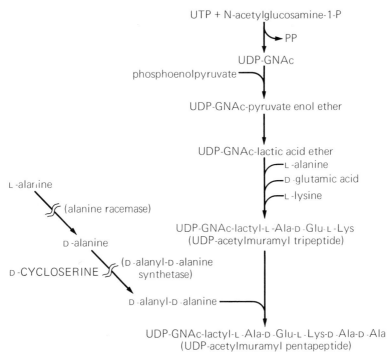

Figure 5-3   The first stage of cell wall synthesis in *S. aureus*. The reactions inhibited by D-cycloserine are indicated by the break marks.

racemase and D-alanyl-D-alanine synthetase. Both enzymes bind the antibiotic 100 times as strongly ($K_i = 5 \times 10^{-5}$ M) as they bind the normal substrate ($K_m = 5 \times 10^{-3}$M).[6]

D-Cycloserine   D-Alanine

(zwitterion forms)

Stage II—Formation of a Linear Peptidoglycan

In the second stage of cell wall synthesis the two uridine nucleotides, UDP-acetylmuramyl pentapeptide and UDP-N-acetylglucosamine, are linked together to form a linear polymer (Figure 5-4). During this stage the cell wall precursor units are attached to the cell membrane. In the first reaction the sugar pentapeptide becomes attached by a pyrophosphate bridge to a phospholipid bound to the cell membrane. Then a second sugar derived from UDP-N-acetylglucosamine is added to form a disaccharide (-pentapeptide)-P-P-phospholipid. In *S. aureus* this molecule is further modified by a series of reactions resulting in the addition of five glycines to the ε-amino group of lysine. In this unusual reaction sequence glycyl-tRNA serves as the amino acid donor molecule.[7] The modified disaccharide is subsequently separated from the phospholipid and is covalently bonded to an acceptor molecule (i.e., pre-existing portions of cell wall) to form a linear peptidoglycan polymer. In the terminal reaction of stage II, the phospholipid carrier molecule with two phosphate groups attached is dephosphorylated with the release of inorganic phosphate. The resulting phospholipid can again bind the end product of stage I synthesis, the UDP-N-acetylmuramyl pentapeptide, and continue on another cycle of the membrane-bound reactions.

During the course of the stage II reactions, the basic repeating units of the cell wall are put together to form a long polymer. All the events up to this point occur either inside the cell or at the cell membrane. It is postulated that the lipid intermediates formed probably represent a mechanism for transporting the prefabricated units of the cell wall through the cell membrane to the exterior site where they are utilized for cell wall synthesis.[5] Three antibiotics inhibit the utilization of the lipid intermediates for the synthesis of the peptidoglycan.

Ristocetin and vancomycin inhibit the reaction in which the finished unit is separated from the membrane-bound phospholipid and attached to the acceptor molecule (Reaction 4, Figure 5-4). Both of these antibiotics inhibit the formation of peptidoglycan from the appropriate second-stage precursors at the same concentration at which they inhibit cell growth.[8] As seen in Table 5-2,

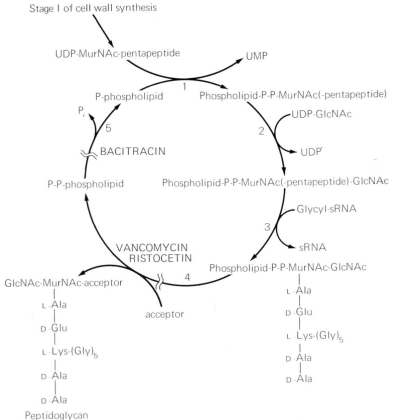

Figure 5-4 The second stage of cell wall synthesis in *S. aureus*. An ATP-requiring amidation of glutamic acid that occurs between reaction 2 and reaction 3 has been omitted. The sites of inhibition by bacitracin, vancomycin, and ristocetin are indicated by the break marks. (Modified from Strominger *et al.*[5])

exposure to penicillin will only inhibit the second-stage process at a concentration of antibiotic more than 6000 times that required to inhibit growth. In the presence of vancomycin or ristocetin, there is a normal synthesis of lipid intermediates, but they cannot be utilized for synthesis of the peptidoglycan (Figure 5-5).

Bacitracin inhibits peptidoglycan synthesis by inhibiting the

Table 5-2 Antibiotic sensitivity of cell growth and of peptidoglycan synthetase in *S. aureus*

Antiobiotics were introduced into cultures of growing cells, and cell growth and peptidoglycan synthetase activity were measured. The enzyme activity was assayed by incubating a particulate enzyme preparation from drug-treated cells with radioactive-labeled UDP-N-acetylmuramyl-pentapeptide and the appropriate substrates and then determining the amount of radioactivity incorporated into peptidoglycan. (From Anderson *et al.*[8])

| Antibiotic | Antibiotic concentration (μg/ml) required for 50 per cent inhibition of: | |
	Growth	Peptidoglycan synthesis by particulate enzyme
Ristocetin	12	12
Vancomycin	6	6
Bacitracin	35	35
Penicillin	0.04	>250

dephosphorylation of lipid pyrophosphate to lipid phosphate (Reaction 5, Figure 5-4), a step essential to the regeneration of the lipid carrier.[10] This is demonstrated by the experiment that provided the data for Table 5-3. Bacitracin inhibited the liberation of inorganic phosphate from lipid pyrophosphate, whereas vancomycin and ristocetin had no effect on this process.

Table 5-3 Effect of antibiotics on the hydrolysis of lipid-P-^{32}P by a particulate enzyme from *M. lysodeikticus*

Particulate enzyme from *M. lysodeikticus* was incubated with lipid-P-^{32}P labeled only in the terminal phosphate. After incubation with and without an antibiotic, lipid phosphate and inorganic phosphate were separated and assayed for radioactivity. Results as cpm of inorganic phosphate released from lipid-P-^{32}P (From Siewert and Strominger.[10])

Antibiotic	Inorganic phosphate recovered (cpm)
None	1040
Bacitracin (153 μg/ml)	361
Vancomycin (40 μg/ml)	1001
Ristocetin (40 μg/ml)	1075

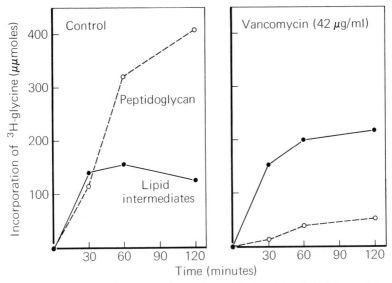

Figure 5-5 Effect of vancomycin on the synthesis of the lipid intermediates and peptidoglycan. A particulate enzyme preparation from *S. aureus* was incubated with ^{3}H-glycine, sRNA, amino acid activating enzymes, and the appropriate substrates for stage II synthesis. The amount of glycine incorporated into peptidoglycan and lipid intermediates was determined at various times in the presence and absence of vancomycin. (From Matsuhashi *et al.*[9])

Stage III—Cross-Linking of the Peptidoglycan

This terminal event in cell wall synthesis takes place outside the cell membrane. There is no ATP available at the extracellular site to act as a source of energy for the reaction, which is a transpeptidation. The energy for the reaction is derived from the peptide bond linking the two terminal D-alanine residues of each polypeptide side chain. As seen in Figure 5-6, the transpeptidase enzyme directs the splitting of the terminal D-alanyl-D-alanyl linkage and forms a peptide bond between the terminal glycine of the pentaglycine side chain and the penultimate D-alanine of an adjacent peptidoglycan strand. Thus each polypeptide side chain of each repeating unit becomes covalently linked to the side chains in two neighboring peptidoglycan strands.

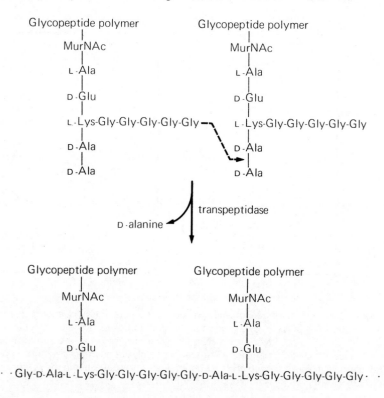

Figure 5-6 The third stage of cell wall synthesis in *S. aureus:* cross-linking of peptidoglycan polymers by the joining of the peptide side chains with the elimination of D-alanine. (Modified from Strominger *et al.* [5])

   The penicillins and the cephalosporins are competitive inhibitors of this transpeptidation. [11] In the presence of penicillin fibrous material, which can be seen by electron microscopy, accumulates at the growing point of the bacterium. [12] These fibers presumably represent the accumulating peptidoglycan strands, which cannot cross-link. The transpeptidase from *E. coli* has been isolated in a cell-free system, and it has been demonstrated that the enzyme is inhibited *in vitro* by several penicillins and a cephalosporin at the same concentrations that inhibit growth *in vivo*. [5] The structure of the penicillins is similar to that of the D-alanyl-

D-alanine terminus of the polypeptide side chain of peptido-glycan.[13] Figure 5-7 shows this similarity in drawings of stereo models of the antibiotic and the dipeptide. The arrows point to the CO-N bond in the β-lactam ring of penicillin and the analogous peptide bond in D-alanyl-D-alanine. Although the precise mechanism of inhibition of the transpeptidase by penicillin is not completely worked out, it appears likely that the penicillin molecule occupies the D-alanyl-D-alanine substrate site of the transpeptidase and becomes covalently bonded to it. This is supported by the observation that penicillin inhibition of transpeptidase is not reversed by washing the particulate enzyme preparation or by digestion with penicillinase.[14] Conversely, the analogous inhibi-

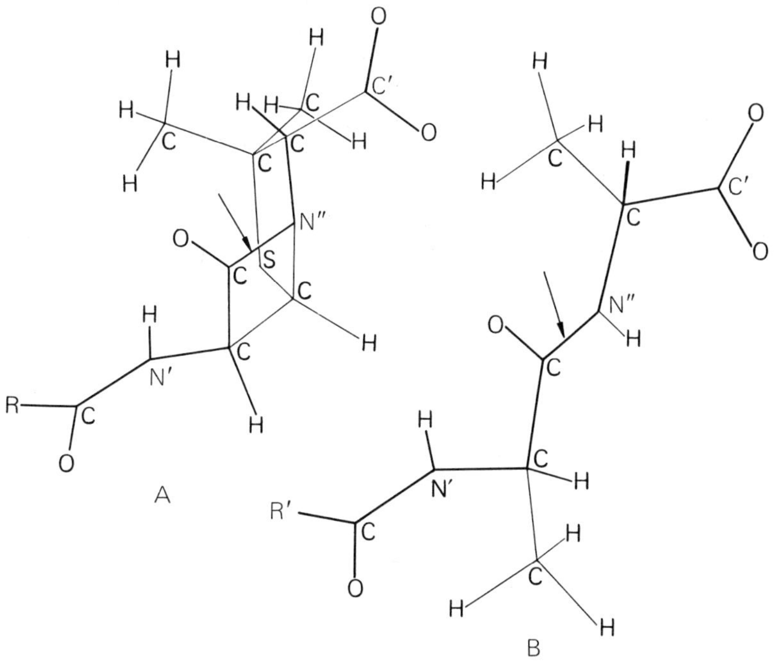

Figure 5-7 Stereomodels of penicillin (A) and of the D-alanyl-D-alanine end of the peptidoglycan strand (B). The arrows indicate the CO-N bond in the β-lactam ring of penicillin and the CO-N bond in the D-alanyl-D-alanine at the end of the peptidoglycan strand. (From Strominger et al.[5]).

tion of D-alanine carboxypeptidase by penicillin is reversed by both washing and penicillinase digestion. Thus the proposal that penicillin occupies the substrate site of the enzyme and that the highly reactive CO-N bond of the β-lactam ring acylates the enzyme and irreversibly inactivates it (Figure 5-8).

Broad-Spectrum Penicillins versus Narrow-Spectrum Penicillins

While most of the penicillins are relatively ineffective in inhibiting the growth of gram-negative organisms, a few (e.g. ampicillin and carbenicillin) are quite effective in treating infections due to certain gram-negative organisms. As all penicillins have the same mechanism of action, it is difficult to explain the large differences in their spectra of action. A particulate preparation of peptidoglycan transpeptidase from a gram-negative organism *(E. coli)* is as sensitive to inhibition *in vitro* by penicillin G as by the broad-spectrum ampicillin.[15] The effective concentration of penicillin G *in vitro* is one-tenth that required to inhibit growth of *E. coli* cells. This might imply that the broad-spectrum antibiotic is a better growth inhibitor of the gram-negative organism because it is better able to reach the transpeptidase enzyme. This postulation

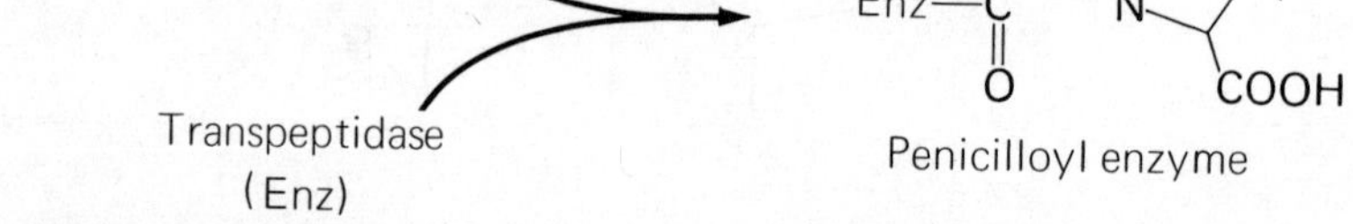

Figure 5-8 Proposed mechanism of transpeptidase inhibition by penicillin. Penicillin occupies the D-alanyl-D-alanine substrate site of transpeptidase, the reactive four-membered (β-lactam) ring is broken by cleavage at the CO-N bond, and the antibiotic becomes linked to the enzyme by a covalent bond. (From Tipper and Strominger.[13])

that gram-negative cells have a permeability barrier that prevents access of penicillin G to the site of action[5], while perhaps important, cannot account entirely for the greater effectiveness of the broad-spectrum antibiotics in these organisms. With methicillin, a narrow-spectrum penicillin, the same high concentration of drug is required to inhibit the *E. coli* particulate enzyme preparation *in vitro* as is required for inhibition of cell growth. When the differences between gram-negative and gram-positive organisms and the biochemical basis for the broad-spectrum effect of some of the penicillins are elucidated, it should be possible to synthesize new penicillins that combine the important properties of broad-spectrum activity and penicillinase insensitivity.

Therapeutic Indications

It is beyond the scope of this text to discuss all the indications for the clinical use of the drugs that inhibit cell wall synthesis. Table 5-4 presents a selected list of infections for which a penicillin is generally considered to be the drug of choice.

Clearly the penicillins are the most important weapons in the physician's armamentarium for the treatment of infectious disease of bacterial origin. The penicillins are used far more frequently than any other group of antibiotics. They are the best drugs for the treatment of infections due to the gram-positive and gram-negative cocci and the gram-positive bacilli. The broad-spectrum antibiotic ampicillin is the current drug of choice for the treatment of infections due to such gram-negative bacilli as *Shigella, Proteus mirabilis,* and *Haemophilus influenzae.*[16] Carbenicillin, also a broad-spectrum agent, is the drug of choice for the treatment of infections due to *Pseudomonas aeruginosa* (often in combination with gentamicin) and *Proteus mirabilis.* When sensitivity tests in bacteria such as the staphylococci reveal resistance to penicillin G, then a penicillinase-resistant penicillin such as methicillin, oxacillin, cloxacillin, or nafacillin generally becomes the drug of choice. Here it must be noted that some strains with an acquired resistance to penicillin G are acquiring resistance to the penicillinase-resistant penicillins as well. Physicians trained during the 1940s and 1950s may have been exposed

Table 5-4   A selected list of agents for which the penicillins are drugs of first choice
(According to recommendations from *The Medical Letter.* [16])

Infecting organism	Drug of choice
Streptococcus	Penicillin G
Enterococcus	Penicillin G* with streptomycin
Pneumococcus	Penicillin G
Staphylococcus aureus	
non-penicillinase-producing	Penicillin G
penicillinase-producing	A penicillinase-resistant penicillin
Meningococcus	Penicillin G*
Gonococcus	Penicillin G
Clostridium (perfringens and tetani)	Penicillin G*
Bacillus anthracis	Penicillin G
Shigella	Ampicillin
Escherichia coli (sepsis)	Ampicillin* or kanamycin*
Proteus mirabilis	Ampicillin or carbenicillin
Pseudomonas aeruginosa	Carbenicillin or carbenicillin plus gentamicin
Bacteroides (respiratory strains)	Penicillin G
Haemophilus influenzae	Ampicillin (parenteral administration for meningitis)
Actinomyces israelii (actinomycosis)	Penicillin G
Treponema pallidum (syphilis)	Penicillin G*
Leptospira	Penicillin G
Mycobacterium balnei	Cycloserine

* Parenteral administration preferred.

to the dogma that certain infections, such as gonococcal infections, are always sensitive to penicillin G and can be treated without sensitivity testing. During the 1960s, however, strains of gonococci emerged that are resistant to penicillin G.

It is safe to say that there is no infection from which a culture can readily be obtained that can be considered properly treated with a penicillin without first attempting to identify the organism and test for sensitivity. Of course, treatment will often start before the results of the culture and sensitivity tests are obtained, and in severe infections (e.g. meningitis, gram-negative sepsis) therapy must be started immediately. But in all cases a rapid culture should be taken before the antibiotic is administered.

On the basis of clinical symptoms, gram strains, or the results of previous culture, it is often clear what the infecting organism and its antibiotic sensitivity are. Even when the organism and its sensitivity appear to be clearly defined, as for example, in a case of sepsis occurring in a patient with a well-characterized urinary tract or surgical wound infection, both blood culture and local culture should be taken before treatment is begun on the basis of clinical judgment.

There is great variability in the sensitivity of many organisms, such as E. coli or Proteus, to the penicillins. These sensitivity changes, from region to region and even from hospital to hospital, mean that a clinician in one area may be able to treat a gram-negative infection with the relatively nontoxic penicillins, while an infection with the same strain of organism in another location might require the use of such toxic drugs as a tetracyline, kanamycin, gentamicin, or a polymyxin. Although recommendations for drugs of choice are readily available, all infecting organisms must be tested for drug sensitivity in order to select the most effective, least toxic drug.

A patient who is allergic to penicillin should, if possible, be given another drug. Yet it may sometimes be best to initiate treatment with penicillin in the face of a history of mild allergic response. There are also unusual circumstances where the benefit of the penicillin therapy may, in the physician's judgment, outweigh the risk for a patient with a history of severe allergic response. It must be remembered that all of the penicillins and the cephalosporins are cross allergic and that no member of either group can be considered a completely safe alternative to another member.

The Penicillins

Many penicillins have been developed, and specific therapeutic advantages are claimed for each preparation. A selected list of penicillins stating their advantages and disadvantages is presented in Figure 5-9. Penicillin G, phenoxymethyl penicillin, and phenethicillin are routinely used to treat infections due to the common, non-penicillinase-producing gram-positive organisms. Phenoxy-

Name	Side chain	Stability in acid	Spectrum of action	Sensitivity to penicillinase	Advantage
Penicillin G	(benzyl, $-CH_2-$ phenyl)	Poor		Sensitive	Cheapest
Phenoxymethyl penicillin	(phenoxymethyl, $-OCH_2-$ phenyl)	Good		Sensitive	Better oral absorption than penicillin G
Methicillin	(2,6-dimethoxyphenyl, OCH_3 ... OCH_3)	Poor (not given orally)		Resistant	For parenteral treatment of infections due to penicillinase-producing organisms
Oxacillin	(5-methyl-3-phenyl-isoxazolyl; $=C-C-CH_3$, $C=N-O$)	Good		Resistant	For oral and parenteral treatment of infections due to penicillinase-producing organisms
Dicloxacillin	(5-methyl-3-(2,6-dichlorophenyl)-isoxazolyl; Cl ... Cl, $=C-C-CH_3$, $C=N-O$)	Good		Resistant	For oral treatment of infections due to penicillinase-producing organisms

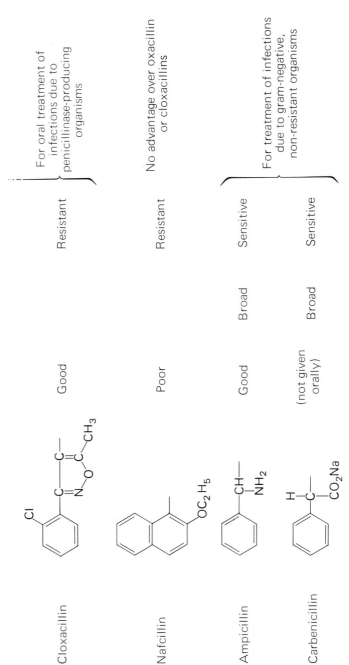

Figure 5-9 Properties and advantages of a selected list of common penicillins.

methyl penicillin and phenethicillin have more stability in acid and achieve higher blood levels by the oral route than penicillin G. This advantage is not so important as it is made out to be in some of the drug literature. Since the penicillins are essentially nontoxic, comparable blood levels can be obtained merely by giving more penicillin G, and when the drug is purchased under its generic name this is far cheaper for the patient. Five principal penicillins are marketed for the treatment of infections with penicillinase-producing organisms.

Because numerous penicillinase-producing pathogens have emerged in recent years, there has been an increasing tendency to treat common infections usually sensitive to penicillin G with one of the penicillinase-resistant penicillins. One example of this practice is the unnecessary use of expensive penicillinase-resistant penicillins in the prophylactic treatment of β-hemolytic streptococcal infection. There is a very low incidence of penicillinase production by streptococci, and the drug of choice is penicillin G. The approximate costs of a ten-day course of treatment with an oral penicillin are compared in Table 5-5. Penicillin G prescribed under the generic name is clearly the cheapest therapy. If penicillinase-producing organisms are encountered, dicloxacillin is reliably absorbed, permitting lower dosage at less cost to the patient.

Pharmacology of Penicillin G

Absorption. Approximately one-third of an oral dose of penicillin G is absorbed from the gastrointestinal tract. Therefore the oral dose must be three times greater than a parenteral dose to achieve the same blood levels. Maximum blood levels are reached in about forty-five minutes. To minimize degradation of penicillin G by acid, this drug should be taken two hours before or three hours after a meal when gastric acidity is lowest. Procaine penicillin G and benzathine penicillin G are poorly soluble in water, and, given intramuscularly, they are absorbed slowly and produce a relatively low concentration of drug that lasts for a day to several days.

Distribution. Penicillin G is distributed widely throughout the body spaces. Significant amounts do not normally pass into the

Table 5-5 Cost of ten-day oral treatment with various penicillins
(From *Handbook of Antimicrobial Therapy.* [17])

Penicillin	Average daily adult dose	Dollar cost to pharmacist of amount required for 10 day's treatment*
Penicillin G—average generic price	1,000,000 units	0.79
(range: 52¢ to $2.68)		
average trade-name price		2.22
(range: $1.32 [Pfizerpen] to $3.12)		
Penicillin V—average generic price	750 mg	2.03
(range: $1.64 to $2.52)		
average trade-name price		2.94
(range: $2.31 [Uticillin VK] to $4.15)		
Phenethicillin—average trade-name price	750 mg	4.26
(range: $4.09 [Darcil] to $4.53)		
Ampicillin—average generic price	1 gm	6.19
(range: $4.72 to $9.98)		
average trade-name price		7.93
(range: $4.54 [Totacillin] to $9.11)		
Hetacillin (Versapen)	1 gm	4.55
Cloxacillin (Tegopen)	1 gm	6.10
Dicloxacillin—average trade-name price	500 mg	5.41
Nafcillin (Unipen)	1 gm	12.00
Oxacillin (Prostaphlin)	1 gm	7.76

* Based on Drug Topics Red Book 1972 listings, for purchase by pharmacist of 100 capsules or tablets where that quantity is available.

cerebrospinal fluid. When the meninges are inflamed, however, the levels in the cerebrospinal fluid are higher.

Metabolism and excretion. We do not know how penicillin is metabolized. Most (80–90 per cent) of an intramuscular dose of penicillin G is excreted by the kidney within an hour and a half. This rapid clearance is accomplished by tubular secretion (about 80 per cent) and by glomerular filtration (about 20 per cent). The tubular secretion mechanism is one shared with such organic acids as phenolsulfonphthalein (PSP) and probenecid. When penicillin was still not readily available, probenecid was sometimes given with penicillin. Probenecid competes for the tubular transport of the penicillin, and longer lasting, higher levels of the drug result. This is no longer necessary. A similar system of active transport for organic acids exists in the choroid plexus. This system transports organic acids like Diodrast and PSP from the cerebrospinal fluid to the blood,[18] and it may well account for the low levels of penicillin seen in the cerebrospinal fluid.

Toxicity. The penicillins have the lowest toxicity of any antibiotic and, in fact, are among the least toxic of all drugs. But with more frequent use of very high doses (in the order of 50 million units) of penicillin, as in prophylaxis against infection during open heart procedures, it has become apparent that neurotoxicity can develop.[19,20] The symptoms are hyperreflexia and seizures.

Toxicity of other drugs that inhibit cell wall synthesis. Several other antibiotics that inhibit cell wall synthesis are quite toxic. Cycloserine can produce severe dysfunction of the central nervous system, including acute psychosis and convulsions. The risk of convulsions is increased by ethyl alcohol. Bacitracin possesses a severe renal toxicity, and hematuria and proteinuria often occur soon after effective antibacterial levels are attained. Extreme care must be taken with the use of this drug, especially with patients with decreased renal function. The most significant reactions with vancomycin involve ototoxicity and nephrotoxicity. Ristocetin produces hematological disturbances (eosinophilia and leukopenia), and because this drug is very irritating thrombophlebitis frequently develops at the site of intravenous injection.

Hypersensitivity Reactions

The incidence of allergic reaction to the penicillins is about 5 per cent in adults. The incidence is higher in people with a history of atopy such as asthma, hay fever, and atopic dermatitis.[21] The reactions encompass virtually every sort of allergic manifestation. Their onset may be immediate, accelerated (occurring 1 to 48 hours after administration), or delayed for several days or even weeks.

Immunochemistry

Before small molecules (such as most drugs) can elicit an immune response, they must become associated in an irreversible manner with large molecules in the host tissues. Antibodies to the complete antigen, the hapten-protein conjugate, then form. The hapten may be either the unaltered drug, a metabolite, or a chemical degradation product. In the case of the penicillins it is clear that penicillin itself is not the form of the molecule that functions as a hapten. Rather, penicillin G can undergo a ring cleavage in solution to form small amounts of several degradation products.[22] One of the products resulting from the nonenzymatic cleavage of the thiazolidine ring is D-benzylpenicillenic acid. This is a very reactive isomer of penicillin, which can react irreversibly with sulfhydryl groups or amino residues in tissue proteins to form hapten-protein conjugates. The proposed mechanism is presented in Figure 5-10. Of primary importance is the reaction of D-benzylpenicillenic acid with the ε-amino group of lysine residues on proteins to form D-benzylpenicilloyl derivatives of tissue proteins, which then function as the complete penicillin antigens.

The results of one experiment supporting the proposal that the D-benzylpenicilloyl-ε-aminolysyl units are the primary antigenic determinants are presented in Figure 5-11. Serum from rabbits, which were exposed to penicillin G, contained an anti-penicillin antibody that precipitated when the serum was incubated with antigen — human gamma globulin containing a number of D-benzylpenicilloyl groups. These antigen-antibody precipitation reactions were carried out in the presence of increasing amounts of penicillin or penicilloylamide compounds to determine what concentration of penicillin G or penicillin derivative effectively competed for the antigen sites on the rabbit anti-penicillin serum antibodies. The more effective a compound was in associating with the antibody (thus preventing precipitation by the gamma globulin antigen) the more closely it would resemble the complete penicillin antigen that elicited antibody production. As seen in Figure 5-11, D-benzylpenicilloly-ε-amino caproate, an analog of the ε-aminolysyl derivative, was effective in blocking the precipitation at one-

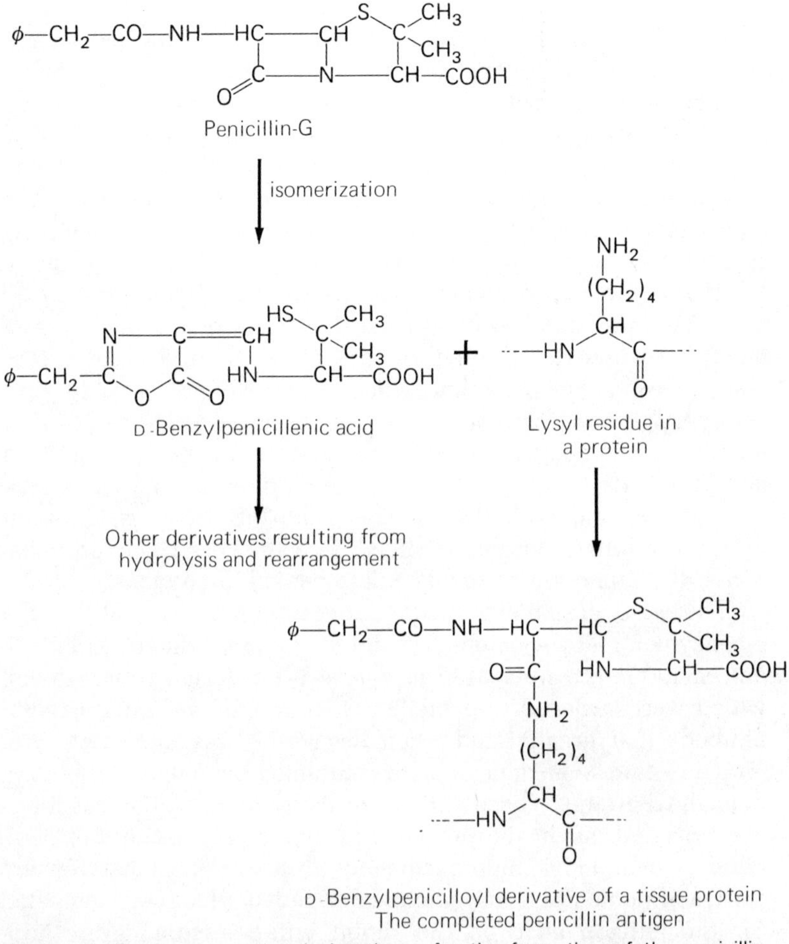

Figure 5-10 Proposed chemical pathway for the formation of the penicillin antigen. A very small percentage of penicillin G is isomerized at physiological pH to D-benzylpenicillenic acid, which then reacts with the ϵ-amino group of lysyl residues in proteins to form the complete penicillin antigen. (From Levine.[22])

hundredth the concentration at which penicillin G or D-benzyl-penicilloic acid were effective. Similar experiments demonstrated that D-benzylpenicilloyllysyl groups were the major antigenic

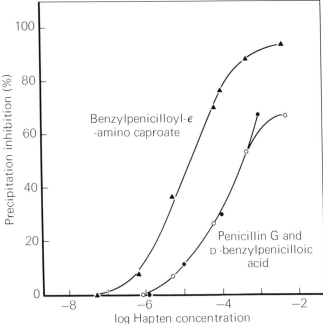

Figure 5-11   Inhibition of antibody precipitation by haptens related to penicillin. Rabbit anti-penicillin G serum was incubated with D-benzylpenicilloyl human
gamma globulin in the presence of various concentrations of D-benzylpenicilloly-
ε-aminocaproate (▲ ------▲), D-benzylpenicilloic acid (● ——●), or penicillin G
(o ——o). The amount of precipitate in each incubation was then assayed. (Data
from Levine and Ovary.[23])

determinants responsible for hypersensitivity to penicillin G in
several allergic patients.[23] The literature on immunochemical
mechanisms in penicillin allergy has been reviewed extensively
by Parker[24] and by Levine.[25]

Apparently allergic responses to commercial penicillin preparations are not always due to complete antigen formed between
penicillin derivatives and tissue protein. Some preparations of
penicillin have been found to contain a high-molecular-weight
material responsible for producing allergic reactions.[26,27] This
antigen may be an impurity carried over from the biosynthetic
process used in production. There is also limited evidence indi-

cating that if allergic patients are given skin tests using fresh preparations of penicillin from which the high-molecular-weight contaminant has been removed, the incidence of reaction decreases.[28]

Skin Testing for Hypersensitivity

A classic method of testing for drug allergy is to inject a small amount of the drug intradermally; if erythema develops, the patient is sensitive. This method of testing with penicillin is unsatisfactory for two reasons: (1) Intradermal injection of penicillin can precipitate a full-blown anaphylactic response in the patient; (2) The results are unreliable. One factor that apparently contributes to the rather high incidence of false negatives is the phenomenon described by the curves in Figure 5-11. A small amount of the penicillin in the test injection is altered and forms the hapten-protein conjugate, but this complete antigen is prevented from reacting with the small amount of antibody in the area of injection because of competition for antibody sites by the relatively large amount of unaltered penicillin. A more reliable test substance than penicillin itself has been developed from the antigenic determinant we have just discussed; it is a penicilloyl derivative of lysine. Penicilloyl-polylysine is a multivalent antigen of approximately 20 lysine residues and 12 to 15 penicilloyl groups per unit. It is not immunogenic, its diffusion from the site of injection is slow because of its molecular size, and systemic response is rare. A small amount of the clear penicilloyl-polylysine solution is administered intradermally, and after 20 minutes the injected area is examined for evidence of a wheal and erythema response. The reaction is graded negative, 2+, or 4+ depending on the magnitude of the response.

The results of this test are more reliable, and the test is certainly much less dangerous than one using the drug itself as the test substance. A positive test reaction, however, is by no means an absolute indication that the patient will have an allergic reaction if he is subsequently treated with penicillin. The data from one survey of the predictive value of penicilloyl-polylysine testing are presented in Figure 5-12. In this survey approximately 0.5 per cent

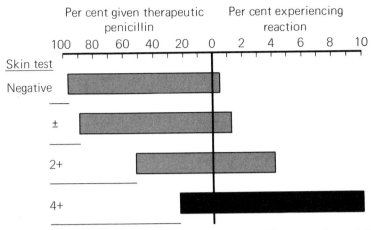

Figure 5-12 Relationship between the results of skin tests with penicilloyl-polylysine and subsequent reaction to penicillin. Skin tests with penicilloyl-polylysine were evaluated by the size of the wheal and by erythema: —, no response; ±, ambiguous response, wheal larger than initial bleb but less than 12 mm in diameter; 2+, positive, wheal 12 to 20 mm in average diameter; and 4+, strongly positive, wheal more than 20 mm in diameter. The positive-responding patients were treated with penicillin only when it was felt that the need outweighed the risk. (From Brown *et al.*[29])

of people who had no reaction on skin testing developed an allergic reaction after therapy with penicillin.[29] Of 206 severely ill patients who had a 4+ response to penicilloyl-polylysine and were treated with penicillin, 21 developed an allergic response. Of the people who had both a positive skin test and a previous history of penicillin sensitivity, 27 per cent who were subsequently treated exhibited allergic symptoms. Also in the same study, 50 per cent of the people who had a positive history of penicillin sensitivity had a negative skin test. This could be explained by the following: (1) the patient may have given an inaccurate history; (2) antibody levels may have declined; (3) the antigenic determinants may have been different; (4) the threshold concentration of antibody required for some systemic allergic responses may be lower than the threshold required for local wheal and erythema. In summary, a positive polylysine test combined with a history of penicillin sensitivity can aid the physician in assessing the allergic state of the individual. It is not an ideal test for determining penicillin sensitivity, and a negative response does not mean that there will not be an allergic reaction on subsequent treatment with penicillin.

Penicillin hypersensitivity may exist in people who have never received penicillin therapeutically. Penicillin is often used to treat infections in cows, and small amounts may be taken into the body from cow's milk. It is hypothesized that such a slight exposure could cause sensitization.

Hypersensitivity to the Cephalosporins

As mentioned previously all penicillins are cross allergenic. A cephalosporin is often recommended as an alternative drug to treat patients allergic to penicillin. This can by no means be done with complete impunity as there is evidence that the cephalosporins demonstrate cross allergenicity with the penicillins.[30] In fact, a severe anaphylaxis following cephalothin administration was seen in a patient who was hypersensitive to penicillin but who had never before been treated with cephalosporins.[31] Whenever possible drugs other than cephalosporins should be used to treat patients allergic to penicillin. Erythromycin for example may be a preferred alternative for the treatment of streptococcal or pneumococcal infections in allergic patients.

Resistance to the Penicillins

Mechanisms of Resistance

When the penicillins first came into wide use in the late 1940s, relatively few infections due to penicillin-resistant gram-positive organisms were encountered. The problem of the selection of resistant strains of organisms such as S. aureus in the presence of the widespread, heavy usage of the penicillins during the 1950s and 1960s is common knowledge and will not be discussed at any length here. It will suffice to say that the use of penicillins when they are not clearly indicated for the treatment of a specific bacterial infection is unwarranted from the standpoint of risk and cost to the patient and contributes heavily to the selection of penicillin-resistant organisms in both hospital patients and outpatients. Resistance to the penicillins results from the production of one of two enzymes by the bacterium (Figure 5-13). By far the most

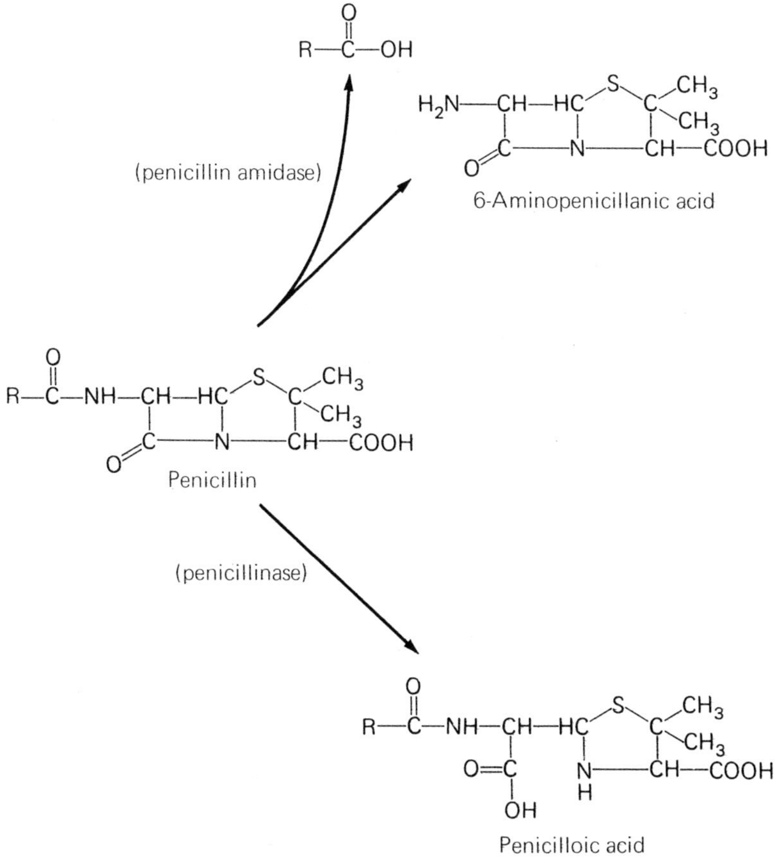

Figure 5-13 Mechanisms of resistance to the penicillins. Resistance to the penicillins usually arises from bacterial production of one of two enzymes—penicillin amidase or penicillinase. Penicillinase production is by far the more common form of resistance.

common mechanism is the production of penicillinase. This enzyme is a β-lactamase, which cleaves the four-membered, β-lactam ring of the penicillin and thereby inactivates the drug. Several types of penicillinase exist, and these can be distinguished from each other by differences in pH optima, immunological differences, and so on. The amount of penicillinase produced by a resistant organism is low under normal growth conditions, but the enzyme may be induced by exposure to penicillins. Penicillins sensitive to digestion by penicillinase and penicillins used to treat penicillinase-producing infections are both able to induce high levels of enzyme activity. The cephalosporins can also induce enzyme activity.[32]

Although the penicillinase enzyme is produced intracellularly, a large amount of it passes through the cell and is released in a free and active form in the growth medium. The cell-bound form is located at the cell surface and is associated with the cell membrane fraction.[33] Vesicular structures in penicillinase-producing cells develop after exposure to the penicillins or cephalothins.[34] These vesicles contain penicillinase at a very high specific activity,[35] and the available evidence indicates that some of the cell-bound enzyme that passes into the growth medium is released from these periplasmic vesicles.[36] In addition to the vesicle depot, a large amount of penicillinase is tightly associated with the plasma membrane itself. The enzyme can also be released from this form into the medium. This membrane-bound form of the enzyme is fully active in hydrolyzing penicillins.[33] Either the penicillinase bound to the membrane or the released penicillinase in the process of diffusing through the extramembranal cell envelope may form an enzyme shield around the cell to protect the trans-peptidase units against attack by penicillin. The membrane-bound penicillinase is of a larger molecular size than the exoenzyme, and it is a more hydrophobic molecule.[37] The conversion of the enzyme from a relatively hydrophobic conformation to one that is more hydrophilic would seem to be essential for the secretion process.

Once outside the cell, the enzyme can inactivate the drug and thereby reduce the antibiotic concentration in the growth medium. In certain mixed infections, penicillinase produced by staphylococci or gram-negative organisms constituting a minor component of the infection may protect a major pathogen, which is sensitive to penicillin. Thus a normally effective dosage regimen may be rendered inadequate in the area of the infection because of penicillinase secreted into the immediate environment. There is one rule of thumb that derives from observations on penicillinase production. It is clear that if one treats an infection with low amounts of penicillin, the drug may indeed destroy some sensitive cells, but those cells that are protected by virtue of their ability to produce even small amounts of penicillinase will be spared and selected for. Therefore, the physician should not prescribe minimally effective doses of this drug. Without affecting the patient adversely, a higher dose will kill those organisms that already possess low levels of resistance and that constitute a population of cells that can rapidly become very difficult to kill.

The Penicillinase-Resistant Penicillins

As one might expect, the effectiveness of a penicillin against penicillinase-producing organisms is an inverse function of its affinity for the penicillinase enzyme. The affinity constants of three penicillins for staphylococcal penicillinase are presented in Table 5-6. It is evident that methicillin, which is used to treat penicillin-resistant infections, has an affinity for the substrate site of penicillinase some four orders of magnitude less than penicillin G, which is readily hydrolyzed. Thus the penicillinase-resistant penicillins are not totally insensitive to penicillinase; rather they

Table 5-6   Affinity of penicillins for S. penicillinase

The K_m was determined for each compound with free penicillinase in the broth from a culture of S. aureus. (From Novick.[38])

Antibiotic	Effectiveness in treatment of penicillinase-producing organisms	K_m (μM)
Penicillin G	Ineffective	2.5
Phenoxymethyl penicillin	Ineffective	3.8
Methicillin	Effective	28,000

are poor substrates, which are consequently hydrolyzed very slowly by the enzyme.[39] It is entirely possible that only minor mutations occurring at the gene locus governing the structure of the substrate site may result in the production of altered penicillinases with the ability to readily hydrolyze the penicillinase-resistant penicillins. Selection of such strains in the hospital environment where large amounts of penicillinase-resistant penicillins are being used might, in a few years, render these drugs useless. Obviously, the penicillinase-resistant penicillins should not be used in an indiscriminate manner. Although they possess a β-lactam ring, the cephalosporins are not substrates (or at least not good substrates) for the penicillinase enzyme, and, therefore, do not demonstrate cross resistance with penicillin G.

Resistance to the Penicillinase-Resistant Penicillins

Resistance to the penicillinase-resistant penicillins has already appeared in the United States and in several clinics in Europe. The methicillin-resistant strains of S. aureus reported in the United States are multiple drug resistant.[40,41] Table 5-7 presents some data from a study of several cases of methicillin-resistant staphylococcal infections at the Boston City Hospital. In the strains tested there was resistance not only to the penicillinase-resistant penicillins but also to the other β-lactam antibiotics and to a number of antibiotics of widely differing structures and mechanisms of action. In the study at Boston City Hospital all strains isolated remained sensitive to vancomycin and bacitracin. But it is easy to visualize the difficulties that can develop when methicillin-resistant, multiple-drug resistant strains of S. aureus are encountered. Therapy is severely hindered when the efficacy of a great many drugs is suddenly diminished.

The mechanism of resistance to methicillin is not clear, but it does not seem to be correlated with penicillinase production.[42] The resistance determinants are carried in a plasmid. If these methicillin-resistant, multiple-drug resistant strains of S. aureus acquire the ability to readily transmit their resistance determinants to strains of ordinarily sensitive organisms, as occurs with

Table 5-7 **Relative sensitivity of methicillin-sensitive and methicillin-resistant strains of *S. aureus* to various antibiotics**
The minimum concentration of antibiotic required to prevent visible growth in cultures of *S. aureus* isolated from patients at the Boston City Hospital was determined. Results as concentration of drug at which growth was totally inhibited in 50 per cent of the strains tested. (Table constructed from data of Barrett *et al.*[41])

| Antibiotic | Antibiotic concentration required for growth inhibition (µg/ml): | | |
	Methicillin-sensitive (291 strains)	Methicillin-resistant (22 strains)	Approximate-fold resistance
Methicillin	1.3	40	34
Cloxacillin	0.24	18	75
Cephalothin	0.24	20	83
Erythromycin	0.24	>100	>400
Tetracycline	1.6	70	44
Chloramphenicol	5	60	12
Vancomycin	2	1.4	0
Bacitracin	20	15	0

resistance transfer factors, then the situation could become very serious. The chance that sudden, widespread, multiple drug resistance could develop in common hospital pathogens such as the staphylococci is an ominous possibility.

References

1. H. W. Florey: *Antibiotics,* Vol. I (ed. H. W. Florey *et al.* New York:) Oxford University Press, 1949.
2. J. Lederberg: Bacterial protoplasts induced by penicillin. *Proc. Natl. Acad. Sci., U.S.* 42:574 (1956).
3. W. D. Donachie and K. J. Begg: Growth of the bacterial cell. *Nature* 227:1220 (1970).
4. S. G. Nathenson and J. L. Strominger: Effects of penicillin on the biosynthesis of the cell walls of *Escherichia coli* and *Staphylococcus aureus. J. Pharmacol. Exp. Therap.* 131:1 (1961).
5. J. L. Strominger, K. Izaki, M. Matsuhashi, and D. L. Tipper: Peptidoglycan transpeptidase and D-alanine carboxypeptidase: penicillin-sensitive enzymatic reactions. *Fed. Proc.* 26:9 (1967).

6. U. Roze and J. L. Strominger: Alanine racemase from *Staphylococcus aureus:* Conformation of its substrates and its inhibitor, D-cycloserine. *Mol. Pharmacol.* 2:92 (1964).

7. M. Matsuhashi, C. P. Dietrich, and J. L. Strominger: Incorporation of glycine into the cell wall glycopeptide in *Staphylococcus aureus:* role of sRNA and lipid intermediates. *Proc. Natl. Acad. Sci. U.S.* 54:587 (1965).

8. J. S. Anderson, M. Mitsuhashi, M. A. Haskin, and J. L. Strominger: Lipid-phosphoacetylmuramyl-pentapeptide and lipid-phospho-disaccharide-pentapeptide: presumed membrane transport intermediates in cell wall synthesis. *Proc. Natl. Acad. Sci. U.S.* 53:881 (1965).

9. M. Matsuhashi, C. P. Dietrich, and J. L. Strominger: Biosynthesis of the peptidoglycan of bacterial cell walls: the role of soluble ribonucleic acid and of lipid intermediates in glycine incorporation in *Staphylococcus aureus. J. Biol. Chem.* 242:3191 (1967).

10. G. Siewert and J. L. Strominger: Bacitracin: an inhibitor of the dephosphorylation of lipid pyrophosphate, an intermediate in biosynthesis of the peptidoglycan of bacterial cell walls. *Proc. Natl. Acad. Sci., U.S.* 57:767 (1967).

11. D. J. Tipper and J. L. Strominger: Biosynthesis of the peptidoglycan of bacterial cell walls: inhibition of cross-linking by penicillins and cephalosporins. *J. Biol. Chem.* 243:3169 (1968).

12. P. Fitz-James and R. Hancock: The initial structural lesion of penicillin action in *Bacillus megaterium. J. Cell Biol.* 26:657 (1965).

13. D. J. Tipper and J. L. Strominger: Mechanism of action of penicillins: a proposal based on their structural similarity to acyl-D-alanyl-D-alanine. *Proc. Natl. Acad. Sci. U.S.* 54:1133 (1965).

14. K. Izaki, M. Matsuhashi, and J. L. Strominger: Biosynthesis of the peptidoglycan of bacterial cell walls: peptidoglycan transpeptidase and D-alanine carboxypeptidase; penicillin-sensitive enzymatic reaction in strains of *Escherichia coli. J. Biol. Chem.* 243:3180 (1968).

15. K. Izaki, M. Matsuhashi, and J. L. Strominger: Glycopeptide transpeptidase and D-alanine carboxypeptidase; penicillin-sensitive enzymatic reactions. *Proc. Natl. Acad. Sci. U.S.* 55:656 (1966).

16. Editorial: Antimicrobial drugs of choice. *Med. Letter* 13:39 (1971).

17. Editorial: Costs of commonly used antimicrobials for acute infections. *Med. Letter* 14 *(Handbook of Antimicrobial Therapy):*50 (1972).

18. J. R. Pappenheimer, S. R. Heisey, and F. F. Jordan: Active transport of Diodrast and phenolsulfonphthalein from cerebrospinal fluid to blood. *Am. J. Physiol.* 200:1 (1961).

19. H. Smith, P. I. Lerner, and L. Weinstein: Neurotoxicity and massive intravenous therapy with penicillin. *Arch. Int. Med.* 120:47 (1967).

20. K. B. Seamans, P. Gloor, A. R. C. Dobell, and J. D. Wyant: Penicillin-induced seizures during cardiopulmonary bypass; a clinical and electroencephalographic study. *New Eng. J. Med.* 278:861 (1968).

21. B. B. Levine, A. P. Redmond, M. J. Fellner, H. E. Voss, and V. Levytska: Penicillin allergy and the heterogeneous immune responses of man to benzylpencillin. *J. Clin. Invest.* 45:1895 (1966).

22. B. B. Levine: Studies on the mechanism of the formation of the penicillin antigen; Delayed allergic cross-reactions among penicillin G and its degradation products. *J. Exptl. Med.* 112:1131 (1960).

23. B. B. Levine and Z. Ovary: Studies on the mechanism of the formation of the penicillin antigen. *J. Exptl. Med.* 114:875 (1961).

24. C. W. Parker: Immunochemical mechanisms in penicillin allergy. *Fed. Proc.* 24:51 (1965).

25. B. B. Levine: Immunochemical mechanisms involved in penicillin hypersensitivity in experimental animals and in human beings. *Fed. Proc.* 24:45 (1965).

26. F. R. Batchelor, J. M. Dewdney, J. G. Feinberg, and R. D. Weston: A penicilloylated protein impurity as a source of allergy to benzylpenicillin and 6-aminopenicillanic acid. *Lancet* 1:1175 (1967).

27. G. T. Stewart: Allergenic residues in penicillins. *Lancet* 1:1177 (1967).

28. E. T. Knudsen, O. P. W. Robinson, E. A. P. Croydon, and E. C. Tees: Cutaneous sensitivity to purified benzylpenicillin. *Lancet* 1:1184 (1967).

29. B. C. Brown, E. V. Price, and M. B. Moore: Penicilloyl-polylysine as an intradermal test of penicillin sensitivity. *J.A.M.A.* 189:599 (1964).

30. S. L. Merrill, A. Davis, B. Smolens, and S. M. Finegold: Cephalothin in serious bacterial infection. *Ann. Int. Med.* 64:1 (1966).

31. J. F. Scholand, J. I. Tennenbaum, and G. J. Cerilli: Anaphylaxis to cephalothin in a patient allergic to penicillin. *J.A.M.A.* 206:130 (1968).

32. D. L. Swallow and P. H. A. Sneath: Studies on staphylococcal penicillinase. *J. Gen. Microbiol.* 28:461 (1962).

33. J. O. Lampen: Cell-bound penicillinase of *Bacillus licheniformis;* properties and purification. *J. Gen. Microbiol.* 48:249 (1967).

34. B. K. Ghosh, M. G. Sargent, and J. O. Lampen: Morphological phenomena associated with penicillinase induction and secretion in *Bacillus licheniformis. J. Bacteriol.* 96:1314 (1968).

35. M. G. Sargent, B. K. Ghosh, and J. O. Lampen: Localization of cell-bound penicillinase in *Bacillus licheniformis. J. Bacteriol.* 96:1329 (1968).

36. M. G. Sargent, B. K. Ghosh and J. O. Lampen: Characteristics of penicillinase release by washed cells of *Bacillus licheniformis. J. Bacteriol.* 96:1231 (1968).

37. M. G. Sargent and J. O. Lampen: A mechanism for penicillinase secretion in *Bacillus licheniformis. Proc. Natl. Acad. Sci. U.S.* 65:962 (1970).

38. R. P. Novick: Staphylococcal penicillinase and the new penicillins. *Biochem. J.* 83:229 (1962).

39. G. N. Rolinson, S. Stevens, F. R. Batchelor, J. C. Wood, and E. B. Chain: Bacteriological studies on a new penicillin-BRL.1241. *Lancet* 2:564 (1960).

40. R. J. Bulger: A methicillin-resistant strain of *Staphylococcus aureus*. *Ann. Int. Med.* 67:81 (1967).

41. F. F. Barrett, R. F. McGehee, and M. Finland: Methicillin-resistant *Staphylococcus aureus* at Boston City Hospital. *New Eng. J. Med.* 279: 441 (1968).

42. S. Seligman: Penicillinase-negative variants of methicillin-resistant *Staphylococcus aureus. Nature* 209:994 (1966).

Chapter 6
Antibiotics that Affect
Membrane Permeability
Amphotericin B
Nystatin
Candicidin
Tyrothricin
Gramicidin
Polymyxin B
Colistin

Introduction

This chapter will deal with the antibiotics that kill bacteria and fungi by virtue of their effect on the permeability of the cell membrane. Some antibiotics (i.e., streptomycin) inhibit cell growth by inhibiting other cellular functions and also affect the cell membrane when they are present in high concentrations. The antibiotics bacitracin, novobiocin, and vancomycin have a locus of action in the bacterial membrane, but their principal effect is to specifically inhibit bacterial cell wall synthesis. The antibiotics to be considered here interact specifically with membranes, and the bulk of the available evidence indicates that this interaction alters the function of the cell membrane in a manner incompatible with the survival of the bacterium or fungus. The two most important groups of these drugs are the polyene antibiotics, which are employed as antifungal agents, and the polymixins, which are used for the treatment of certain gram-negative bacterial infections.

Structures and Physical Properties

The polyene antibiotics are a large group of compounds, many of which are too toxic to be used in therapy. The two most clinically important compounds are amphotericin B and nystatin. The polyenes are large molecules with a hydroxylated portion, which is hydrophilic, and a portion containing four to seven conjugated double bonds, which is lipophilic. The exact structure of most of these compounds is not yet known, and the structure of filipin (an agent too toxic for clinical use) is given here as an example of this class of drugs. The presence of both a hydrophilic and a lipophilic portion in these molecules may be essential for their

Filipin
(a polyene antibiotic)

action in membranes. The unsaturated chromophore region is subject to photo-oxidation, and this contributes to the instability of these compounds in solution. This lipophilic portion also dictates a poor solubility in aqueous media. The instability of the molecules and their solubility characteristics make the administration of these drugs difficult. This problem will be discussed later in the chapter.

The gramicidins are macrocyclic polypeptides that affect the permeability of both natural and model membranes.[1] Tyrothricin is a mixture of gramicidin and another polypeptide, tyrocidine. These compounds are used in the treatment of certain superficial bacterial infections of the skin.

Of the polymyxin group of antibacterial agents, polymyxin B and colistin (polymyxin E) are the least toxic and the only ones used clinically. They contain both hydrophilic and hydrophobic portions and behave as cationic surface-active compounds at physiological pH. The antibacterial activity of the polymyxins is decreased in the presence of anionic compounds such as soap.

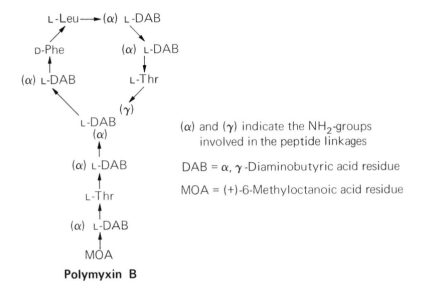

(α) and (γ) indicate the NH_2-groups involved in the peptide linkages

DAB = α, γ-Diaminobutyric acid residue

MOA = (+)-6-Methyloctanoic acid residue

Polymyxin B

Mechanism of Action

The Effect on Cell Permeability—An Explanation of the Cell Killing Effect

Research on the mechanism of action of the polyene antibiotics has been reviewed by Lampen[2] and by Kinsky.[1,3] Early experiments demonstrated that exposure of intact sensitive yeast cells to nystatin or amphotericin B affected a number of biochemical functions, including respiration and glycolysis. Investigators found that adding K^+ or NH_4^+ to the buffer solution in which the yeast cells were suspended prevented the inhibition of glycolysis that occurs at neutral pH.[4] The amount of nystatin taken up by the yeast cell was not altered by NH_4^+ or K^+, and nystatin treatment rapidly depleted intracellular potassium. These observations suggested that inhibition of glycolysis was secondary to the loss of K^+ resulting from a nystatin-induced change in membrane permeability. The demonstration that polyenes did not inhibit glycolysis by yeast extracts or respiration by yeast mitochondrial suspensions supported this conclusion.[2] Indeed, the polyenes have not been shown to inhibit the function of any enzyme system *in vitro.*[2]

Although the effect of the polyenes on glycolysis in intact cells can be reversed by potassium or ammonium ions, their fungicidal action is not reversed.[4] This could be explained by the leakage of other cellular components needed for cell survival but not for glycolysis. When polyene antibiotics are added to yeast cell cultures there is a marked decrease in dry weight of the cells and a rapid leakage of a number of small molecules from the cell (including nucleotides, amino acids, inorganic phosphate, and phosphorylated and free sugars).[5,6] These changes are accompanied by a decreased density of the cell cytoplasm as viewed by electron microscopy[7] and a rapid loss of integrity of fungal protoplasts.[8] The sequelae of the polyene-induced change in cellular permeability would seem to account for the fungicidal action of this group of antibiotics.

The polymyxins, which are bactericidal for a number of gram-negative bacilli, also cause leakage of small molecules such as phosphate and nucleosides from sensitive bacteria. The extent of the leakage as measured by the amount of the material of small molecular size appearing in the growth medium is proportional to the killing effect of the drug.[9] Changes in cellular permeability as a result of exposure to polymyxin have also been demonstrated with a dye compound. The dye N-tolyl-α-naphthylamine-8-sulfonic acid fluoresces under ultraviolet light when it is bound to protein. *Pseudomonas* cells exposed to the dye did not fluoresce; however, when a polymyxin was added to the cell suspension, the permeability characteristics of the cell exterior were altered, the dye was permitted to penetrate the cell membrane, and fluorescence resulted from association of the dye with cellular protein.[10] This evidence for a change in the permeability of bacterial cells in the presence of polymyxins is supported by a number of other studies, which have been reviewed by Sebek.[11]

The cell-killing effect of the polyene and polymyxin groups of antibiotics does not require growth of the organism. This stands in contrast to the penicillins, for example, which only have a killing effect on growing organisms.

The Site of Action—The Cell Membrane

The polyene antibiotics are bound only to cells sensitive to their killing effect.[12] These drugs are bound by isolated cell walls and protoplast membranes derived from yeasts, but they are not taken up by bacteria. They can be extracted from the cell with organic solvents, suggesting that the binding is not covalent. That the binding is of high affinity is implicit in the finding that bound radioactive-labeled nystatin cannot be readily displaced by adding unlabeled drug to the medium. Virtually all of the polyene antibiotic bound by protoplasts is found in the cell membrane.[13]

As will become clear in a moment, the specificity of polyene action is defined by the association of the drug with the membranes of sensitive cells. These drugs inhibit the growth of fungi, protozoa, and algae, but bacteria neither bind the drugs nor are they sensitive to them. This difference in the sensitivity of different organisms is determined by the presence of sterols in their cell membranes. In sensitive yeast cells, for example, nystatin is distributed in various subcellular fractions in direct proportion to sterol content.[13] The higher algae contain sterols in their membranes and are sensitive to the polyenes. The blue-green algae do not contain sterols and are insensitive. Bacteria do not have sterols in their cell membranes, and even bacterial protoplasts will not bind polyenes.[14]

The sterol requirement for polyene sensitivity, has been demonstrated even more directly. If membranes from sensitive cells that bind nystatin are extracted with ethanol-acetone, the membranes' ability to bind nystatin is abolished (see Table 6-1). The binding capacity can be partially restored by incubating the extracted particles with ergosterol. One of the clearest demonstrations of the correlation between sterol in the cell membrane and sensitivity to the polyene antibiotics was carried out with *Mycoplasma laidlawii*. This saprophytic PPLO organism, in contrast to

Table 6-1   The effect of sterol on the ability of a particulate fraction from *Neurospora crassa* to bind nystatin

A particulate fraction was prepared from pulverized, lyophylized, mycelial mats of *Neurospora crassa* by high speed centrifugation. A portion was extracted with ethanol-acetone, and reconstituted particles were prepared by adding the ethanol-acetone extract or ergosterol back to the extracted particulate fraction. The reconstituted particles were then dried, suspended in buffer, and assayed for their capacity to bind nystatin at a concentration of 10 μg/ml. Values represent μg nystatin bound by equivalent 0.4 ml aliquots of particulate fraction per hour. (Data from Kinsky.[14])

Particle treatment	Addition to particles	Nystatin bound
None	None	13.3
Extracted	None	0
Extracted	Extract	10.1
Extracted	Ergosterol	6.8

most mycoplasma, does not require sterols for growth.[15] In a sterol-free medium these organisms are resistant to polyene antibiotics, but when they are grown in a cholesterol-containing medium they incorporate sterol into the membrane and are sensitive to amphotericin B[16] and filipin[17] (see Table 6-2).

Further definition of the mechanism of action of the polyenes and other antibiotics that affect membrane function is limited by our understanding of the fundamental structure and action of biological membranes. One of the areas of research designed to promote such understanding is the study of synthetic membrane systems. The effects of the polyenes on a number of model membranes such as lipid monolayers, bilayers, and liposomes have been investigated.[1] Some of the most intriguing work in this area concerns the effect of the polyenes on the rate of release of small ions and glucose from liposomes. Liposomes are artificial spherules of phospholipid formed in this instance by mixing lecithin and dicetyl phosphate in the presence or absence of cholesterol. The lipids are permitted to swell in the presence of a small molecule like glucose. The resulting spherules, which contain the sequestered markers, are then dialyzed to eliminate soluble, (extraspherular) glucose from the suspending buffer. Test substances such as the polyene antibiotics can then be added to the liposome

Table 6-2 **Interconversion of *Mycoplasma laidlawii* between sensitivity and resistance to amphotericin B by growth in the presence and absence of cholesterol**

Mycoplasma laidlawii were grown in medium with (sensitive, S cells) and without (resistant, R cells) 20 μg/ml cholesterol. Both types of cells were harvested, washed, suspended in cholesterol-free medium, and assayed for viability with and without 25 μg/ml of amphotericin B. Cholesterol was then added to the R cells, and each parent culture was divided in half for further incubation at either 4° or 37° C. At the end of this second incubation viability tests were performed as before. *Mycoplasma laidlawii* has a generation time of about 2 hours; therefore, if the drug had no effect on cell growth during the 2-hour incubation in the presence of amphotericin B, the number of cells would be expected to double and approach 200 per cent of the initial viability assay. If the drug had a killing effect, then the per cent survivors would be less than 100 per cent (that is, less than the initial viability assay carried out before exposure to the drug). Growing the R cells at 37° C in cholesterol medium makes them drug sensitive, while the S cells are made drug insensitive by growth at 37° C without cholesterol.

Cell type	Per cent survivors after a 2-hour exposure to amphotericin B
S cells	2
R cells	200
S cells incubated in cholesterol-free medium for 2 hours at	
37° C	150
4° C	5
R cells incubated in cholesterol-containing medium for 2 hours at	
37° C	3
4° C	180

suspension, and the rate of release of sequestered glucose from the trapped to the free form can be measured as a function of both sterol content and antibiotic concentration. It has been demonstrated that the polyenes increase the rate of release of glucose[18] and also of small ions such as $CrO_4^=$ and $H_2PO_4^-$ from phospholipid spherules[19] that contain a sterol (see Figure 6-1). In the absence of a sterol there is little effect. Thus an *in vitro* system has been prepared that mimics some of the characteristics of the response of the far more complex biological membranes to the polyenes.

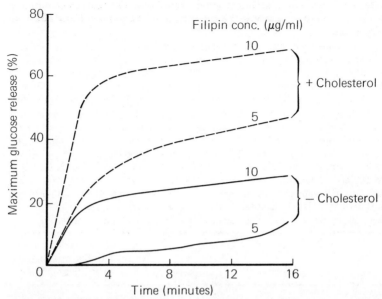

Figure 6-1 The effect of a polyene antibiotic on the release of glucose from liposomes made with and without cholesterol. Liposomes were prepared from egg lecithin, dicetyl phosphate, and glucose in the presence or absence of cholesterol. After dialysis to remove free glucose, filipin was added to equivalent suspensions of liposomes, and the release of sequestered glucose to the free form was measured by a spectrophotometric assay. The rate of release and the extent of release are much larger in the liposomes containing cholesterol (dotted line). (Figure adapted from Kinsky et al.,[18] Fig. 8.) Similar results have been obtained for the effect of nystatin and amphotericin B on the release of $CrO_4^=$ and $H_2PO_4^-$ from liposomes prepared with and without a sterol.[19]

If the presence of sterols in a membrane is a determinant for sensitivity to the polyene antibiotics, then, as mammalian cell membranes contain sterols, one might expect that these drugs would have an effect on the permeability of host cells. This is indeed the case. The polyene antibiotics have been shown to rapidly lyse human erythrocytes suspended in isotonic saline.[20] This effect is inhibited by serum. It has been demonstrated that filipin can induce pits in erythrocyte membranes as well as in lecithin-cholesterol dispersions.[21] These pits can be demonstrated by electron microscopy. The formation of pits in the phospholipid dispersions is dependent on the presence of cholesterol. What then is the basis for the selective toxicity of the polyenes for fungi? The answer to this question is by no means clear. First, it should be noted that these are very toxic drugs. They have a very low therapeutic index. Second, the composition of cell membranes varies from one organism or cell type to another. It has been suggested that sensitivity to the polyenes may depend on the phospholipid to sterol ratio in the membrane,[22] which may differ in host cells and fungi.

The polymyxins have been shown to associate with the cell membrane. Newton demonstrated that when *Pseudomonas aeruginosa* or *Bacillus megaterium* were exposed to a fluorescent DANSyl-derivative of polymyxin, the drug accumulated in the periphery of the cell.[23] Protoplasts obtained from such cells also fluoresced, and, after disruption, the drug was recovered in the fraction containing the cell membrane. The molecular association of the polymyxins with cell membranes has not been characterized in any detail. The drug-membrane interaction does not require the presence of a sterol as with the polyene antibiotics, and no data are available that demonstrate why these drugs are effective against gram-negative bacilli but generally inactive against other bacteria.

Potentiation of the Antifungal Effects of Other Drugs by Amphotericin B

The clinical usefulness of some drugs is limited because the cytoplasmic membrane is not permeable to them. It is possible that agents that alter cellular permeability could be used to increase the intracellular concentration of these poorly penetrating drugs. This possibility is suggested by the observation that amphotericin B potentiates the antifungal effects of rifampicin and 5-fluorocytosine.[24] Rifampicin (see Chapter 1) is used primarily as an antibacterial drug. It is not particularly effective against yeasts. In the presence of low concentrations of amphotericin B, however, rifampicin has a potent antifungal effect *in vitro*. A similar antifungal synergism of amphotericin B with 5-fluorocytosine has also been demonstrated. 5-Fluorocytosine is a halogenated pyrimidine (available in the United States for investigational use) that has been shown to inhibit fungal growth.[25,26] The ability of amphotericin B to potentiate the effects of these two compounds is probably due to its effect on the permeability of the yeast cell membrane, permitting increased penetration of the other drugs.[24] Presumably the increased antifungal effect of the drug combination would be accompanied in the patient by an increased toxicity to host tissues. In the case of rifampicin, however, there may not be a severe toxic effect on the host cells. The possibility that one drug may be used to reversibly alter cellular permeability in order to allow another drug to achieve effective intracellular concentrations is an intriguing concept which may find future clinical application.

Therapeutic Indications

The Polyene Antibiotics

The treatment of fungal infection may be divided into two therapeutic problems, the treatment of deep infection and the treatment of superficial infection. Amphotericin B is the only effective drug available for treating deep fungal disease, such as fungal pneumonia, bone infections, fungal meningitis, and disseminated fungal infection. Some of the fungal infections for which amphotericin B is the drug of choice are listed in Table 6-3.[27] Amphotericin B has also been reported to be effective in the treatment of American (mucocutaneous) leishmaniasis.[28]

The treatment of deep fungal infection is a very difficult therapeutic problem. In such cases amphotericin B is given intravenously. The tolerance to amphotericin B varies substantially from patient to patient, and because of the extensive toxicity and side effects therapy is instituted at a lower dosage than the maintenance dose. The manufacturer recommends an initial dose of 0.25 mg/kg. This dose is then increased gradually. There is no fixed maintenance dosage. The dose arrived at is often about 1.0 mg/kg daily.[29] The only way to tell if enough drug is being given is to test the ability of the patient's serum to kill the fungus *in vitro*. A rational, controlled therapy can then be aimed at achiev-

Table 6-3   Drugs of choice for the treatment of selected fungal infections[27]

Infecting fungus	Drug of choice	Alternative
Dermatophytes	Griseofulvin	No systemic alternative
Epidermophyton		Topical agents such as
Microsporon		undecenylic acid
Trichophyton		and tolnaftate
Candida albicans		
Superficial	Nystatin (topical)	
Intestinal	Nystatin (oral)	
Systemic infection	Amphotericin B	
Histoplasma capsulatum	Amphotericin B	None
Aspergillus	Amphotericin B	None
Cryptococcus neoformans	Amphotericin B	None
Mucor	Amphotericin B	None
Coccidioides immitis	Amphotericin B	None
Blastomyces dermatitidis	Amphotericin B	Hydroxystilbamidine
(N. American)		
Blastomyces braziliensis	Amphotericin B	A sulfonamide
(S. American)		
Sporotrichum schenkii		
Localized	An iodiode	Amphotericin B; griseofulvin
Disseminated	Amphotericin B	

ing a plasma concentration approximately two times higher than that demonstrated as effective *in vitro*.[30] Many clinicians prefer to administer double dosages of the drug every other day, finding that appropriate serum concentrations can be maintained and the patient can tolerate therapy better than when he receives the drug on a daily basis.[31] Therapy continues for a number of weeks. The drug is generally not discontinued until the patient is asymptomatic and has had at least two successive negative cultures.

Superficial fungal infections may be treated topically with a number of drugs, including nystatin and amphotericin B. Some of the other drugs used for treating superficial infection (griseofulvin, tolnaftate, and undecenylic acid) will be discussed in the last section of this chapter. Although nystatin has the same mechanism of action as amphotericin B, it is less potent than the latter compound and is given only topically. The main use for this drug is in the treatment of superficial infection with *Candida albicans*. *Candida* infection of the skin and cornea is treated with nystatin given as an ointment, a powder, or an ophthalmic solution. Vaginal moniliasis is treated topically with vaginal suppositories. Oral nystatin prepared as a slurry is useful for the treatment of moniliasis of the oropharynx (thrush), and it is used in tablet form for the treatment of intestinal or anal candidiasis. Since nystatin is not absorbed from the gastrointestinal tract, its oral administration for intestinal candidiasis constitutes a local use of the drug. Amphotericin B may also be administered topically for candidiasis, but nystatin is preferable.

The incidence of systemic candidiasis increases in persons who have Hodgkin's disease or lymphoproliferative and myeloproliferative disorders and in patients who are receiving antibiotics (superinfection) or immunosuppressive drugs.[32] The therapy of choice for deep *Candida* infection is amphotericin B given intravenously.

For an extensive review of fungal diseases and their treatment the reader is referred to a complete text on this subject.[33]

The Polymyxins

The principal therapeutic role of the polymyxins is in the treatment of infection due to gram-negative organisms. Although other less toxic drugs are the drugs of choice here, polymyxin B is frequently a useful alternative, particularly in infection with *Pseudomonas aeruginosa*. Carbenicillin or a combination of carbenicillin and gentamicin are the drugs of choice for treatment of infections due to *Pseudomonas*. Polymyxin B is the drug of choice for the treatment of infection with enteropathogenic strains of *E. coli*.[27] It is given topically for superficial infection due to gram-negative organisms. Some of the infecting organisms in addition to *Pseudomonas* that respond well to polymyxin B are *E. coli*, *Klebsiella*, and *Enterobacter*. Colistin (Polymyxin E) has the same therapeutic indications as polymyxin B.

Pharmacology of the Polyenes and Polymyxins

The Polyenes

Absorption and method of administration. Nystatin is administered primarily topically, and this use of the antibiotic is associated with a very low incidence of side effects and no sensitivity reactions. It is never given intramuscularly and only rarely intravenously.

Amphotericin B is poorly absorbed from the gastrointestinal tract. Several attempts have been made to employ amphotericin B orally, but the drug blood levels achieved are low and inconsistent.[31,32] The oral route is used in special instances, as in the treatment of cutaneous blastomycosis. Systemic fungal disease requires intravenous therapy. The drug alone is essentially insoluble in water; therefore, it is brought into a colloidal dispersion with sodium deoxycholate. The drug-deoxycholate mix is supplied as a dry powder, which is first suspended in sterile water and then added to a 5 per cent solution of dextrose. As the drug will precipitate from saline solutions, they should never be employed. The personnel administering this drug must be cautioned to watch for precipitate formation. If a precipitate forms, the solution should be immediately discarded. The solution should be kept from light while it is being infused because the drug in solution can be degraded by light. Perhaps by virtue of its effect on cell membranes, amphotericin B causes thrombophlebitis. The risk of this complication can be lowered by using a small needle and a very slow drip. As the course of therapy is often long, the physician can preserve the maximum amount of vein for future infusion by alternating therapy between arms and by starting the infusion site distally and moving it proximally if necrosis of the veins takes place.

The levels of drug in the spinal fluid after intravenous administration are very low compared to the blood levels.[34] For fungal meningitis the drug is given intrathecally, often in combination with intravenous therapy. Intrathecal administration can cause headache, pain in the extremities, sensory loss, and chemical meningitis. Intrathecal administration is carried out every other day, and often the route of injection (intracisternal or intra-spinal) is alternated. Because of its physical properties, its toxic-ity, and the difficulty of determining appropriate serum levels, amphotericin B is one of the most difficult of all drugs to admin-ister.

Distribution and excretion. The data available on distribution of amphotericin B in both man and animals are very limited. Most of the work has been carried out in humans and has involved measur-ing blood and cerebrospinal fluid levels by bioassay techniques after intravenous administration. It is very difficult to interpret data gathered by withdrawing a sample of blood and determin-ing the antifungal activity of the serum. When properly con-trolled such measurements will give a fairly good indication of the amount of free drug present in the serum but not of the total drug. Drug bound to β-lipoprotein in the serum,[31] for example, would not be included. Sterols in the serum inhibit the effect of the polyenes on fungi,[36] and it is possible that such assays may vary considerably according to the patient's serum cholesterol content. These studies are therefore inadequate if one is trying to answer the pharmacological question—What is the distribution of the drug? On the other hand, they are the best method available for determining the answer to the therapeutically important ques-tion—What is the level of antifungal activity achieved in the serum? Even bioassay methods can give results that are in error. The values will be too high, for instance, if the assay conditions allow dissociation of a drug from the serum-bound to the biolog-ically active, free form.[37]

Bindschadler and Bennett have carried out serum bioassays for amphotericin B after infusion of the drug at various doses every day or every other day.[31] They demonstrated that at the end of an infusion no more than 10 per cent of the biologically active drug could be found in the serum, and no more than 40 per cent by calculation, in the extracellular fluid. Only a small percentage of the drug was removed by excretion during the period of the drug infusion. The investigators noted that as the dose of the drug was increased inactivation and/or storage mechanisms increased also. After cessation of therapy the drug could be detected in the serum for three weeks, a finding confirmed by other studies. The results of Bindshadler and Bennett's study are consistent with the hypothesis that amphotericin B is rapidly sequestered in the body and then slowly released from its depot into the blood. It is possible that this depot consists of the cell membranes that contain sterols and bind the polyenes.

No data are available to demonstrate that the concentration of free antibiotic in infected tissues parallels the concentration in the patient's serum. With intravenous administration it is clear that the concentrations achieved in the cerebrospinal fluid and other body spaces, such as the pleural space, are much lower than the blood concentrations.

Toxicity. When given orally for the treatment of intestinal candidiasis, nystatin may cause nausea, vomiting, and diarrhea. When given topically there are essentially no side effects. The grave side effects accompanying administration of this drug by injection effectively prohibit its intramuscular or intravenous use.

The intravenous use of amphotericin B is associated with a wide variety of side effects. Virtually every patient is affected by one or more toxic phenomenon. In one study 27 of 29 patients experienced fever.[38] Other common side effects include anorexia, headache, nausea, vomiting, abdominal pain, and phlebitis. Less commonly patients will experience chest pains and rhythm changes, generalized pain, fatigue, and transitory radiculitis caused by leakage during intrathecal therapy. Prolonged usage is sometimes associated with a normocytic, normochronic anemia. Low serum potassium and magnesium are also sometimes associated with long-term treatment. This may be due both to disturbances in renal function and to diarrhea.

Amphotericin B is nephrotoxic. In one study of 56 patients elevated blood urea nitrogen values were observed in 93 per cent, and 83 per cent had high serum creatinine values.[39] The extent of permanent renal damage with total intravenous doses under 4 gm is not clear but with doses over 5 gm residual damage is seen. The mechanism of this renal toxicity is not known. It has been demonstrated that, as one would expect from its mechanism of action in fungal membranes, amphotericin B markedly increases the permeability of cells of the toad bladder to small ions.[40,41] But it is not clear whether this effect is related to permanent damage to renal function. This action may be at least partly responsible for the hypokalemia and hypomagnesemia that amphotericin B can produce. Tubular lesions associated with calcium deposition are also seen in gross section.[39]

In view of the problems of administration and toxicity, a number of precautions should be observed when amphotericin B is given intravenously. The drug should be used only for severe deep fungal infection. It should not be used when positive skin or serological tests alone are present without symptomatology indicating potentially fatal fungal infection. It should be used only with hospitalized patients. Before therapy is begun the physician should obtain a complete hemogram, urinalysis, liver function tests, serum potassium, and BUN. During therapy these tests should be performed at least weekly, and BUN should be determined two to three times weekly. The total daily dose should never exceed 1.5 mg/kg.

The Polymyxins

Absorption, distribution, and excretion. Neither polymyxin B nor colistin is absorbed from the gastrointestinal tract. For systemic use these drugs are administered intramuscularly or intravenously. Intramuscular injection is painful, and some preparations of colistin contain a local anesthetic. When polymyxin B is given intramuscularly, a local anesthetic can be added to the injection solution. Intravenous polymyxin B cannot be mixed with cephalothin, chloramphenicol, heparin, or the tetracyclines.[42] Excretion of the polymyxins is predominantly renal. In the presence of renal impairment the dose of these antibiotics must be reduced.

Toxicity. The polymyxins are nephrotoxic drugs. It has been reported that at intramuscular doses below 2.5 mg/kg/day polymyxin B sulfate does not have a significant nephrotoxic effect.[43] With higher doses nephrotoxicity is seen. This rule of thumb cannot be relied upon, and all patients receiving the drug intramuscularly or intravenously should have frequent urinalysis and BUN performed. It has also been reported that there is no difference between the toxicity of colistin and polymyxin B when one takes into account the fact that the former has a less potent antibacterial effect and must be used in larger amounts.[44] Studies of renal function in dogs, however, indicate that colistin may have less of a nephrotoxic effect than polymyxin B.[45] The possibility that sodium sulfomethyl-colistin is less nephotoxic than the sodium sulfomethyl derivative of polymyxin B or polymyxin B sulfate deserves further consideration.

Parenteral administration of polymyxin is often accompanied by paresthesias of the distal extremities and lips, which diminish as the drug is excreted. Fever, dizziness, ataxia, and drowsiness also occur. Intravenous administration of the polymyxins can on rare occasion produce a neuromuscular blockade with respiratory paralysis that can be reversed by supportive therapy. The paralysis does not respond to neostigmine, but calcium gluconate may be helpful.[46]

Other Drugs Used to Treat Superficial Fungal Infection (Griseofulvin)

Introduction

The dermatophytes and yeasts such as *Candida albicans* are responsible for most superficial fungal infections. The dermophytic infections are treated either with topical drugs, such as undecenylic acid and tolnaftate, or with the systemic agent griseofulvin (Table 6-3). Griseofulvin has been isolated from a number of molds of the genus *Penicillium*. The drug is inactive against bacteria, yeasts, and fungi that cause systemic disease, and its use in the chemotherapy of infection is limited to the treatment of dermatophytic infections.

Griseofulvin

Although it is not clear whether griseofulvin as it is used in therapy has a predominantly fungistatic or fungicidal action, experiments with cultured fungi demonstrate that it can act as a fungicide. For griseofulvin to exert a killing effect, the organism must be growing.[47] The drug is concentrated as much as 100-fold by *Microsporum gypseum*.[48] The uptake of griseofulvin by fungi is energy dependent, and it is correlated with the sensitivity of the organism to the drug.[49] Exposure of fungi to griseofulvin results in the alteration of many biochemical functions and in gross morphological changes. Unfortunately, the data do not yet permit a coherent hypothesis for a mechanism of action. The extensive and confusing literature on griseofulvin has been reviewed in detail elsewhere.[35,50,51]

Pharmacology

Absorption, distribution, and metabolism. Griseofulvin is essentially insoluble in water. Absorption of the drug from the gastrointestinal tract is enhanced by employing the ultra fine particle form. Absorption is increased when the drug is taken with a fatty meal.[52]

Part of the absorbed drug is bound to keratin as it is being laid down by the dividing cells of the skin, nailbeds, and hair follicles, and the fungi are not able to grow in the griseofulvin-containing layer of skin, hair, or nail. But fungi in cell layers laid down before griseofulvin therapy was initiated are not affected. Thus the duration of therapy with griseofulvin is controlled by the rate for the complete turnover of the cells in the infected area. In most areas of the skin this is ten days to three weeks. Once griseofulvin therapy is started for infection of the skin or hair it should be continued for a minimum of four weeks. The skin of the palms and soles requires six to eight weeks for regeneration. The longest courses of therapy are required for infection of the nails. Infection of the finger nails requires therapy for three to six months and infection of the toe nails six to twelve months and sometimes longer. The symptoms of the fungal infection are usually relieved after a few days, even though much longer periods are required for eradication of the fungus. This antibiotic has not proved very effective when given topically.

Metabolism of griseofulvin is principally by demethylation in the liver. In the rat the rate of metabolism of griseofulvin is somewhat increased by phenobarbital,[53] a drug that induces activity of the hepatic microsomal drug metabolizing system. Concomitant administration of clinically usual doses of phenobarbital results in a significant reduction of the blood levels of griseofulvin in man. It has been presumed that the decreased blood level is primarily due to an increased rate of metabolism. However, studies in patients receiving griseofulvin intravenously or orally indicate that the major effect of phenobarbital is to decrease the gastrointestinal absorption of griseofulvin.[54] Griseofulvin itself apparently causes an increased rate of metabolism of the coumarin anticoagulants and diminishes the effect of these drugs. Because of poor absorption from the gut, the bulk of orally administered griseofulvin is excreted in the feces. The drug is excreted in the urine in a biologically inactive form.

Toxicity. Griseofulvin is a very safe drug. The most common side effect is headache, which occurs in about 10 to 15 per cent of patients. The headache usually disappears within a few days despite continuation of therapy. Lapses of memory and impairment of judgment have been reported to occur, and this contraindicates the use of the drug in pilots and bus drivers. Griseofulvin causes skin rashes and, in rare cases, photosensitivity. Gastrointestinal distress is an occasional side effect. The drug apparently increases porphyrin excretion in mice, and it has been reported to increase fecal porphyrin execretion in man.[55] The increased porphyrin metabolism results from the induction of increased levels of δ-aminolevulinic acid synthetase, a rate-limiting enzyme in porphyrin metabolism.[56] The status of the effect of griseofulvin on porphyrin levels in humans is not clear,[57] but the drug is not used in people with porphyria. As with any antibiotic, superinfection can occur (particularly with *Candida*).

Griseofulvin in high doses causes metaphase arrest in mammalian cells growing *in vitro*. The gross effect is similar to that produced by colchicine; the mitotic spindle is disrupted.[58] The mechanism of the effect is unknown, but it is clearly not the same as that of colchicine.[59] Like colchicine, griseofulvin has an anti-inflammatory effect, and it is effective in the treatment of acute gouty arthritis and the shoulder-hand syndrome of rheumatoid arthritis. As with any drug inhibiting mammalian cell division, there was initially some concern over the possibility that griseofulvin might have an adverse effect on the hematopoeitic system and on spermatogenesis. The available evidence, however, supports the conclusion that griseofulvin at the doses used clinically does not visibly affect either process.[33] It is nevertheless prudent to withhold the drug from pregnant women, especially during the first trimester of gestation.

Undecenylic Acid and Tolnaftate

Several compounds are employed for the topical treatment of superficial fungal infections. In addition to those already discussed (nystatin, amphotericin B, and candicidin), two others are effective agents. Undecenylic acid is one of a number of fatty acids possessing anti-fungal activity. The reason for this efficacy is unknown. Undecenylic acid is sold in various proprietary preparations for the treatment of tinea pedis (athlete's foot). Tolnaftate is used in the treatment of a wider spectrum of dermatophytic infections. It is quite effective in the treatment of infection with *Trichophyton rubrum*, a fungus that is often resistant to other topical agents and to griseofulvin.

References

1. S. C. Kinsky: Antibiotic interactions with model membranes. *Ann. Rev. Pharmacol.10:119 (1970).*

2. J. O. Jampen: "Interference by polyenic antifungal antibiotics (especially nystatin and filipin) with specific membrane functions" in *Biochemical Studies of Antimicrobial Drugs,* ed. by B. A. Newton and P. E. Reynolds. London: Cambridge University Press. 1966, pp. 111–130.

3. S. C. Kinsky: "Polyene antibiotics" in *Antibiotics I* ed. by D. Gottlieb and P. D. Shaw. New York: Springer-Verlag, 1967, pp. 122–141.

4. F. Marini, P. Arnow, and J. O. Lampen: The effect of monovalent cations on the inhibition of yeast metabolism by nystatin. *J. Gen. Microbiol.* 24:51 (1961).

5. S. C. Kinsky: Alterations in the permeability of Neurospora crassa due to polyene antibiotics. J. Bacteriol. 82:889 (1961).

6. D. Gottlieb, H. E. Carter, J. H. Sloneker, L. C. Wu, and E. Gaudy: Mechanisms of inhibition of fungi by filipin. Phytopathology 51: 321 (1961).

7. G. R. Gale: Cytology of Candida albicans as influencd by drugs acting on the cytoplasmic membrane. J. Bacteriol. 86:151 (1963).

8. S. C. Kinsky: Effect of polyene antibiotics on protoplasts of Neurospora crassa. J. Bacteriol. 83:351 (1962).

9. B. A. Newton: The release of soluble constituents from washed cells of Pseudomonas aeruginosa by the action of polymyxin. J. Gen. Microbiol. 9:54 (1953).

10. B. A. Newton: Site of action of polymyxin on Pseudomonas aeruginosa; antagonism by cations. J. Gen. Microbiol. 10:491 (1954).

11. O. K. Sebek: "Polymyxins and circulin" in Antibiotics I ed. by D. Gottlieb and P. D. Shaw. New York: Springer-Verlag, 1967, pp. 142–152.

12. J. O. Lampen and P. M. Arnow: Significance of nystatin uptake for its antifungal action. Proc. Soc. Exptl. Biol. Med. 101:792 (1959)

13. J. O. Lampen, P. M. Arnow, Z. Borowska, and A. I. Laskin: Location and role of sterol at nystatin-binding sites. J. Bacteriol. 84:1152 (1962).

14. S. C. Kinsky: Nystatin binding by protoplasts and a particulate fraction of Neurospora crassa, and a basis for the selective toxicity of polyene antifungal antibiotics. Proc. Natl. Acad. Sci. 48:1049 (1962).

15. S. Razin, M. Argaman, and J. Avigan: Chemical composition of Mycoplasma cells and membranes. J. Gen. Microbiol. 33:477 (1963).

16. D. S. Feingold: The action of amphotericin B on Mycoplasma laidlawii. Biochem. Biophys. Res. Commun. 19:261 (1965).

17. M. W. Weber and S. C. Kinsky: Effect of cholesterol on the sensitivity of Mycoplasma laidlawii to the polyene antibiotic filipin. J. Bacteriol. 89:306 (1965).

18. S. C. Kinsky, J. Haxby, C. B. Kinsky, R. A. Demel, and L. L. M. Van Deenen. Effect of cholesterol incorporation on the sensitivity of liposomes to the polyene antibiotic, filipin. Biochim. Biophys. Acta 152:174 (1968).

19. G. Weissmann and G. Sessa: The action of polyene antibiotics on phospholipid-cholesterol structures. J. Biol. Chem. 242:616 (1967).

20. S. C. Kinsky: Comparative responses of mammalian erythrocytes and microbial protoplasts to polyene antibiotics and vitamin A. Arch. Biochem. Biophys. 102:180 (1963).

21. S. C. Kinsky, S. A. Luse, D. Zopf, L. L. M. Van Deenen, and J. Haxby: Interaction of filipin and derivatives with erythrocyte membranes and lipid dispersions; electron microscopic observations. Biochim. Biophys. Acta 135:844 (1967).

22. R. A. Demel, F. J. L. Crombag, L. L. M. Van Deenen, and S. C. Kinsky: Interaction of polyene antibiotics with single and mixed lipid monolayers. Biochim. Biophys. Acta 150:1 (1968).

23. B. A. Newton: A fluorescent derivative of polymyxin; its preparation

and use in studying the site of action of the antibiotic. *J. Gen. Microbiol.* 12:226 (1955).

24. G. Medoff, G. S. Kobayashi, C. N. Kwan, D. Schlessinger, and P. Venkov: Potentiation of rifampicin and 5-fluorocytosine as antifungal antibiotics by amphotericin B. *Proc. Natl. Acad Sci. U.S.* 69:196 (1972).

25. S. Shadomy, H. J. Shadomy, J. A. McCay, and J. P. Utz: In vitro susceptibility of *Cryptococcus neoformans* to amphotericin B, hamycin, and 5-fluorocytosine. *Antimicrob. Ag. Chemother.* 8:452 (1968).

26. S. Shadomy: Further in vitro studies with 5-fluorocytosine. *Infect. Immun.* 2:484 (1970).

27. Editorial: Antimicrobial drugs of choice. *Med. Letter* 13:39 (1971).

28. S. A. P. Sampaio, J. T. Godoy, L. Paiva, N. L. Dillon, and C. S. Lacaz: The treatment of American (mucocutaneous) leishmaniasis with amphotericin B. *Arch. Dermatol.* 82:627 (1960).

29. V. T. Andrioli and H. M. Kravetz. The use of amphotericin B in man. *J.A.M.A.* 180:269 (1960)

30. D. J. Drutz, A. Spickard, D. E. Rogers, and M. G. Koenig: Treatment of disseminated mycotic infections. *Am. J. Med.* 45:405 (1968).

31. D. D. Bindschadler and J. E. Bennett: A pharmacologic guide to the clinical use of amphotericin B. *J. Infect. Dis.* 120:427 (1969).

32. P. D. Hart, E. Russell, and J. S. Remington: The compromised host and infection. II. Deep fungal infection. *J. Infect. Dis.* 120:169 (1969).

33. G. Hildick-Smith, H. Blank, and I. Sarkany: *Fungus Diseases and Their Treatment*, Boston: Little, Brown, 1964.

34. D. B. Louria: Some aspects of absorption, distribution and excretion of amphotericin B in man. *Antibiotic Med. Clin, Ther.* 5:295 (1958).

35. H. M. Kravetz, V. T. Andriole, M. A. Huber, and J. P. Utz: Oral administration of solubilized amphotericin B. *New Eng. J. Med.* 265:183 (1961).

36. D. Gottlieb, H. Carter, J. H. Sloneker, and A. Amman: Protection of fungi against polyene antibiotics by sterols. *Science* 128:361 (1958).

37. B. T. Fields, J. H. Bates, and R. S. Abernathy: Amphotericin B serum concentrations during therapy. *Appl. Microbiol.* 19:955 (1970).

38. J. H. Seabury and H. E. Dascomb: Experience with amphotericin B. *Ann. New York Acad. Sci.* 89:202 (1960).

39. W. T. Butler, J. E. Bennett, D. W. Alling, P. T. Wertlake, J. P. Utz, and G. J. Hill: Nephrotoxicity of amphotericin B; early and late effects in 81 patients. *Ann. Int. Med.* 61:175 (1964).

40. I. Singer, M. M. Civan, R. F. Baddour, and A. Leaf: Interactions of amphotericin B, vasopressin, and calcium in toad urinary bladder. *Am. J. Physiol.* 217:938 (1969).

41. A. L. Finn: Effects of potassium and amphotericin B on ion transport in the toad bladder. *Am. J. Physiol.* 218:463 (1970).

42. Editorial: Incompatibility of drugs for intravenous administration. *Med. Letter* 9:67 (1967).

43. E. M. Yow and J. H. Moyer: Toxicity of polymyxin B. *Arch. Int. Med.* 92:248 (1953).

44. N. M. Nord and P. D. Hoeprich: Polymyxin B and colistin, a critical comparison. *New Eng. J. Med.* 270:1030 (1964).

45. J. Vinnicombe and T. A. Stamey: The relative nephrotoxicities of polymyxin B sulfate, sodium sulfomethyl-polymyxin B, sodium sulfomethyl-colistin (colymycin), and neomycin sulfate. *Invest. Urol.* 6: 505 (1969).

46. L. A. Lindesmith, R. D. Baines, D. B. Bigelow, and T. L. Petty: Reversible respiratory paralysis associated with polymyxin therapy. *Ann. Int. Med.* 68:318 (1968).

47. E. J. Foley and G. A. Greco: Studies on the mode of action of griseofulvin. *Antibiotics Annual,* p. 670 (1959–60).

48. M. A. El-Nakeeb and J. O. Lampen: Uptake of griseofulvin by the sensitive dermatophyte, *Microsporum gypseum. J. Bacteriol.* 89:564 (1965).

49. M. A. El-Nakeeb and J. O. Lampen: Uptake of griseofulvin by microorganisms and its correlation with sensitivity to griseofulvin. *J. Gen. Microbiol.* 39:285 (1965).

50. J. O. Lampen, W. L. McLellan and M. A. El-Nakeeb: Antibiotics and fungal physiology. *Antimicrob. Agents Chemother.* 5:1006 (1965).

51. K. J. Bent and R. H. Moore: "The mode of action of griseofulvin" in *Biochemical Studies of Antimicrobial Drugs,* ed. by B. A. Newton and P. E. Reynolds. London: Cambridge University Press. 1966, pp. 82–110.

52. R. G. Crounse: Effective use of griseofulvin. *Arch. Dermatol.* 87:86 (1963).

53. D. Busfield, K. J. Child, and E. G. Tomich: An effect of phenobarbitone on griseofulvin metabolism in the rat. *Brit. J. Pharmacol.* 22:137 (1964).

54. S. Riegelman, M. Rowland, and W. L. Epstein: Griseofulvin-phenobarbital interaction in man. *J. Am. Med. Assoc.* 213:426 (1970).

55. C. Rimington, P. N. Morgan, K. Nicholls, J. D. Everall, and R. R. Davies: Griseofulvin administration and porphyrin metabolism. *Lancet* 2:318 (1963).

56. S. Granick: Induction of the synthesis of δ-aminolevulinic acid synthetase in liver parenchyma cells in culture by chemicals that induce acute porphyria. *J. Biol. Chem.* 238:2247 (1963).

57. H. Blank: Antifungal and other effects of griseofulvin. *Am. J. Med.* 39:831 (1965). The literature concerning the effect of griseofulvin on porphyrin metabolism in man is confusing. It is discussed in detail in this paper.

58. S. E. Malawista, H. Sato, and K. G. Bensch: Vinblastine and griseofulvin reversibly disrupt the living mitotic spindle. *Science* 160:770 (1968).

59. L. Wilson: Properties of colchicine binding protein from chick embryo brain. Interactions with vinca alkaloids and podophyllotoxin. *Biochemistry* 9:4999 (1970).

Part II
Drugs Employed in the Treatment of Parasitic Disease

The parasitic diseases, which are prevalent under conditions of crowding, poverty, and poor sanitation, constitute one of the major health problems of man. Parasitic infestations generally are not responsible for producing a fulminant, life-threatening situation. Rather they are chronic in nature, and, in hyperendemic areas where there is substantial undernutrition as well, the chronic disability may have far-reaching effects on the society. In many areas of the world chronic parasitic infestation is accepted as a part of life by the rural population. Large numbers of people living under conditions of poor sanitation in tropical areas may be infested simultaneously with a number of different parasites. Children are, as a rule, more frequently affected than adults. Because of a lack of acquired humoral and tissue immunity, the morbidity and mortality is also greater in children. Particularly in the developing countries in the tropics the constant infestation and accompanying malnutrition may result in a decreased intellectual function in the people who grow up under these conditions. This in turn may seriously affect the rate at which the people in these areas can acquire the technical skills to provide better living standards that would contribute greatly to the solution of the problem of parasitic disease. A circular process is thus set up by the presence of parasitic infestation where the debilitating physical and mental effects contribute to a decreased capacity for food production, mass sanitary improvement, and other corrective measures. The successful control of parasitic disease is one of the major goals of the health professions in the last quarter of this century.

Chapter 7
The Chemotherapy of Malaria

Introduction

Malaria is still one of the major health concerns of the world, affecting millions of people annually. However, the great progress made in the eradication of the disease from most of Europe and North America and in the reduction of the incidence of the disease in Africa, Asia, and South America establishes the fight against malaria as one of the major achievements in the public health field. It has taken place at many levels. The greatest contribution made in the control of the disease has been in the effort to control the mosquito vector. Thus in a very real sense the chemical that has been most effective in controlling the incidence of malaria is DDT. Another level of attack has been, of course, the development of drugs that specifically act on the parasite in the patient.

For centuries the mainstay of antimalarial therapy was quinine. The fascinating history of this drug is well worth reading.[1] The access to and control of quinine production has had considerable influence on world history over the past four hundred years; malaria has literally determined the fates of nations. The possession of antimalarial drugs and the development of new, more effective antimalarials has been and still is intimately bound up with the establishment of national spheres of influence, which have risen and declined over the past two hundred years. The young male American physician encounters malaria largely in connection with American military activity abroad. A great portion of the current research on antimalarial drugs is funded or carried out by the military.

The Disease

Malaria is characterized clinically by paroxysms of severe chills, fever, and profuse sweating. These episodes occur at reasonably well-defined intervals determined by the life cycle of the invading plasmodium (Fig. 7-1). When untreated, after recovery from the acute attack, the disease often becomes chronic with repeated relapses. Malaria can confer a low grade but specific immunity on the host.[3] However, the immunity is generally of short duration, and a person can have repeated attacks within a short period of time. The disease is the result of infestation with protozoa of the genus *Plasmodium*. There are more than forty species of the genus *Plasmodium* of which only four affect man—*P. vivax, P. falciparum, P. malariae,* and *P. ovale.* Malaria caused by the last organism is rare, and in this chapter only the first three will be discussed. The organisms are transmitted to man in the saliva of the female *Anopheles* mosquito. The lapse between the invasion time and the onset of clinical symptoms varies according to the species of the plasmodium, as does the frequency of the febrile paroxysms. As summarized in Table 7-1, the most common type of malaria is the tertian variety, caused by *P. vivax*, which is distinguished by febrile paroxysms occurring every other day. The second most common, and the type producing the severest symptomatology, is caused by *P. falciparum.* This form is called malignant tertain malaria, and it is characterized by paroxysms of somewhat longer duration occurring at irregular intervals. Quartan malaria is caused by *P. malariae.* This is the least common of the three and is generally characterized by fever spikes occurring every seventy-two hours.

The Life Cycle of the Parasite

In order to understand the rationale behind the therapy of malaria, it is necessary to understand the life cycle of the plasmodium. The various stages are presented in schematic form in Figure 7-2. The vector for this disease, the female *Anopheles* mosquito, becomes a carrier of the plasmodium by ingesting the blood of a host that contains the male and female sexual forms of the parasite. In the stomach of the mosquito the male gametocyte produces hairlike bodies that detach and fertilize the female gametocyte forming the zygote. The parasite then penetrates the stomach wall and forms a cyst on its outer surface. Numerous cell divisions

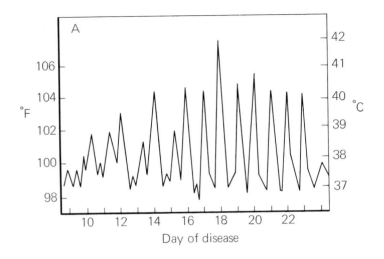

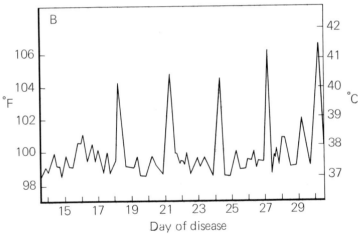

Figure 7-1   A. Temperature chart of a patient with vivax malaria. Both tertian (every other day) and quotidian (every day) fever patterns can be seen. B. Temperature chart of a patient with quartan malaria demonstrating fever spikes with two days between each episode. (From Coggeshall[2] in Beeson and McDermott: *Textbook of Medicine.* 1963.)

Table 7-1 Some characteristics of the three common malarias

Common name	Agent	Frequency of occurrence	Latency after infestation	Frequency of febrile paroxysms	Severity
Tertian malaria	*Plasmodium vivax*	Most common	26 days	Every 2 days	Mild
Malignant tertian (estivoautumnal)	*Plasmodium falciparum*	Less common	~12 days	Irregular	Severe
Quartan malaria	*Plasmodium malariae*	Least common	18–40 days	Every 3 days	Intermediate

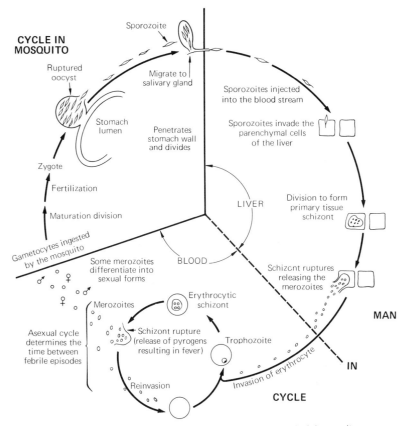

Figure 7-2 Schematic diagram of the life cycle of the malarial parasite.

take place producing an oocyst containing thousands of sporozoites. The cyst bursts, releasing the sporozoites into the body
cavity. The sporozoites migrate to the salivary glands, and, when
the mosquito bites a suitable host, some of the sporozoites are
injected into the bloodstream. The sporozoites rapidly disappear
from the blood and appear within the parenchymal cells of the
liver. Inside the liver cells they divide, forming an hepatic (exo-
erythrocytic) schizont containing numerous merozoites. The different latency times for the disease are defined by variations in the
length of this hepatic phase. The patient is asymptomatic during

this time. After this period the affected hepatic cells burst, releasing merozoites into the bloodstream. Some of these may reinvade the liver cells, producing secondary hepatic schizonts, but the vast majority invade the erythrocytes where they again multiply asexually. A mature erythrocytic schizont is formed, which then ruptures, and again merozoites are released. The rupture of the parasitized erythrocyte is accompanied by the release of pyrogenic substances causing the rapid rise in body temperature. The released merozoites have two fates. The asexual forms can reinvade erythrocytes giving rise to continued cycles of division and rupture. The length of the interval between fever paroxysms is determined by the rate at which this synchronized intra-erythrocytic growth takes place. A few of the merozoites produced with each erythrocyte cycle undergo a sexual division to form the male and female gametocytes, which are then ingested by the mosquito, and the life cycle in the vector is continued.

The Therapeutic Rationale

The erythrocytic stages of the plasmodium cycle are the most sensitive to antimalarial drugs. The exo-erythrocytic (liver) stage is more difficult to treat, while the sporozoites injected by the mosquito into the bloodstream are not sensitive to any of the antimalarial drugs. As the sporozoite is not affected, it is not possible to prevent viable plasmodia from reaching the liver. Therefore, therapy must be directed toward the hepatic or the erythrocytic stages of the parasite cycle. Unfortunately effective treatment of the erythrocytic stage of the cycle, although it will make the person asymptomatic, often does not get rid of the parasite completely. When therapy is stopped the symptoms can resume because merozoites are released into the bloodstream from the liver. To completely rid the body of the plasmodium it is necessary in many cases to administer drugs that are effective against the hepatic forms of the parasite. Often, however, when a person will remain in an area where malaria is endemic and continual reinvasion is a virtual certainty, it is not reasonable to attempt complete eradication of the parasite from the body. In this case therapy is aimed at suppressing the symptomatology by inhibiting the erythrocytic stages of the cycle.

The drug regimens employed to achieve these various therapeutic goals are presented in Table 7-2. Chloroquine, which is active only against the erythrocytic stages of the plasmodia, is employed on an acute basis for therapy of the acute attack and on a once a week basis over long periods for suppression of malarial attacks. Primaquine is effective against the hepatic forms of the parasite. It is employed to rid the body of the organism in radical cure and has also been used for prophylaxis. However, the routine use of primaquine for chemoprophylaxis in people who reside in endemic areas is not a good idea, as it favors the selection of resistant strains.

There are two characteristics of P. falciparum that modify treatment. On rupture of the hepatic schizont the merozoites of this organism are less likely to reinvade the liver and spleen and cause secondary tissue schizonts. As a result, successful treatment of the initial acute attack often results in complete eradication of the organism from the patient. A second characteristic of P. falciparum is that it becomes resistant to drug therapy much more readily than the other strains. As stated by Hunsicker, "Falciparum malaria has proved to be the Staphylococcus aureus of the malarias, and has demonstrated its ability to develop resistance to all the agents currently in use."[4] When an acute attack of falciparum malaria does not respond to chloroquine therapy promptly, it must be presumed that the organism is resistant to this drug. In this case therapy must be changed to a triple-drug regimen. When falciparum malaria is contracted in an area in which resistance is prevalent, treatment should be initiated with the triple-drug regimen. The therapy with the highest rate of cure (95–98 per cent)[5] in chloroquine-resistant malaria consists of treatment with quinine plus pyrimethamine plus either a sulfonamide or a sulfone. The biochemical basis for this particular combination of agents will be explained under sections concerned with the individual groups of drugs.

Table 7-2 Drugs of choice for the treatment of malaria

Drug dosages and therapeutic schedules are mentioned only where they illustrate the application of principles discussed in the text.

Therapeutic goal	Drug of choice	Alternative	Comments
Prophylaxis Prevention of disease by use of drugs effective against the exo-erythrocytic stage.	Primaquine Effective against all plasmodia	Pamaquine Pyrimethamine ⎱ *P. falci-* Chloroguanide ⎰ *parum* only	Exposure of large numbers of people who are resident in endemic areas to these drugs for prophylactic purposes should be discouraged. It increases the rate of selection of resistant organisms. Prophylaxis is most useful for a visitor
Treatment of the acute attack			
Uncomplicated attack	Chloroquine phosphate (oral) (1 gm, then 0.5 gm in 6 hours, then 0.5 gm daily for 2 days)	Amodiaquine	With *P. falciparum* if there is no response in 12 hours, switch to triple-drug therapy (quinine sulfate, pyrimethamine, and sulfadiazine or Dapsone) for resistant strains
Severe attack (all except *P. falciparum*)	Chloroquine hydrochloride (IM) 250 mg every 6 hours	None	Switch to oral medication as soon as possible
Chloroquine-resistánt falciparum malaria	Quinine sulfate plus pyrimethamine plus either sulfadiazine or Dapsone		For treatment of severe illness it is necessary to give quinine dihydro-chloride 600 mg in 300 ml of normal saline intravenously over no less than 30 minutes. This is repeated every 6 to 8 hours until oral therapy is possible

Table 7-2 *continued*

Therapeutic goal	Drug of choice	Alternative	Comments
Supression Suppression of disease while remaining in an endemic area	Chloroquine (500 mg weekly)	Amodiaquine	
Radical cure Eradication of persistent exo-erythrocytic parasites after clinical cure. Only in infestation with *P. vivax* and *P. malariae*	Primaquine	None	*Plasmodium falciparum* does not readily reinvade tissue cells to cause secondary tissue schizonts after rupture of primary schizont

Antimalarials Effective against Erythrocytic Forms of the Plasmodium

4-Aminoquinolines

Structures

The two most widely used 4-aminoquinolines are chloroquine and amodiaquine. They are very effective against the asexual erythrocytic forms of both P. vivax and P. falciparum. They are also active against the sexual forms of P. vivax but not those of P. falciparum. These drugs are virtually inactive against the hepatic forms of the plasmodia.

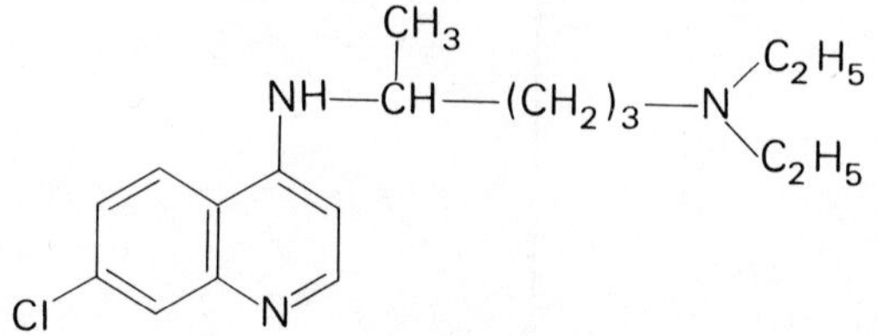

Chloroquine

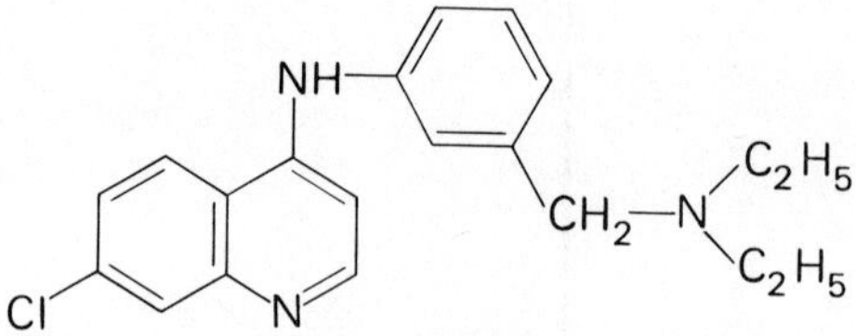

Amodiaquine

Mechanism of Action

There is a great deal of difference between studying the mechanism of action of a growth-inhibiting agent in bacteria and in an intracellular parasite such as the plasmodium. Compared to bacteria much less is known about the biochemistry of the various protozoa, and it is difficult to set up good experimental systems with which to study mechanisms of drug action in these organisms in vitro. Chloroquine in high concentrations kills some bacteria.

It is therefore not surprising that many of the experiments that have elaborated on early observations that chloroquine and quinine decrease the incorporation of radioactive phosphate into nucleic acids in plasmodia[6] were carried out in bacterial systems. At present, the best evidence available from all systems supports the hypothesis that the schizontocidal effect of the 4-aminoquinolines and the cinchona alkaloids (i.e. quinine) is due to the ability of these compounds to bind to native DNA and inhibit nucleic acid synthesis in the dividing organism.

When a culture of Bacillus megaterium is exposed to chloroquine at 10^{-3} M, there is a rapid killing effect preceded by an inhibition of nucleic acid and protein synthesis.[7] The bactericidal effect, however, is observed at a concentration of drug in the order of one thousand times the maximum therapeutic concentration achieved in plasma during therapy of the acute malarial attack, 10^{-6} M.[8] It is impossible to assume that effects observed in bacteria at concentrations of drug lethal for the patient represent the same events responsible for the therapeutic effect of the drug in the treatment of malaria. An experimental model has been developed, however, that permits the investigator to study drug effects in a plasmodium that is growing in synchrony in vitro.[9] Plasmodium knowlesi is a parasite that normally infests monkeys. This organism has a complete erythrocytic cycle of twenty-four hours. Erythrocytes harvested from heavily infested monkeys during the first three or four hours of the erythrocytic cycle are suspended in a culture medium with radioactive precursor molecules. The development of the plasmodium is followed morphologically and can be correlated with the rate of nucleic acid and protein synthesis during the different stages of growth. As nonnucleated erythrocytes do not synthesize nucleic acids or significant amounts of protein, the incorporation of labeled substrates reflects plasmodial metabolism. The relationships of macromolecular synthesis to the erythrocytic growth stages of the parasite are presented in Figure 7-3.

If chloroquine is added to this culture system, the synthesis of both plasmodial nucleic acids and protein is inhibited.[10] Nucleic acid synthesis is inhibited more than is protein synthesis. The maximal effect of chloroquine on DNA synthesis occurs at a con-

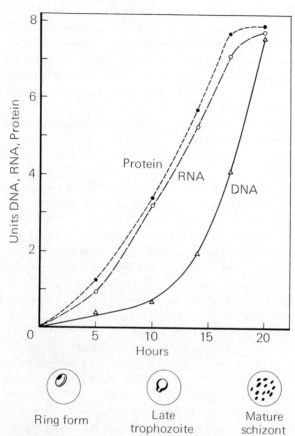

Figure 7-3 The synthesis of nucleic acids and proteins at various stages of the erythrocytic cycle of *Plasmodium knowlesi*. Erythrocytes obtained from an infested monkey are suspended in a culture medium. Radioactive orotic acid or leucine is added to replicate cultures, and the cumulative incorporation of radioactivity into the isolated macromolecules is assayed at various times. One unit of the ordinate is equivalent to 75 cpm per culture for DNA, 300 cpm per culture for RNA, and 450 cpm per culture for protein. Incorporation into DNA, RNA, and protein of uninfected control cultures has been subtracted. The drawings below the graph are made from photomicrographs of Giemsa-stained cells taken at the corresponding times of the culture period noted on the abcissa (Adapted from Polet and Barr.[9])

centration in the culture medium of approximately 10^{-6} M. Thus, the drug is maximally effective in the *in vitro* system at the same concentration as that employed therapeutically. But this concentration of chloroquine is only about one-hundreth that required to demonstrate similar effects in bacteria and in purified nucleic acid synthesizing systems prepared from bacteria. This discrepancy between the concentration of drug required to inhibit the parasite and the concentration required to demonstrate chloroquine effects on bacterial enzyme systems is resolved by the demonstration that the concentration of drug in parasitized erythrocytes is one hundred times that of the plasma.[11] Thus the concentration of total drug in the parasitized erythrocyte is about 10^{-4} M at therapeutic levels. It is not known if the drug is actively transported into the parasitized erythrocyte or whether there is free diffusion followed by binding to the parasite inside the cell. In fact it is not known whether the concentration mechanism is a function of the parasite alone or of the whole parasitized erythrocyte.[11]

The ability of chloroquine to inhibit nucleic acid synthesis can be demonstrated in purified systems where DNA or RNA synthesis is carried out under the direction of DNA template and a purified polymerase enzyme from *E. coli*.[12] The dose-response curve for chloroquine inhibition of DNA synthesis promoted by the bacterial enzyme is seen in Part A of Figure 7-4. There are three major components to this reaction system: the enzyme, the DNA template, and the nucleoside triphosphate precursors. Chloroquine could inhibit the system by interacting with any of these components. If chloroquine inhibits DNA synthesis by decreasing the effectiveness of the enzyme or the DNA template, then the addition of that component in large amounts to the system might reverse the chloroquine effect. Part B of Figure 7-4 shows that the effect of chloroquine is reversed as larger amounts of DNA template are added to the enzyme reaction. Changing the amount of enzyme had no effect on the extent of inhibition. It was demonstrated that the added DNA primer overcame the chloroquine inhibition in a competitive manner. The same observations made in the DNA polymerase reaction were also made with an RNA

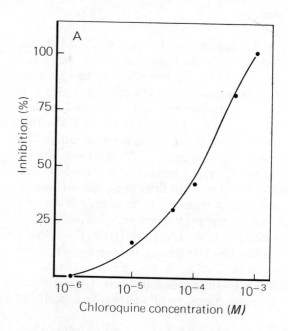

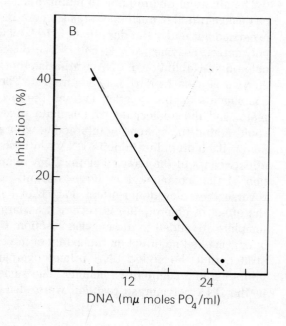

polymerase reaction system, although RNA synthesis was some-what less sensitive to the drug. These experimental results are consistent with the conclusion that chloroquine inhibits nucleic acid synthesis by affecting the ability of DNA to act as a template. The receptor for chloroquine in the cell is DNA. The interaction of chloroquine with DNA has been demonstrated by a number of physical methods. Chloroquine, for example, can alter the temperature at which native, double-stranded DNA uncoils to form denatured, single-stranded DNA (Figure 7-5).[13] This indicates a strong binding between the drug and the receptor. The strong interaction between chloroquine and DNA can be recorded as a change in the absorption spectrum of the drug.[14] This effect can be seen in Figure 7-6. It seems clear that chloroquine is interca-lated between the stacked base pairs of the double-stranded DNA helix.[15] Studies on the association of chloroquine with synthetic polynucleotides such as poly A and poly G suggest that the drug interacts preferentially with the purines (adenine and guanine) rather than the pyrimidines (cytidine and thymine).[14] The interac-tion of chloroquine with free nucleotides can be recorded as alter-ations in the nuclear magnetic resonance spectrum of the drug.[16] Again, such interactions are strong with the purines but minimal with the pyrimidines. Although the cellular receptor is the complex molecule DNA, it may be possible to study at least part of the drug receptor interaction in a simple solution of the drug and AMP or GMP.

DNA is composed of four nucleotides present in various propor-tions depending on the type of organism from which it is derived. The basic composition of the molecule is quite similar in the para-site and in the cells of the host. One might reasonably expect that a small molecule like chloroquine, which binds to the DNA

Figure 7-4   A. Inhibition of DNA synthesis by chloroquine. DNA polymerase purified from *E. coli* was incubated with purified *E. coli* DNA, the four nucleotide triphosphates, and various concentrations of chloroquine. The amount of radio-active dATP incorporated into DNA was assayed after 20 minutes. (The figure was constructed from data presented in tabular form by Cohen and Yielding,[12] Table 1.) B. The effect of DNA primer concentration on the inhibition of *E. coli* DNA polymerase by 10^{-4} *M* chloroquine. DNA assays were carried out as above with increasing concentrations of primer DNA. (From Cohen and Yielding.[12])

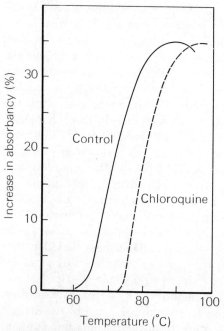

Figure 7-5 The effect of chloroquine on the thermal dissociation of calf thymus DNA. Calf thymus DNA is heated slowly in the presence or absence of 5×10^{-6} M chloroquine. As the DNA is heated it uncoils, and the two strands separate. The single-stranded, denatured DNA formed absorbs a greater amount of light at 260 $m\mu$ than the comparable quantity of DNA in the native, double-stranded form. This change from double-stranded to single-stranded DNA is recorded on the ordinate of the figure as a percentage increase in absorbancy at 260 $m\mu$. When chloroquine is bound to the DNA, the strands are held together at temperatures that cause almost complete separation in the control. (From Cohen and Yielding.[13])

of the parasite, would also bind in a similar manner to DNA in the cells of the host. Chloroquine might then be expected to inhibit the growth of such rapidly dividing cell systems as bone marrow, skin, or endothelium of the gastrointestinal tract. What then is the basis for the selective toxicity of chlorquine? The drug inhibits cell replication and nucleic acid synthesis in cultured mammalian cells at a concentration of 10^{-5} to 10^{-4} M. [17] This concentration is roughly one hundred times the schizontocidal concentration. The parasitized erythrocytes are able to concentrate chloroquine so that its intracellular level is many times the plasma concentration. It has been suggested that the selective toxicity of chloroquine is due to this selective concentration of the drug.[10,11] This may not account entirely for the selective effect of the drug because it has been clearly demonstrated that chloroquine is extensively bound in the tissues of the host as well.[18] The level of the drug at therapeutic doses in the spleen and liver of mice, for example, is

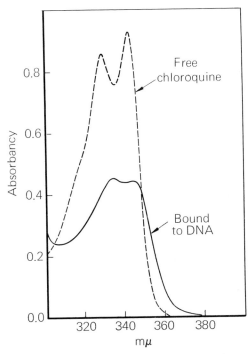

Figure 7-6 Change in the absorption spectrum of chloroquine resulting from the interaction of the drug with DNA. The dotted line represents the absorption spectrum of 4.8×10^{-5} M chloroquine in 15 mM potassium phosphate buffer, pH 5.9, at 22°C. In the presence of calf thymus DNA (solid line) there is binding of the drug and the bound form of the drug is less able to absorb light energy. (From Cohen and Yielding.[13])

approximately one-third that in the parasitized erythrocytes of the same animals.[11] It is not clear whether such a difference is enough to account for the therapeutic index of the drug. Similarly, the same study showed that the level of the drug in the erythrocytes of mice parasitized with a strain of the plasmodium resistant to chloroquine was only 50 per cent of the amount present in erythrocytes containing the sensitive strain. This apparent decrease in ability to concentrate the drug in the parasitized erythrocyte may account in part for the resistance to chloroquine.

Tissue Binding

It is known that chloroquine binds to serum proteins[18] and to RNA[19] as well as to DNA. At therapeutic concentrations chloroquine is bound to all three of these cell components. The sequestration of chloroquine in the patient's cells is responsible for two clinically important phenomena that must be considered in administering the drug. When initiating therapy with chloroquine, it is necessary to administer a loading dose that is twice the maintenance dose. This is done to saturate tissue binding and to reach effective free drug levels. For suppressive therapy, a maintenance dose of 500 mg is given only once a week. The long interval between doses is necessary because the drug has a half-life of several days. The long half-life is due to a slow release from tissue-binding sites. When the drug is withdrawn, several weeks pass before it disappears from the tissues. Quinine also binds to DNA, but the avidity of the binding in the tissues is much less than that of chloroquine. Quinine has a short half-life, and no priming dose is required. Quinacrine, a polycyclic drug employed in the treatment of helminthic infestations, binds to DNA and inhibits nucleic acid synthesis. This yellow compound is bound in tissues to a greater extent than chloroquine.[18] During therapy, the tissue-bound drug produces a yellowish discoloration of the skin.

Pharmacology

Absorption, distribution, and excretion. Chloroquine and amodiaquine are both absorbed rapidly from the gastrointestinal tract. Chloroquine is distributed widely in the body with extensive tissue binding. Chloroquine is metabolized by the liver microsomal drug metabolizing system. In the presence of an inhibitor of this metabolizing system, SKF-525A, plasma concentrations of the drug are prolonged.[20] This is an important observation because it allows one to predict that the plasma level of free chloroquine may be depressed if the patient is being treated concomitantly with any of the growing number of drugs known to induce the hepatic drug metabolizing system. This consideration is not crucial in short-term treatment of the acute malarial attack, but it should be kept in mind during suppressive therapy, when low blood levels of the free drug are maintained for long periods of time. The kidney is primarily responsible for eliminating the metabolized products of chloroquine from the body.

Toxicity and side effects. Chloroquine is a safer drug than the studies of its mechanism of action would predict. In doses used for treatment of acute attacks, it can cause dizziness, headache, difficulty in accommodation, itching, vomiting, and skin rashes. At the low blood levels of drug employed for suppressive therapy the drug does not have significant toxicity. With the use of high doses of chloroquine for prolonged periods in the treatment of intestinal amebiasis, lupus erythematosis, and discoid lupus, toxic effects in the skin, blood, and eyes have been noted. Skin eruptions, photosensitivity, alopecia, and bleaching of the hair can occur. Occasionally there is leukopenia.

Ocular damage can take the form of a temporary, reversible blurring of vision, and with large doses there may be severe eye damage and even permanent blindness. The cause of the retinopathy resulting from chloroquine treatment is not known.[21] Chloroquine is localized in the melanin-containing areas of the eye,[22] and it binds extensively to preparations of choroidal melanin both in vivo and in vitro.[23] The drug binds to melanin in the skin as well,[24] and studies of the binding of iodoquine (the iodine-containing analog of chloroquine) to purified melanin and DNA suggest that chloroquine may bind even more strongly to melanin than to nucleic acid.[25] It is not known whether the avid association of the drug with the retinal pigment is in some way responsible for the retinopathy. The retinal lesion appears as a hyperpigmentation of the macula surrounded by a zone of depigmentation that in turn is encircled by another ring of pigment. This bull's-eye lesion is pathognomonic of chloroquine retinopathy.[26] It has been reported that the lesion can occur months after cessation of chloroquine therapy.[27]

There is a form of toxicity that should be considered when any drug that interacts with DNA is given to large populations on a chronic basis—the compound may be mutagenic. Chloroquine, amodiaquine, quinacrine, and quinine all interact with DNA and are employed chronically in large populations. Many agents of similar structure, such as the acridine dyes that intercalate between the base pairs in DNA, are potent mutagens and carcinogens.

Cinchona Alkaloids

The cinchona alkaloids are all compounds isolated from the bark of the cinchona tree. The most important member of the group is quinine. Until the 1920s, when more potent synthetic antimalarials were first introduced, the cinchona alkaloids were the only specific antimalarial drugs. The use of quinine in antimalarial therapy would probably be merely of historical interest if it were not for the recent development of resistance to the more potent drugs in P. falciparum. For reasons that are unknown, resistance has not readily developed to quinine,[28] and, in spite of its lesser potency, the drug has again found a role in the treatment of malaria.

Quinine

Mechanism of action. Quinine has a structure similar to the 4-aminoquinolines, and like chloroquine it binds directly to DNA and inhibits nucleic acid synthesis.[29] Quinine does not interact with the DNA receptor in precisely the same way that chloroquine does, but the effects seem to be similar.

Absorption, distribution, and excretion. Quinine sulfate is well absorbed from the gastrointestinal tract, and it should not be given by intramuscular or subcutaneous injection. Quinine hydrochloride is the form of the drug employed for intravenous administration. Quinine is widely distributed in the body; however, it does not accumulate in the tissues like chloroquine. Most of the quinine is metabolized in the liver, primarily by hydroxylation, and the hydroxylated products are rapidly excreted by the kidney.[30] The rapid metabolism and excretion define a short half-life for the drug, and to obtain a maximum therapeutic effect in treating the acute malarial attack it must be given every six to eight hours.[31]

Toxicity. Quinine has a large number of pharmacological effects. The effects of quinine on the central and peripheral nervous system and the cardiovascular system will not be considered here except as they relate to the toxicity observed when the drug is used in the treatment of malaria. The administration of quinine in high doses for treatment of the acute malaria attack is often accompanied by tinnitus, blurred vision, nausea, headache, and decreased hearing acuity. This symptom complex is similar to salicylism and is called cinchonism. Sometimes these symptoms become so severe that therapy must be withdrawn. Permanent damage to vision, balance, and hearing can result. In high concentrations quinine, like its dextro-isomer quinidine, can directly depress the myocardium. Quinine also causes vasodilation by a direct effect on vascular smooth muscle. During intravenous therapy, high blood levels of quinine are achieved; as a result of the myocardial depression and vasodilatation, the patient can go into shock. The drug therefore must be given very slowly when the intravenous route is employed.

Quinine can cause contraction of uterine muscle, and it has been used in medicine to stimulate contraction during labor. It does not have significant effect until labor has begun. At toxic

doses, quinine can cause abortion. It is unclear whether the aborti-
facient effect is due to an action on the uterus or whether it is due
to fetal poisoning. If other antimalarial drugs can be used, quinine
should not be given to pregnant women. Quinine is rarely responsible for causing hemolysis and bone-marrow depression. Occasional rashes and photosensitivity reactions occur during quinine
therapy. Patients who have a history of cardiac arrythmia, episodes of hemolysis, tinnitus, or optic neuritis should be treated
with other drugs if possible. Quinine has the poorest ratio between
therapeutic potency and toxicity of all the antimalarial drugs.

Antimalarials Effective against Exo-Erythrocytic Forms of the Plasmodium

8-Aminoquinolines

The only commonly employed member of the 8-aminoquinoline
group is primaquine. Other drugs in this group include pamaquine
and quinocide. The ring structure of these drugs is the same as
that of chloroquine, and as one would expect they bind to DNA.[32]

Primaquine

However, the similarity between the two groups of compounds
seems to end here. The 8-aminoquinolines are effective against
the exo-erythrocytic stages of the parasite. They have no activity
against the erythrocytic forms of the parasite, but they do kill
the sexual forms in the blood. Their mechanism of action is unknown. There is evidence that primaquine may become associated
with the mitochondria of the exo-erythrocytic forms of plasmodia
growing in culture[33] and that exposure to primaquine causes the
mitochondria to swell and become vacuolated.[34] These experi-

ments are not definitive, and there is no suggestion that the primary effect of the drug is in the mitochondrion.

Pharmacology

Primaquine is rapidly absorbed from the gastrointestinal tract.
All of the 8-aminoquinolines are metabolized rapidly. It is clear
that at least for pamaquine and pentaquine the metabolites are
more potent antimalarials than the parent compounds.[35][36] This
would also seem to be the case with primaquine. Peak plasma
concentrations of primaquine are achieved four to six hours after
drug administration, but the prophylactic effect of a single dose
of the drug is maximal when it is administered twelve hours before
infestation.[36] The difference between the time of peak plasma
levels of the unaltered drug and peak therapeutic effect may be
due to the fact that more active forms of the drug are being produced by metabolism in the patient. The 8-aminoquinolines do not
bind in the tissues like the 4-aminoquinolines. As a result of their
rapid metabolism, the rapid renal excretion of the metabolites,
and the lack of tissue binding, these drugs have a relatively short
half-life in the body and are administered daily.

Toxicity. Primaquine has a good therapeutic index. The ratio of
the maximum tolerated dose to the smallest dose capable of preventing nearly all relapses is about ten. The same ratio for pamaquine is one.[37] For this reason pamaquine is no longer employed.
With primaquine there are occasional symptoms of gastrointestinal distress, and leukopenia is sometimes observed at high doses,
but the most important side effect is hemolytic anemia, which
occurs in certain primaquine-sensitive people.

Primaquine Sensitivity

While most patients tolerate primaquine quite well, in about
5 to 10 per cent of Negro males therapeutic doses can precipitate
an acute hemolytic anemia. This response is also seen rarely in
darker-hued Caucasians (such as Indians), in Asians, and in people
living in the countries bordering the Mediterranean.[38] People who
are primaquine sensitive have a genetically determined deficiency

of glucose-6-phosphate dehydrogenase (G6PD) in their erythrocytes. This enzyme (Figure 7-7) is responsible for the oxidation of glucose-6-phosphate to 6-phosphogluconic acid. This reaction is necessary to produce NADPH, which functions as a proton donor in the glutathione reductase reaction. In this second reaction, reduced glutathione is produced from oxidized glutathione. For reasons that are unknown, reduced glutathione seems to be necessary for the maintenance of erythrocyte integrity. The hemolysis seen in the reduced glutathione-deficient state is apparently the result of an increased susceptibility of the erythrocyte to mechanical breakage. A metabolite of primaquine acts in the erythrocyte as an oxidizing agent and converts reduced glutathione to oxidized glutathione.[39] With a deficiency of G6PD the cell is unable to produce enough NADPH to regenerate the reduced form of glutathione and hemolysis takes place.

In addition to hemolysis, patients who are deficient in glucose-6-phosphate dehydrogenase may develop methemoglobinemia on treatment with primaquine. Methemoglobin can be converted to hemoglobin by four known systems. One of these systems derives its reduced equivalents from NADPH, and another is a nonenzymatic process in which the proton donor is reduced glutathione.[40] As illustrated schematically in Figure 7-7, this side effect of the drug can also be explained on the basis of G6PD deficiency.

Glucose-6-phosphate dehydrogenase deficiency is inherited as a sex-linked trait. Primaquine is not the only drug that causes hemolysis in people who have this enzyme deficiency. A number of drugs including the sulfonamides, the cinchona alkaloids, the 4-aminoquinolines, and chloramphenicol can produce hemolytic anemia in these people.[41] A reasonably simple test has been devised to detect G6PD deficiency.[42] It consists of measuring the glutathione content in erythrocytes after incubation with acetylphenylhydrazine, one of the most effective of the hemolytic compounds. The results of such a test are presented in Figure 7-8. Before exposure to acetylphenylhydrazine the erythrocytes from normal controls and G6PD-deficient individuals contain the same amount of reduced glutathione. After two hours of incubation in the presence of the oxidant, the erythrocytes from the G6PD-deficient individuals have a much lower level of reduced glutathione. This type of clinical test is helpful in identifying potential reactors.

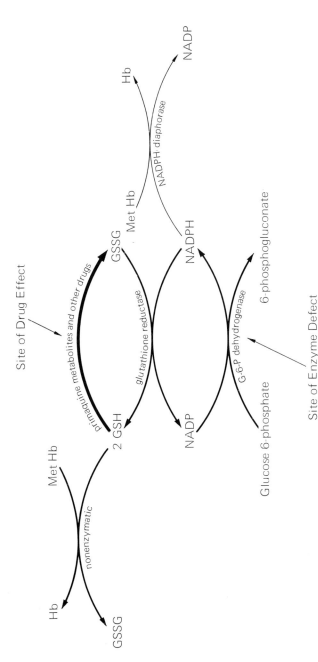

Figure 7-7 Schematic diagram of the principal reactions related to the hemolysis and methemoglobinemia that occur in primaquine-sensitive patients. In the presence of primaquine metabolites and a number of other drugs reduced glutathione (GSH) is converted to oxidized glutathione (GSSG). In erythrocytes from normal individuals the GSH level is maintained at a constant amount by the glutatione reductase reaction which requires NADPH. The principal source of NADPH in the cell is the glucose-6-phosphate dehydrogenase (G6PD) reaction. In primaquine-sensitive individuals G6PD activity is low, and the cell consequently cannot provide enough NADPH to keep up the levels of GSH in the presence of hemolyzing drugs. The depressed levels of GSH apparently render the erythrocyte susceptible to mechanical breakage. Low amounts of both NADPH and GSH in the cell may contribute to the methemoglobinemia occasionally observed in these patients.

169

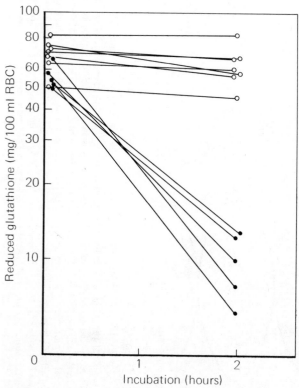

Figure 7-8   The reduced glutathione (GSH) stability test for primaquine sensi-tivity. Assays for GSH were performed on blood samples from seven non-sensitive (o-o and five primaquine-sensitive subjects (●-●). The erythrocytes were then incubated in the presence of acetylphenylhydrazine for two hours, and the GSH assay was repeated. (From Beutler.[42])

Antimalarials that Inhibit Both Erythrocytic and Exo-Erythrocytic Forms of the Plasmodium

The Inhibitors of Folic Acid Synthesis

Introduction

Several compounds that inhibit the synthesis of folic acid have been developed for antimalarial use; these include pyrimethamine, trimethoprim, chloroguanide, and cycloguanil pamoate. Of this

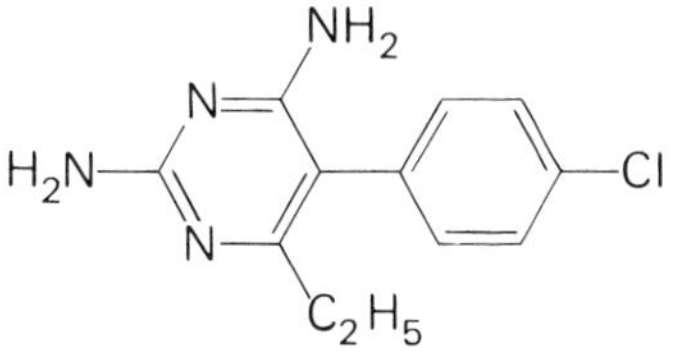

Pyrimethamine 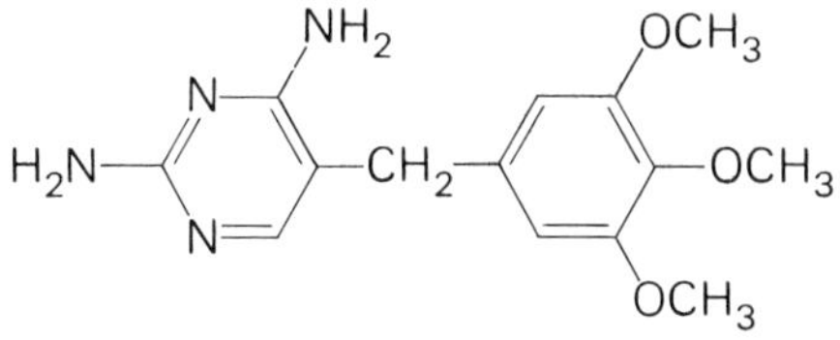   **Trimethoprim**

group, pyrimethamine receives the widest clinical application. These drugs are schizontocidal for both the erythrocytic and exo-erythrocytic forms of *P. falciparum*. There is some effect on the exo-erythrocytic forms of *P. vivax* but not enough to make the drugs useful in the radical cure of malaria caused by this organism.

Chloroguanide is less potent than pyrimethamine, and there is good evidence that chloroguanide itself is not the active form of the drug. It was demonstrated some time ago that chloroguanide has no effect on the exo-erythrocytic forms of *P. gallinaceum in vitro*. When the drug was incubated with minced liver tissue, however, it proved to be very effective.[43] The active dihydrotriazine metabolite produced by the liver is a closed ring form that has a structure similar to that of pyrimethamine (Figure 7–9).

Mechanism of Action

Originally synthesized as a thymine analog, pyrimethamine was found to have an antifolic acid activity. The early investigations of the mechanism of action were carried out in bacteria and indicated that pyrimethamine inhibits synthesis of the reduced forms of folic acid.[44] Recently it has been demonstrated that

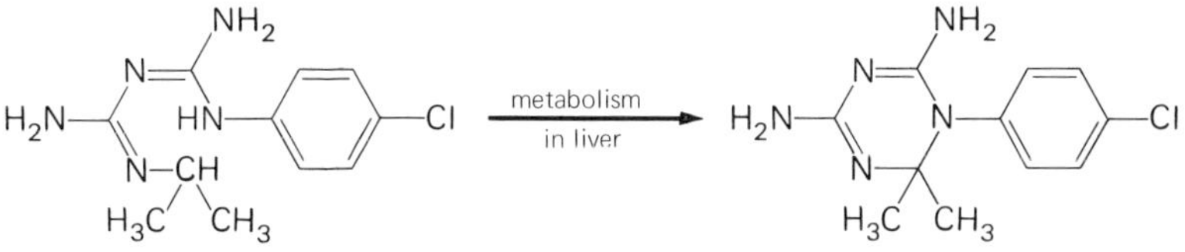

Chloroguanide   metabolism in liver →   Dihydrotriazine metabolite (active form of drug)

Figure 7-9 Chloroguanide is inactive as an antimalarial compound until it is altered by ring closure in the body to form the active dihydrotriazine metabolite.

plasmodia synthesize dihydrofolate *de novo* in much the same way as bacteria.[45] Dihydrofolate is then reduced under the direction of dihydrofolate reductase to tetrahydrofolate. This is the form of the compound that can function as the one-carbon carrier molecule required for the synthesis of thymidine and the purines. Pyrimethamine inhibits the dihydrofolate reductase enzyme isolated from *P. berghei* in a competitive manner.[46] Thus the drug interacts with its receptor, the reductase enzyme, at binding points in common with the natural substrate dihydrofolate. In Figure 7-10 the structure of pyrimethamine is redrawn to show the similarity between the drug and the pteridine portion of dihydrofolate.

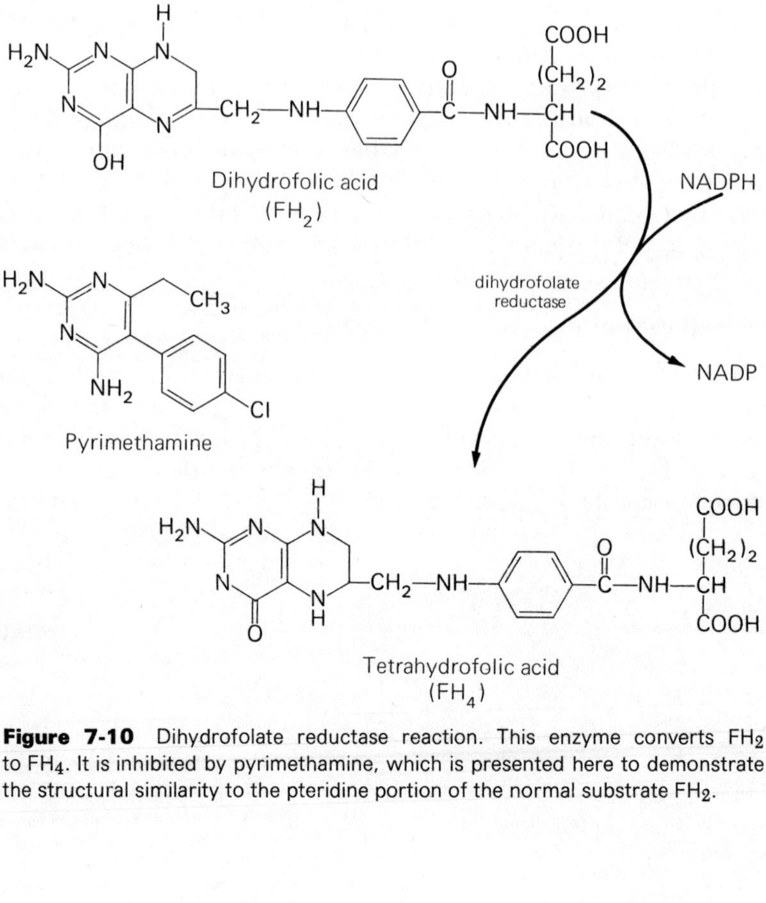

Figure 7-10 Dihydrofolate reductase reaction. This enzyme converts FH_2 to FH_4. It is inhibited by pyrimethamine, which is presented here to demonstrate the structural similarity to the pteridine portion of the normal substrate FH_2.

The reduction of folic acid compounds is a necessary step in the normal biochemistry of the host as well as the plasmodium. Inhibition of this enzyme by the drug would be expected to have a severe adverse effect in the patient (easily demonstrated with other antifolates such as methotrexate). However, pyrimethamine and the other drugs of this class are selectively toxic to the plasmodium. A concentration of only 5×10^{-9} M is sufficient to inhibit the enzyme from *P. berghei,* whereas a concentration of 10^{-6} M is required to inhibit the dihydrofolate reductase enzyme in mouse erythrocytes.[47] There is, therefore, a difference of 200-fold in the sensitivity of these two enzymes. This difference in sensitivity is probably due to differences in the amino acid sequence at the binding site for the drug.

There is a way in which the selectivity of pyrimethamine action can be enhanced clinically. The plasmodium, like many of the bacteria, must synthesize dihydrofolate directly. These organisms cannot take up and utilize folate or the one-carbon-charged forms of reduced folate such as folinic acid.[45] The mammalian cell of course cannot synthesize folate and must utilize the compound provided from external sources. Therefore, to protect against hematological toxicity folinic acid (N^5-formyl-tetrahydrofolic acid) is given daily to the patient. This prevents toxicity in the host by providing a compound that bypasses the blocked reaction but cannot modify the therapeutic response because it does not enter the plasmodium.

Combination Therapy with Sulfones and Sulfonamides

As the plasmodium must synthesize dihydrofolic acid, drugs such as the sulfonamides and sulfones which compete for the utilization of para-aminobenzoic acid in that synthetic pathway should be effective antimalarial agents. When used alone these drugs are not potent antimalarials but when used in combination with the inhibitors of dihydrofolate reductase they are therapeutic. A combination of two inhibitors is likely to produce a synergistic effect when the two drugs act at different points on the same metabolic pathway (see Figure 7-11). A combination of a sulfonamide or a sulfone with an inhibitor of dihydrofolate reductase is

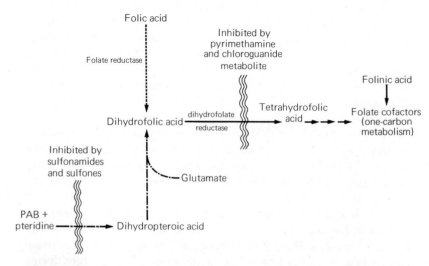

Figure 7-11 Schematic representation of sites of action for inhibitors of dihydrofolate synthesis and reduction. Reactions occurring in parasite only (____. ____. ____), man only (. . .), and parasite and man (____).

synergistic in antimalarial therapy.[48] This is clear from the experiment presented in Figure 7-12, which demonstrates that the presence of very low concentrations of sulfadiazine markedly reduces the amount of pyrimethamine required for therapeutic effect. This is the biochemical basis for the use of these agents together in the treatment of chloroquine-resistant falciparum malaria.

Resistance to Pyrimethamine

Many plasmodia can develop resistance to pyrimethamine.[49] There are a number of ways in which this resistance could develop. In one study it was demonstrated that resistant plasmodia contained more reductase than sensitive cells.[46] The enzyme isolated from these resistant cells was also found to have a much lower affinity for the drug. Thus resistance arose in this particular case by selection of organisms with an increased content of structurally altered dihydrofolate reductase as a result of mutation in the gene or genes controlling the synthesis of this enzyme.

Another study has provided evidence suggesting that pyrimethamine resistance can be transferred from one species of plasmodium to another.[50] In this study pyrimethamine-resistant *Plasmodium vinckei* and pyrimethamine-sensitive *P. berghei* were inoculated simultaneously into mice, and both organisms were allowed to multiply. Both plasmodia were then transferred from the mice to a hamster that was subsequently treated with high doses of pyrimethamine. Since *P. vinckei* is not able to grow in hamsters, the hamster can serve as a biological filter to select for *P. berghei* that have become drug resistant. Drug-resistant *P. berghei* were recovered from the hamster. The dihydrofolate

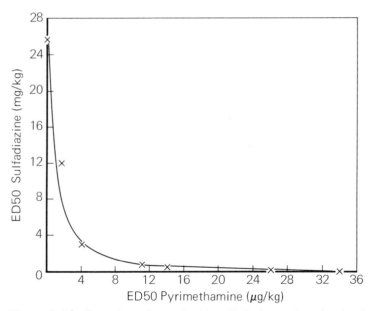

Figure 7-12 Synergism observed with sulfadiazine and pyrimethamine in chicks infested with *P. gallinaceum.* The figure presents the doses of pyrimethamine and sulfadiazine, administered both singly and together in various proportions, which were required to reduce parasitemia to 50 per cent of controls. (From Rollo.[48])

reductase enzyme prepared from these newly resistant plasmodia behaved similarly to the altered enzyme of the original drug-resistant *P. vinckei.* Thus it is postulated that there was transfer of genetic material from the drug-resistant to the drug-sensitive plasmodium. The mechanism by which transfer took place is not known; however, the observation is similar to the infectious type of drug resistance described in Chapter 1 where resistance information contained in episomes is transferred from one type of bacterium to another. Mixed malarial infections do occur in humans, and it is possible that resistance may be transferred in the patient.

Pharmacology

Pyrimethamine and chloroguanide are absorbed well from the gastrointestinal tract. Pyrimethamine is bound in the tissues to a greater extent than is chloroguanide, and it is extensively metabolized. As mentioned earlier in this chapter, chloroguanide is metabolized to at least one active metabolite. Excretion is predominantly renal. About 60 per cent of the chloroguanide is excreted as the parent compound and about 40 per cent as its metabolites.[51] Because tissue binding is less and excretion by the kidneys is more rapid, the effect of chloroguanide lasts a shorter time than the effect of pyrimethamine. For this reason, and because of its higher potency, pyrimethamine is the more popular drug. Pyrimethamine is secreted in human milk, and breast feeding yields suppressive levels of the drug in the infant.[52] Cycloguanil pamoate, a repository preparation of the dihydrotriazine metabolite of chloroguanide, has been developed. A single intramuscular dose of this compound will protect experimental animals and man for weeks against clinical attack.[53]

The toxicity of pyrimethamine is quite low. Gastrointestinal distress is occasionally observed. Rarely, high doses given to children can cause convulsions. There is occasional bone-marrow depression that can be reversed by administration of citrovorum factor (folinic acid). This marrow-depressant effect of pyrimethamine has been exploited with the use of higher doses in the treatment of polycythemia rubra vera. The drug is contraindicated during pregnancy.

References

1. M. B. Kreig: "The incredible history of quinine." in *Green Medicine*. New York; Rand McNally, 1964, pp. 165–206.
2. L. T. Coggeshall: "Malaria" in *Textbook of Medicine*, ed. by P. B. Beeson and W. McDermott. Philadelphia: W. B. Saunders, 1963, pp. 383–389.
3. I. N. Brown: Immunological aspects of malaria infection. *Adv. Immunol.* 11:267 (1969).
4. L. G. Hunsicker: The pharmacology of the antimalarials. *Arch. Int. Med.* 123:645 (1969).
5. T. W. Sheehy and R. C. Reba: Treatment of chloroquine resistant *Plasmodium falciparum* infections in Vietnam. *Ann. Int. Med.* 66:616 (1967).
6. K. A. Schellenberg and G. R. Coatney: The influence of antimalarial drugs on nucleic acid synthesis in *Plasmodium gallinaceum* and *Plasmodium berghei*. *Biochem. Pharmacol.* 6:143 (1961).
7. J. Ciak and F. E. Hahn: Chloroquine: Mode of action. *Science* 151:347 (1966).
8. A. S. Alving, L. Eichelberger, B. Craige, R. Jones, C. M. Whorton, and T. N. Pullman: Studies on the chronic toxicity of chloroquine (SN-7618). *J. Clin. Invest.* 27 Suppl. :60(1948).
9. H. Polet and C. F. Barr: DNA, RNA, and protein synthesis in erythrocytic forms of *Plasmodium knowlesi*. *Am. J. Trop. Med. Hyg.* 17:672 (1968).
10. H. Polet and C. F. Barr: Chloroquine and dihydroquinine; *In vitro* studies of their antimalarial effect upon *Plasmodium knowlesi*. *J. Pharm. Exp. Ther.* 164:380 (1968).
11. P. B. Macomber, R. L. O'Brien and F. E. Hahn: Chloroquine: Physiological basis of drug resistance in *Plasmodium berghei*. *Science* 152:1374 (1966).
12. S. N. Cohen and K. L. Yielding: Inhibition of DNA and RNA polymerase reactions by chloroquine. *Proc. Natl. Acad. Sci.* 54:522 (1965).
13. S. N. Cohen and K. L. Yielding: Spectrophotometric studies of the interaction of chloroquine with deoxyribonucleic acid. *J. Biol. Chem.* 240:3123 (1965).
14. L. W. Blodgett and K. L. Yielding: Comparison of chloroquine binding to DNA, and polyadenylic and polyguanylic acids. *Biochim. Biophys. Acta* 169:451 (1968).
15. M. Waring: Variation of the supercoils in closed circular DNA by binding of antibiotics and drugs: Evidence for molecular models involving intercalation. *J. Mol. Biol.* 54:247 (1970).
16. H. Sternglanz, K. L. Yielding, and K. M. Pruitt: Nuclear magnetic resonance studies of the interaction of chloroquine diphosphate with adenosine 5'-phosphate and other nucleotides. *Mol. Pharmacol.* 5:376 (1969).

17. J. D. Gabourel: Effects of hydroxychloroquine on the growth of mammalian cells *in vitro*. *J. Pharm. Exp. Ther.* 141:122 (1963).

18. R. W. Berliner, D. P. Earle, J. V. Taggart, C. G. Zubrod, W. J. Welch, N. J. Conan, E. Bauman, S. T. Scudder, and J. A. Shannon: Studies on the chemotherapy of human malarias: VI. The physiological disposition, antimalarial activity, and toxicity of several derivatives of 4-aminoquinoline. *J. Clin. Invest.* 27:Suppl. 98 (1948).

19. J. L. Irvin, E. M. Irvin, and F. S. Parker: The interaction of antimalarials with nucleic acids. *Science* 110:426 (1949).

20. L. E. Gaudette and G. R. Coatney: A possible mechanism of prolonged antimalarial activity. *Am. J. Trop. Med. Hyg.* 10:321 (1961).

21. H. E. Hobbs, A. Sorsby, and A. Freedman: Retinopathy following chloroquine therapy. *Lancet* 2:478 (1959).

22. H. Bernstein, N. Zvaifler, M. Rubin, and A. M. Mansour: The ocular deposition of chloroquine. *Invest. Ophth.* 2:384 (1963).

23. A. M. Potts: The reaction of uveal pigment *in vitro* with polycyclic compounds. *Invest. Ophth.* 3:405 (1964).

24. W. M. Sams and J. E. Epstein: The affinity of melanin for chloroquine. *J. Invest. Derm.* 45:482 (1965).

25. M. Blois: Melanin binding properties of iodoquine. *J. Invest. Derm.* 50:250 (1968).

26. A. L. Scherbel, A. H. Mackenzie, J. E. Nousek, and M. Atdjian: Ocular lesions in rheumatoid arthritis and related disorders with particular reference to retinopathy. *New Eng. J. Med.* 273:360 (1965).

27. R. P. Burns: Delayed onset of chloroquine retinopathy. *New Eng. J. Med.* 275:693 (1966).

28. L. H. Schmidt: Chemotherapy of the drug-resistant malarias. *Ann. Rev. Microbiol.* 23:427 (1969).

29. F. E. Hahn, R. L. O'Brien, J. Ciak, J. L. Allison, and J. G. Olenick: Studies on modes of action of chloroquine, quinacrine, and quinine and on chloroquine resistance. *Military Med.* 131:1071 (1966).

30. B. B. Brodie, J. E. Baer, and L. C. Craig: Metabolic products of the cinchona alkaloids in human urine. *J. Biol. Chem.* 188–567 (1951).

31. R. D. Powell: The chemotherapy of malaria. *Clin. Pharm. Ther.* 7:48 (1966).

32. L. P. Whichard, C. R. Morris, J. M. Smith, and D. J. Holbrook: The binding of primaquine, pentaquine, pamaquine, and plasmocid to deoxyribonucleic acid. *Mol. Pharmacol.* 4:630 (1968).

33. M. Aikawa and R. L. Beaudoin: *Plasmodium fallax*: High-resolution autoradiography of exoerythrocytic stages treated with primaquine *in vitro*. *Exp. Parasit.* 27:454 (1970).

34. M. Aikawa and R. L. Beaudoin: Morphological effects of 8-aminoquinolines on the exoerythrocytic stages of *Plasmodium fallax*. *Military Med.* 134:986 (1969).

35. D. J. Taylor, E. S. Josephson, J. Breenberg, and G. R. Coatney: The *in vitro* activity of certain antimalarials against erythrocytic forms of *Plasmodium gallinaceum. Am. J. Trop. Med. Hyg.* 1:132 (1952).

36. A. S. Alving, R. D. Powell, G. J. Brewer, and J. D. Arnold: "Malaria, 8-aminoquinolines and haemolysis" in *Drugs, Parasites and Hosts,* ed. by L. G. Goodwin and R. H. Nimmo-Smith. Boston: Little, Brown, 1962, pp. 83–111.

37. J. H. Edgcomb, J. Arnold, E. H. Yount, A. S. Alving, and L. Eichelberger: Primaquine, SN13272, a new curative agent in vivax malaria: A preliminary report. *J. Nat. Malaria Soc.* 9:293 (1950).

38. E. Beutler: The hemolytic effect of primaquine and related compounds; a review. *Blood* 14:103 (1959).

39. I. M. Fraser and E. S. Vesell: Effects of metabolites of primaquine and acetanilid on normal and glucose-6-phosphate dehydrogenase deficient erythrocytes. *J. Pharm. Exp. Ther.* 162:155 (1968).

40. P. S. Gerald and E. M. Scott: "The hereditary methemoglobinemias" in *The Metabolic Basis of Inherited Disease,* ed. by J. B. Stanbury, J. B. Wyngaarden and D. S. Fredrickson, New York: McGraw-Hill, 1966 p. 1095.

41. P. A. Marks and J. Banks: Drug-induced hemolytic anemias associated with glucose-6-phosphate dehydrogenase deficiency; a genetically heterogeneous trait. *Ann. N.Y. Acad. Sci.* 123:198 (1965).

42. E. Beutler: The glutathione instability of drug sensitive red cells; A new method for the *in vitro* detection of drug sensitivity. *J. Lab. Clin. Med.* 49:84 (1957).

43. F. Hawking and W. L. M. Perry: Activation of paludrine. *Brit. J. Pharmacol.* 3:320 (1948).

44. R. C. Wood and G. H. Hitchings: Effect of pyrimethamine on folic acid metabolism in *Streptococcus faecalis* and *Escherichia coli. J. Biol. Chem.* 234:2377 (1959).

45. R. Ferone and G. H. Hitchings: Folate cofactor biosynthesis by *Plasmodium berghei.* Comparison of folate and dihydrofolate as substrates. *J. Protozool* 13:504 (1966).

46. R. Ferone: Dihydrofolate reductase from pyrimethamine-resistant *Plasmodium berghei. J. Biol. Chem.* 245:850 (1970).

47. R. Ferone, J. J. Burchall, and G. H. Hitchings: *Plasmodium berghei* dihydrofolate reductase; isolation, properties, and inhibition by antifolates. *Mol. Pharmacol.* 5:49 (1969).

48. I. M. Rollo: The mode of action of sulfonamides, proguanil and pyrimethamine on *Plasmodium gallinaceum. Brit. J. Pharmacol.* 10:208 (1955).

49. G. H. Hitchings: Pyrimethamine: The use of an antimetabolite in the chemotherapy of malaria and other infections. *Clin. Pharm. Ther.* 1:570 (1960).

50. R. Ferone, M. O'Shea, and M. Yoeli: Altered dihydrofolate reductase

associated with drug-resistance transfer between rodent plasmodia. *Science* 167:1263 (1970).

51. C. G. Smith, J. Ihrig, and R. Menne: Antimalarial activity and metabolism of biguanides. *Am. J. Trop. Med. Hyg.* 10:694 (1960).

52. D. F. Clyde: Prolonged malaria prophylaxis through pyrimethamine in mother's milk. *East African Med. J.* 37:659 (1960).

53. G. R. Coatney, P. G. Contacos, J. S. Lunn, J. W. Kilpatrick, and H. A. Elder: The effect of a repository preparation of the dihydrotriazine metabolite of chlorguanide, CI-501, against the Chesson strain of *Plasmodium vivax* in man. *Am. J. Trop. Med.* 12:504 (1963).

Chapter 8
Chemotherapy of Protozoal and Helminthic Diseases

Introduction

The incidence of parasitic disease will surely decline as improvements in economy, nutrition, and sanitary standards continue, particularly in the nations of Africa, Asia, and South America. During the next few generations, however, parasitic diseases will have to be attacked on a worldwide scale in much the same way that malaria has been. Large-scale programs of chemotherapy are important in controlling some of these parasitic diseases but probably have less impact than efforts devoted to the control of vectors, elimination of reservoirs of infestation, and amelioration of the poor sanitary conditions and living conditions responsible for transmission of parasites.

The problem of the chemotherapy of parasitic diseases is complicated by a number of factors. First, the size of the population infested with parasites or living in areas where parasitic diseases are endemic is huge. For example, in Egypt, according to recent estimates, there are 14 million people out of a total population of 30 million infested with schistosomes.[1] The estimated economic cost to the country, to say nothing of the human misery, is about 560 million dollars per year. It has also been estimated that the completion of the Aswan dam (a project that will provide new breeding grounds for the snail reservoir of these parasites) will add 2,650,000 new cases to this total, raising the infested portion of the population from 47 to 57 per cent.

Second, therapy is complicated by the fact that quite often individuals are infested with several organisms simultaneously. To provide these people with appropriate medical care it is necessary to carry out numerous diagnostic and follow-up laboratory tests and institute multiple-drug therapy. After this is done in a careful way, the person often returns to an environment where multiple parasites are endemic, and optimum conditions for recurrent infestation exist.

Third, many people are used to being infested and are not well enough educated to understand and be conscientious in following the treatment recommendations of the physician. This is linked to the problem that health workers (often from an alien culture) are sometimes considered outsiders whose efforts are felt as threatening to well-established life patterns.

At present, there are no immunization procedures for protection against protozoal and helminthic disease.[2] The physician must rely on the drugs discussed in this chapter for treatment of these conditions. Not a great deal is known about the mechanisms of action or mechanisms behind the toxic effects and side effects of most of these drugs.

The Chemotherapy of Protozoal Infestations

Amebiasis

The Disease

Amebiasis results from infestation by the protozoan *Entamoeba histolytica*. The disease occurs in all parts of North America and throughout the world. As with malaria and many other parasitic diseases, it is important to know the life cycle of the protozoan and the normal progression of the disease process in order to understand the therapy. Man is the principal host and the main source of infestation by *E. histolytica*. The patient becomes infested by ingesting mature cysts which are resistant to the acidic environment of the stomach and pass to the small intestine (Figure 8-1). The cyst disintegrates in the small intestine, releasing four amebas which divide to form eight trophozoites. The trophozoites pass into the large intestine where they may live and multiply for a time in the crypts of the bowel. Some of the trophozoites are able to invade the intestinal epithelium, and encystation and ulceration of the intestinal wall takes place. The presence of bacteria is required for survival of the protozoan in the intestine of the host. Although diarrhea is often seen, ulceration does not usually result in prolonged diarrhea or abdominal pain. Indeed many affected

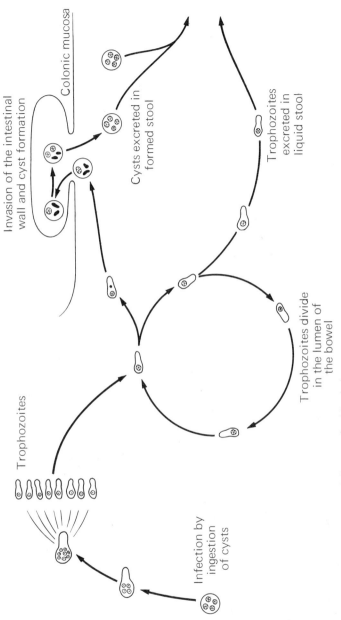

Figure 8-1 Life cycle of *Entamoeba histolytica*.

Colonic mucosa

Invasion of the intestinal wall and cyst formation

Cysts excreted in formed stool

Trophozoites excreted in liquid stool

Trophozoites

Trophozoites divide in the lumen of the bowel

Infection by ingestion of cysts

patients have no complaints. The cysts formed from the tropho-zoites on the surface of the colon are passed in formed stools. Thus people readily become asymptomatic carriers of the disease by passing the cyst forms in the stool for long periods of time. Patients with active diarrhea do not spread the disease because the trophozoites are not able to mature into the active cyst forms in the hyperactive bowel. The lesions produced by E. histolytica are primarily located in the large bowel, although secondary sys-temic invasion can occur. The organisms may pass up the portal vein to the liver producing hepatitis and abscess formation. Encystation rarely occurs in organs other than the liver.

A large and confusing number of therapeutic regimens have been employed in the treatment of amebiasis. The advantages and drawbacks of each drug regimen have been comprehensively reviewed by Marsden and Schultz.[3] For the treatment of mild intestinal infestation or for eradication of the asymptomatic carrier state, diiodohydroxyquin is the drug of choice (Table 8-1).[4] Recent experience indicates that metronidazole is the best drug for treatment of severe intestinal disease (dysentery) and hepatic abcess.[5] Severe intestinal disease can also be treated with emetine or dehydroemetine, usually in combination with an antibiotic. While the emetines have a direct amebicidal effect on the trophozoites, the role of the antibiotics in this case is interest-ing for, with the exception of paromomycin (Chapter 3), which has been demonstrated to have a direct amebicidal effect in vitro,[6] the antibiotics do not affect the amebae directly but inhibit the growth of the amebas by reducing the bacterial population of the bowel. The amebas are dependent upon bacteria in the bowel for growth.[7] The treatment of choice for hepatic amebiasis has been the combination of dehydroemetine and chloroquine. Chloroquine is not effective in the treatment of intestinal amebiasis; it is con-centrated in the liver (Chapter 7) and is almost as effective as emetine in the treatment of the hepatic disease.[3] Metronidazole has been reported to be very effective in the treatment of liver abscess.[8,9] As it is less toxic than dehydroemetine, metronida-zole is now a better candidate for drug of choice for the hepatic disease.

Table 8-1   Drugs used to treat protozoal diseases
(A selected listing according to recommendations from *The Medical Letter.*[4])

Infesting organism	Drug of choice	Alternative
Entamoeba histolytica		
Mild or asymptomatic intestinal disease	Diiodohydroxyquin	
Severe intestinal disease	Metronidazole	Dehydroemetine dihydrochloride or paromomycin
Hepatic abscess	Metronidazole	Dehydroemetine dihydrochloride plus chloroquine phosphate
Dientamoeba fragilis	Diiodohydroxyquin	A tetracycline
Giardia lamblia	Quinacrine hydrochloride	Metronidazole
Trichomonas vaginalis	Metronidazole	Topical agents (e.g. arsenicals or hydroquinones)
Balantidium coli	Oxytetracycline	Diiodohydroxyquin
Pneumocystis carinii	Pentamidine isethionate	Pyrimethamine plus sulfadiazine
Toxoplasma gondii	Pyrimethamine plus triple sulfonamide	None
Leishmania donovani (kala azar, visceral leishmaniasis)	Antimony sodium gluconate	Pentamidine isethionate
Leishmania tropica (oriental sore, cutaneous leishmaniasis)	Antimony sodium gluconate	
Leishmania braziliensis (American mucocutaneous leishmaniasis)	Antimony sodium gluconate	Amphotericin B
Trypanosoma gambiense	Pentamidine isethionate	Suramin
Trypanosoma rhodesiense (Either one in late disease with central nervous system involvement)	Suramin Melarsoprol	Pentamidine isethionate Tryparsamide plus suramin

Drugs Employed in the Treatment of Amebiasis

Diiodohydroxyquin

There are three iodinated 8-hydroxyquinolines that are effective in the treatment of intestinal amebiasis: diiodohydroxyquin, iodohydroxyquin, and chiniofon. Diiodohydroxyquin causes less gastrointestinal irritation than the others and is more frequently employed in North America. These compounds are amebicidal, and their mechanism of action is not known. Diiodohydroxyquin is taken orally and very little of the drug is absorbed into the systemic circulation.

Diiodohydroxyquin

Diiodohydroxyquin acts only on amebas in the gastrointestinal tract (Table 8-2), and it is used only in the treatment of mild or asymptomatic intestinal infestation. Other drugs effective against intestinal forms, such as tetracycline, are sometimes given with diiodohydroxyquin. The use of tetracycline here should be dis-

Table 8-2 **The site of action of the antiamebic drugs**

| Drug | Effective against: | |
	Intestinal disease	Hepatic abscess
Metronidazole	+	+
Dehydroemetine and emetine	+	+
Niridazole	+	+
Diiodohydroxyquin	+	−
Arsenicals (glycobiarsol and carbasone)	+	−
Antibiotics (paromomycin)	+	−
Chloroquine	−	+

couraged as there is a risk of superinfection (Chapter 4). Diiodo-hydroxyquin has a good chemotherapeutic index. Occasional diarrhea, nausea, and vomiting occur as well as skin rashes and anal pruritis. Although the systemic absorption of this iodinated drug is limited, slight enlargement of the thyroid gland is occasionally observed. The drug should not be given to people who have known iodine sensitivity.

Metronidazole

Most of the therapeutic experience with metronidazole has been in the treatment of trichomonal vaginitis. Until this compound was introduced, trichomoniasis was treated with a variety of topical agents. Complete cure of the disease was difficult to achieve, and recurrent infestation often occurred as a result of reintroduction of the parasite by the sexual partner. Metronidazole given orally to both partners has proved to be a very effective therapy for trichomoniasis.[10]

Metronidazole has only recently been employed for the treatment of severe intestinal amebiasis and hepatic abscess, and very good cure rates have been reported in these conditions.[5,8,9,11] Metronidazole has a great advantage over the other systemic amebicides (niridazole, emetine, and dehydroemetine) in that it is not cardiotoxic.

$$H-C-N$$
$$O_2N-C-N \diagdown C-CH_3$$
$$CH_2CH_2OH$$

Metronidazole

Metronidazole is trichomonacidal and amebicidal. Its mechanism of action is unknown. The drug is given orally. In most cases absorption from the gastrointestinal tract is good, but therapeutic failure as a result of poor intestinal absorption has been reported.[12] Most of the drug is excreted in the urine as unchanged metronidazole, a glucuronide, and several oxidation products.[13]

Metronidazole frequently causes nausea and headache and

occasional vomiting, diarrhea, weakness, paresthesias, vertigo, stomatitis, and leukopenia. In a large sampling of people being treated with metronidazole it was noticed that one side effect was the occurrence of unpleasant sensations when patients drank alcohol. It has been suggested that this is due to the fact that the drug inhibits alcohol dehydrogenase, one of the enzymes responsible for alcohol metabolism. However, the enzyme inhibition reported occurs only at drug concentrations much higher than those obtained clinically.[14] This side effect has led to the doubtfully beneficial use of metronidazole in the treatment of alcoholism.[15] It has been found that use of the drug in combination with disulfiram results in acute psychosis.[16]

Resistance to metronidazole has been reported,[17] but it is not a common problem in the treatment of *Trichomonas vaginalis* infestation. Metabolism of the drug by intestinal or vaginal bacteria can be a cause of treatment failure.[17] Because of its high therapeutic activity, low toxicity, and the apparent low rate of emergence of resistant protozoa, the use of metronidazole in antiprotozoal therapy will probably increase over the next few years. A great deal more information must be obtained on the biochemistry, pharmacology, and clinical usefulness of this very promising drug.

Dehydroemetine and Emetine

Emetine has been the mainstay of treatment of severe intestinal and extraintestinal amebiasis for centuries. Dehydroemetine is less cardiotoxic than emetine,[18] but both drugs are nevertheless very toxic agents and should not be used for the treatment of mild infestations. Metronidazole is less toxic than the emetine compounds, and experience with this drug has been extensive enough to relegate the emetine compounds to the position of drugs of second choice.

In the treatment of hepatic abscess the combination of an emetine and chloroquine is more effective and relapses occur less often than with either drug alone.[19]

The emetines kill the trophozoite forms of the amebas directly, but they are not very active against the cyst form of *E. hystolytica* in the intestinal wall. We do not know the precise mechanism of action of the emetines on the amebas, but a number of studies carried out with mammalian cells may begin to describe the biochemical events underlying both the amebicidal and the toxic effects.

Emetine is structurally similar to cycloheximide (Figure 8-2), an antibiotic that inhibits protein synthesis in mammalian cells, certain yeasts, protozoa, and plants.[20] Cycloheximide, like emetine, is not active against *E. coli*.[21] When emetine is added to human cells in culture there is a rapid inhibition of protein synthesis and a lesser and delayed effect on RNA synthesis (Figure 8-3).[22] There is also a rapid inhibition of DNA synthesis, but this is most probably secondary to a primary effect on protein synthesis, for in animal cells protein synthesis is required for concurrent synthesis of DNA. The precise mechanism of inhibition of protein synthesis has not been determined, but the available evidence points to an inhibition of translocation (Figure 2-2).

As mentioned in the discussion of chloroquine (Chapter 7), it is not possible to assume that the effect of a drug in a mammalian or bacterial system represents the primary biochemical insult in a protozoan. In this case, however, the observations in HeLa cells

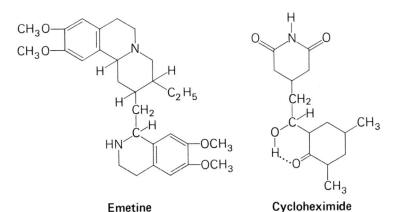

Emetine   Cycloheximide

Figure 8-2 Structures of emetine and cycloheximide. The dotted line between the ketone and hydroxyl groups of cycloheximide represents hydrogen bonding. The similarity of structure between the glutarimide antibiotics like cycloheximide and the ipecac alkaloids (emetine) was demonstrated by Grollman.[20]

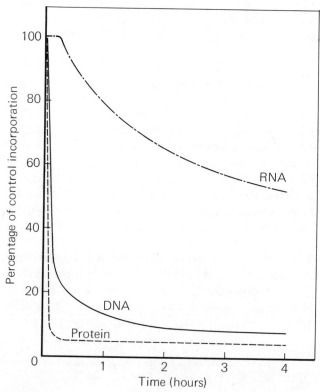

Figure 8-3 The effect of emetine on the synthesis of protein, RNA, and DNA in HeLa cells. HeLa cell suspensions were incubated with emetine ($10^{-6}M$) and radioactive precursors of DNA, RNA, and protein. The amount of incorporation was determined for ten-minute periods and is expressed as a percentage of the incorporation seen in control suspensions without the drug. (Redrawn from Grollman.[22])

may be related to the antiamebic effect, since emetine has been reported to inhibit protein synthesis in cultures of *E. histolytica*.[22] Similarly, emetine has been shown to decrease the rate of incorporation of amino acids into protein in the rat myocardium.[23] Although it has not yet been demonstrated that this is a specific effect, it may turn out that the toxic effect of the emetines on the myocardium can be attributed to their effects on macromolecular synthesis (although certainly there are many other possible explanations). If the toxic and therapeutic effects are the result of inhibition of the same biochemical process in the parasite and the host, then one would predict that the emetines would have a very low chemotherapeutic index or that some other factor contributes to the differential toxicity of the drug for the parasite as opposed to the host. In the case of emetine the former is certainly true. It is difficult to treat a patient with emetine without observing drug-related abnormalities in cardiovascular function (in one study 83 per cent of 93 patients being treated for amebiasis demonstrated some cardiovascular toxicity[24]).

Emetine and dehydroemetine are administered subcutaneously or intramuscularly. Oral administration is not employed, as it often produces nausea and vomiting. Because of the cardiotoxicity, the intravenous route is contraindicated. Animal studies indicate that more emetine is concentrated in the liver, kidney, spleen, and lung than in heart muscle.[25] The relative sensitivity of the heart to the toxic effects of the emetines therefore cannot be explained on the basis of selective concentration in that organ, but concentration of the drug in the liver may very well contribute to its efficacy in treating hepatic amebiasis. Emetine is excreted almost entirely by the kidney. The rate of excretion is slow, and high drug levels can readily build up in the body. The total dosage administered must therefore be carefully monitored. The drug is given at a dose of 1 mg/kg (up to a maximum of 65 mg) for no more than ten days. This total dosage limit should not be exceeded.

Injection of the emetines is often accompanied by pain, tenderness, and muscle weakness at the site of injection. Nausea and vomiting is occasionally observed. Emetine can induce diarrhea. This effect, as well as the hypotensive effect of emetine, may occur as a result of a blockade of the sympathetic nervous system.[26] The cardiotoxic effects of emetine include tachycardia, precordial pain, dyspnea, abnormalities in the electrocardiogram, and congestive heart failure that can lead to death. Electrocardiographic abnormalities such as lengthening of the P-R and Q-T intervals, ST elevation, T wave inversion, and abnormal rhythms occurred in approximately 50 per cent of the patients in one study.[24] The electrocardiographic changes rarely regress unless the drug is discontinued. Both electrocardiographic changes and signs of myositis may appear after cessation of therapy. The neuromuscular effect, characterized by general muscle weakness, is probably due in most cases to direct action on the muscle. True neuritis probably does not occur.

It is clear that certain precautions in patient management are warranted in view of the toxicity of the emetines. An electrocardiogram should be taken before therapy is initiated and repeatedly thereafter. The patient should remain sedentary during therapy and for a while thereafter. Emetine should not be used in patients with heart disease unless absolutely necessary—that is if metronidazole or chloroquine are ineffective. It is not difficult to understand the enthusiasm that metronidazole, a less toxic drug, now commands. Some research findings indicate that dehydroemetine is less cardiotoxic than emetine, but there have been conflicting reports concerning its relative therapeutic potency.

Other Amebicidal Drugs

Chloroquine. Chloroquine is concentrated in the liver and is an effective hepatic amebicide. It is largely ineffective against intestinal amebiasis; however, it is often given in conjunction with intestinal amebicides in the treatment of amebic dysentery to kill any trophozoites that might be carried to the liver. The mechanism of action, pharmacology, toxicity, and side effects of chloroquine were reviewed in Chapter 7.

The arsenicals. Carbasone and glycobiarsol are pentavalent arsenicals that have been employed in the treatment of mild intestinal amebiasis in combination with other intestinal amebicides. These pentavalent arsenicals are used less often now in the treatment of amebiasis. They are not converted to inorganic arsenic in the body and are thus reasonably safe. The arsenical group of drugs is considered in greater detail in the next section of this chapter.

Niridazole. This new drug is an effective oral agent for the treatment of hepatic amebiasis. Cure rates are apparently equivalent to those produced by emetine. Niridazole is also effective in the treatment of intestinal disease. The drug will probably not be very important in the treatment of amebiasis, as it produces slight electrocardiographic changes more frequently than emetine (although, in contrast to emetine, serious cardiotoxicity has not been observed).[27] Its usefulness in the treatment of amebiasis will probably be restricted to treatment of hepatic abscess. This compound will be considered again with the anti-schistosomal drugs.

The Blood and Tissue Flagellates (Leishmaniasis and Trypanosomiasis)

The Diseases

There are three principal diseases caused by *Leishmania:* visceral leishmaniasis (kala azar), the result of infestation with *L. donovani;* cutaneous leishmaniasis (oriental sore), *L. tropica;* and American mucocutaneous leishmaniasis, *L. braziliensis.* The *Leishmania* organisms, which assume the flagellated form in the insect vector and in culture, are ovoid unflagellated organisms in man; they are transmitted from a reservoir of numerous species of small animals and rodents to the human host by the bite of sandflies of the genus *Phlebotomus.* Visceral leishmaniasis is a disease of gradual onset characterized by fever, weight loss, hepatosplenomegaly, lymphadenopathy, hemorrhage, and hepatic malfunction. When untreated, this disease is fatal in a high percentage of cases (90 per cent in adults). Cutaneous leishmaniasis is characterized by a superficial ulceration of the skin at the site of the bite. The organism can be identified in scrapings from the edge of the ulcerations, which are prone to superinfection. American mucocutaneous leishmaniasis occurs in several different forms. There may be extensive ulceration of the mucous membrane of the mouth, palate, pharynx, and nose. Progressive and grossly disfiguring erosion takes place.

Trypanosomiasis also occurs in three forms. The first two forms produce a similar clinical picture, and both are called African trypanosomiasis (sleeping sickness). One form is caused by *Trypanosoma gambiense*, the other by *T. rhodesiense.* They are transmitted to humans by the bite of an infected *Glossina* (tsetse fly). The first stage of the disease is characterized by invasion of the lymphatic system with lymphadenopathy, hepatosplenomegaly, intermittent febrile attacks, dyspnea, and tachycardia. The chronic, sleeping-sickness stage is initiated by invasion of the central nervous system. This stage is marked by headache, increasing mental dullness and apathy, and disturbances in coordinated nervous functions. In the final stages of progression the patient sleeps continually, emaciation becomes profound, and coma and death result. Although the symptomatology of the two diseases is similar, the symptoms develop sooner, and the disease progresses more rapidly with *T. rhodesiense*. The third form of the disease, called South American trypanosomiasis (Chagas' disease), is caused by *T. cruzi* and is transmitted to man by reduviid bugs. These organisms evoke a symptom complex quite unlike the African trypanosomes, and there is at present no satisfactory treatment for the condition.

The drug of choice for the treatment of all three forms of leishmaniasis is antimony sodium gluconate, a pentavalent antimonial. The antimonials are also used extensively for the treatment of schistosomiasis and they are discussed in the section on the treatment of fluke infestations later in this chapter. American mucocutaneous leishmaniasis can also be treated with amphotericin B (Chapter 6) or cycloguanil pamoate (Chapter 7). Both *L. donovani* infestation and the two forms of African trypanosomiasis are effectively treated with pentamidine isethionate.

Pentamidine Isethionate

Pentamidine is one of a number of diamidine compounds, including propamidine and stilbamidine, which have trypanosomicidal activity. The drug is useful both in the treatment of early trypanosomiasis before central nervous system involvement and in chemoprophylaxis. The experience of the American physician with this drug has been primarily in the treatment of infestation by *Pneumocystis carinii*. This protozoan produces a pneumonitis in infants, children with hypogammaglobulinemia, and patients with malignant disease or organ transplants who are receiving immunosuppressive therapy. The use of pentamidine isethionate in the treatment of this difficult disease has been reviewed by Western et al.[28] The mechanism of action of pentamidine is unknown.

$$H_2N-C(=NH)-\text{(aryl)}-O-(CH_2)_5-O-\text{(aryl)}-C(=NH)-NH_2$$

Pentamidine

Pentamidine is administered parenterally. In mice the drug is eliminated by the kidneys primarily in the unchanged form.[29] The extent and nature of its metabolism in man are not known. The drug is bound in body tissues, the highest levels being found in the kidney, a localization that may contribute to its renal toxicity. The drug is excreted over an extended period of time, and it can be found in tissues such as the liver, kidney, and adrenals months after treatment has stopped. Pentamidine does not enter the central nervous system to any extent. Therefore, it cannot be employed in treating trypanosomiasis during the later phases of the disease marked by central nervous system involvement.

The administration of pentamidine is frequently accompanied by pain at the injection site and sometimes followed by abscess formation and tissue necrosis. The drug is quite toxic. In one survey, for example, 69 out of 164 patients experienced side effects.[28] Immediate reactions including hypotension, tachycardia, and vomiting are frequently seen. Liver and renal toxicity occur occasionally. Pentamidine can cause hypoglycemia, an important effect to remember in the treatment of the diabetic.

Suramin

Suramin is a compound developed from a group of nonmetallic dyes, such as trypan blue, that are known to have trypanocidal activity. Its mechanism of action is unknown. Suramin is the drug of choice for T. rhodesiense infestation and it is also effective in the treatment of infestation by one of the filaria, Onchocerca *volvulus.* In the latter case it is employed in combination with or following a course of diethylcarbamazine. The drug is not well absorbed from the gastrointestinal tract and is therefore administered parenterally. It does not penetrate into the central nervous system and in the treatment of trypanosomiasis with central nervous system involvement an arsenical must also be employed. The drug binds tightly to proteins, a predictable effect for a dye derivative. It persists in the circulation for a long time because it binds tightly to plasma protein. The slow release from plasma protein as well as the slow excretion by the kidney permit the drug to be administered on a weekly basis for the treatment of *O. volvulus* infestation and on a bimonthly basis for chemoprophylaxis of sleeping sickness.

Suramin is given slowly by the intravenous route. As some people demonstrate an intolerance to the drug (nausea and vomiting and occasionally an immediate reaction leading to shock and loss of consciousness), a 100- to 200-mg test dose is given initially. If this is not attended by severe reaction, a dose of 1 gm is given on days 1, 3, 7, 14, and 21 in the therapy of sleeping sickness and at weekly intervals for *O. volvulus* infestation. If there is intolerance to the test dose therapy should not be initiated. The basis of the intolerance is not known. As the drug is toxic to the kidney, frequent urinalyses should be performed during therapy; the presence of renal disease is a contraindication to the use of this drug. Suramin has a number of other side effects including rashes, photophobia, and a curious hyperesthesia of the palms and soles.

The Arsenicals

The arsenical drugs have played a pioneering role in the development of the concept of selective toxicity in chemotherapy. The previous wide use of these drugs in the treatment of syphilis ended with the development of the penicillins. Because of their toxicity their use in all but the meningoencephalitic stages of trypanosomiasis has been discontinued, and pentamidine and suramin are used instead.

The arsenicals, like the antimonials, are produced in trivalent (melarsoprol) and pentavalent (tryparsamide) forms. The penta-

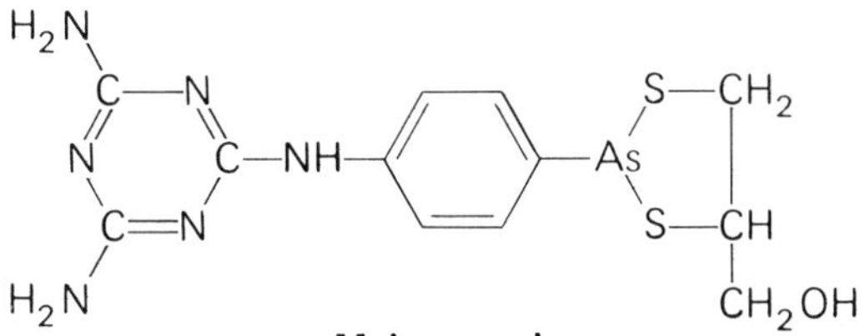

Melarsoprol

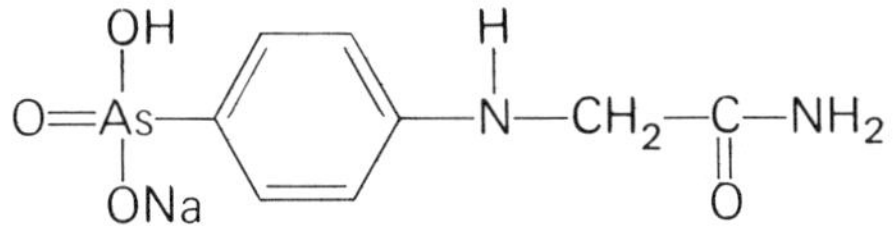

Tryparsamide

valent arsenicals are probably not trypanocidal until they have been converted to the trivalent form. The arsenicals probably are trypanocidal by virtue of the fact that they interact with sulfhydryl (-SH) groups in proteins. The integrity of -SH groups is essential in maintaining the appropriate structure and function of a number of enzymes in the cell. The inhibition of enzyme function, not only in energy production processes but also in other key cellular reactions, is the probable basis of the trypocidal action.

Given a nonspecific mechanism of action such as this, it would be predicted that the arsenicals are very toxic drugs and that any selective toxicity would be based on different concentrations of the drugs in the cells of the parasite and of the host. The first prediction is true; side effects are common with the trivalent arsenicals. Resistance to the arsenical drugs can occur, and it has been postulated that the parasites become resistant because they take up less of the drug. The basis of the selective toxicity of these agents is simply not clear, but a differential permeability between the host cells (or the resistant parasites) and the sensitive trypanosomes seems to be a possible explanation.

Pentamidine and suramin are less toxic agents and are the drugs of choice for the treatment of the early stages of trypanosomiasis. Melarsoprol and tryparsamide penetrate into the cerebrospinal fluid, and they are the agents of choice for the treatment of try-panosomal meningoencephalitis. Carbasone and glycobiarsol are pentavalent arsenicals formerly employed in the treatment of mild intestinal amebiasis.

Melarsoprol and tryparsamide are administered intravenously. The use of melarsoprol is often accompanied by side effects, among which are hypertension, abdominal pain and vomiting, albuminuria, and peripheral neuropathy. A serious and poten-tially fatal side effect is the development of a reactive encephalo-pathy. Melarsoprol should be given only to hospitalized patients. Tryparsamide is somewhat less toxic but also less potent. An important side effect of this drug is a disturbance of vision that can result in blindness. Tests of visual field and acuity should be conducted before and during therapy if the condition of the patient permits an accurate assessment.

The Chemotherapy of Helminthic Disease

Introduction

The helminthic, or worm, diseases are caused by members of two phyla. The nematodes (roundworms) belong to the phylum Nemathelminthes. Diseases caused by this group of organisms include, for example, ascaris, whipworm, pinworm, and hook-worm infestations, trichinosis, and elephantiasis. The cestodes, or tapeworms, and the trematodes, a group including the various flukes (e.g., the schistosomes), are both members of the phylum Platyhelminthes (flatworms). These worms are multicellular or-ganisms that possess crude organ systems. They have complex life cycles that usually include a stage of development in the human intestinal tract.

The interaction between the drugs used to treat helminth disease and the biochemistry of the worms has been reviewed by Saz and Bueding.[30] Bueding has made some observations about the basis of anthelminthic chemotherapy that are well worth pre-senting here.[31] The pathogenic forms of most of the worm infesta-tions amenable to chemotherapy are the adult, nongrowing stages of the parasite's life cycle. Therefore, drugs which are inhibitors of growth would not be expected to be particularly useful as anthelminthic agents. There are two processes in the worm sensitive to chemotherapeutic attack: the mechanisms essential for the motor activity of the organisms and the reactions that generate metabolic energy. The selective effect of the anthelminthic drugs is sometimes based on differences between the biochemistry of the host and the parasite. In other cases where there is no selective toxicity, the parasite is exposed to high concentrations of the agent in its intestinal habitat by the use of orally administered, nonabsorbable drugs. The discussion of the drugs used to treat the worm infestations will expand upon these observations.

Drugs Employed in the Treatment of Fluke and Tapeworm Disease (Flatworm Infestations)

Schistosomiasis

Schistosomiasis is one of the most prevalent diseases of man, and is therefore one of the most serious health problems in the world today. Schistosomes are multicellular flukes with primitive excretory, nervous, and circulatory systems and specialized organs of reproduction. These organisms penetrate the skin of the human host and migrate to the liver via the bloodstream, residing for a time in the hepatic vessels. After a few weeks a retrograde migration to various areas of the abdominal vascular plexuses occurs; S. hematobium lives in the venules of the vesicle plexus and S. mansoni and S. japonicum in the mesenteric veins. Here the organisms mate, depositing eggs that are excreted in the urine and feces. The reservoir for these parasites is the fresh water snail. The disease symptomatology is protean in nature and cannot be described in a few words. In the early stages of infestation, chemotherapy is very successful. If the disease has been present for some time, however, the intestine and particularly the liver become fibrosed, and chemotherapy cannot reverse the pathology.

The Organic Antimonials

A number of antimonial compounds have been employed in the treatment of schistosomiasis and leishmaniasis (Table 8-3). They include such pentavalent antimonials as antimony sodium gluconate and meglumine antimoniate and such trivalent antimonials as stibophen, antimony dimercaptosuccinate, and antimony potassium tartrate. The trivalent antimonials are active both *in vivo* and *in vitro*. The pentavalent compounds are much less active in cultures of trypanosomes[32] and leishmania[33] than the trivalent antimonials. In addition, there is a long lag period between the administration of the pentavalent antimonials to animals and the appearance of a detectable trypanocidal effect.[34] These observations indicate that the pentavalent arsenicals are activated by metabolism to the trivalent compounds in the host. It has been demonstrated that 25 per cent of the antimony recovered from the livers of mice treated with pentavalent antimony sodium gluconate is in the trivalent form.[35] Thus the capacity for metabolic conversion to the trivalent form clearly exists.

Antimony sodium gluconate
(a pentavalent antimonial)

Antimony potassium tartrate
(a trivalent antimonial)

Mechanism of action. The biochemical locus of action of the antimonials is well defined. These drugs inhibit glycolysis in the parasite by inhibiting phosphofructokinase, a rate-limiting enzyme in the pathway for the anaerobic metabolism of glucose. The survival of certain organisms like *Schistosoma mansoni* depends

Table 8-3   Drugs used to treat flatworm infestations
(A selected listing according to recommendations from *The Medical Letter.*[4])

Infesting organism	Drug of choice	Alternative
Flukes (Trematodes)		
Schistosoma haematobium	Niridazole or stibophen	Lucanthone (only for children under 16) Antimony sodium dimercaptosuccinate
Schistosoma mansoni	Stibophen or antimony sodium dimercaptosuccinate	Lucanthone (only for children under 16) Niridazole
Schistosoma japonicum	Antimony potassium tartrate	Stibophen Antimony sodium dimercaptosuccinate
Clonorchis sinensis (liver fluke)	Chloroquine phosphate	Bithionol
Paragonimus westermani (lung fluke)	Bithionol	Chloroquine phosphate
Fasciola hepatica (sheep liver fluke)	Emetine hydrochloride or dehydroemetine dihydrochloride	Bithionol Chloroquine phosphate
Tapeworms (Cestodes)		
Taenia saginata (beef tapeworm) *Diphyllobothrium latum* (fish tapeworm)	Niclosamide or quinacrine hydrochloride	Aspidium oleoresin (very toxic) or paromomycin
Taenia solium (pork tapeworm)	Quinacrine hydrochloride	Aspidium oleoresin (very toxic) or paromomycin
Hymenolepis nana (dwarf tapeworm)	Niclosamide	Quinacrine hydrochloride

almost entirely on the anaerobic metabolism of carbohydrate. The rate of utilization of glucose in schistosomes is very high. The mature S. mansoni, for example, can metabolize in one hour an amount of glucose equal to one-fifth its dry weight.[36] Inhibition of this metabolism results in the death of the parasite. Concentrations of trivalent antimonials in the range of the therapeutic

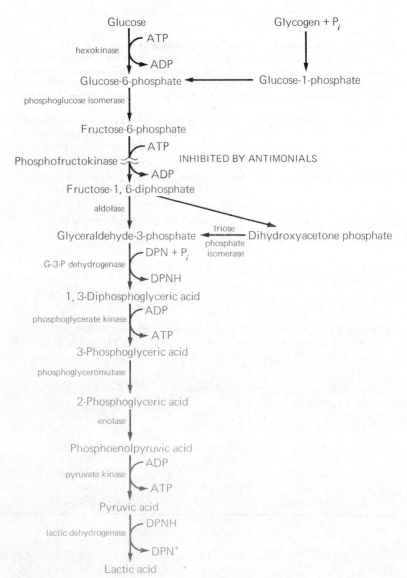

Figure 8-4 Embden-Meyerhof-Parnas scheme of glycolysis. The trivalent arsenicals inhibit the production of energy and lactate from glucose by anaerobic glycolysis by inhibiting the enzyme phosphofructokinase in the parasite.

dose inhibit glycolysis in the intact schistosome[36] and in subcellular extracts prepared from the worm.[37]

The activity of the glycolytic pathway (Figure 8-4) can be easily assayed in schistosome homogenates by measuring the rate of production of lactic acid from glucose. When glucose or fructose-6-phosphate is added to a broken cell homogenate of schistosomes the rate of production of lactic acid is inhibited by the trivalent antimonials. However, when fructose-1,6-diphosphate is provided as the substrate, lactic acid production is unaffected by the drugs (Figure 8-5).[37] This indicates that it is the conversion of fructose-6-phosphate to fructose-1,6-diphosphate, the reaction catalyzed by phosphofructokinase, that is inhibited by the drug. If purified mammalian phosphofructokinase is added to a schistosome ho-

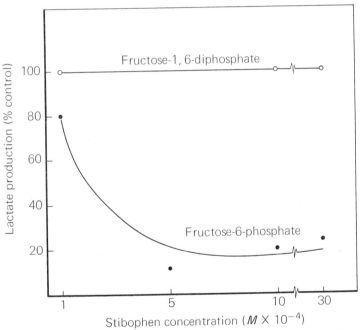

Figure 8-5 Effect of stibophen (a trivalent antimonial) on lactic acid production from fructose-6-P and fructose-1,6-diphosphate by schistosome extracts. (From Mansour and Bueding.[37])

mogenate inhibition of lactate production from glucose by trivalent antimonials is reversed (Table 8-4).[38] As the partially purified mammalian enzyme is not inhibited by the antimonials, it appears that the basis for the selective toxicity of the parasite versus that of the host rests on a difference in the sensitivities of the two phosphofructokinases to the drugs. Although phosphofructokinase has been purified from mammalian sources, the enzyme has not been purified from schistosomes, and the mechanism of the drug inhibition has not been elaborated in detail.

An interesting change in the location of schistosome organisms in the body occurs when doses of antimonials that are sublethal to the worms are administered. About an hour after a single dose of an antimonial drug is administered to mice infected with S. mansoni, the worms have shifted from the mesenteric veins to the liver.[39] Later, the organisms migrate back to the mesenteric veins. This reverse migration is correlated with a return of their phosphofructokinase activity to normal levels.[30] The reason for this shift of the organism in response to anti-schistosomal drugs is not completely clear. It seems probable that the organisms require energy

Table 8-4 **Effect of an antimonial drug and mammalian phosphofructokinase on lactic acid production by homogenates of Schistosoma mansoni**

Replicate samples of a homogenate of S. mansoni were incubated for 30 minutes at 37°C with glucose and ATP. Stibophen ($1 \times 10^{-4}M$), potassium antimony tartrate ($5 \times 10^{-5}M$), or phosphofructokinase (PFK) from rabbit muscle (0.5 units/ml) were added. At the end of the incubation period, lactic acid was assayed, and the results are expressed as μmoles lactic acid produced per milligram of protein in 30 minutes. (Data from Beuding and Mansour,[38] Table I.)

Additions	Production of lactate from glucose
None	1.2
Stibophen	0.4
PFK (rabbit muscle)	2.0
Stibophen + PFK	1.9
Potassium antimonial tartrate	0.4
Potassium antimonial tartrate + PFK	1.7

to attach to the mesenteric vessels and to move against the direction of blood flow, and that when the anaerobic energy production mechanism is inhibited, they are passively carried to the liver with the normal portal blood flow.

Pharmacology and toxicity. The organic antimonials are administered by intramuscular or slow intravenous injection. Antimony potassium tartrate is given only by the intravenous route; it is both the most therapeutically potent and the most toxic and irritating of the antimonials. Great care must be taken during its administration so that extravasation into perivascular tissue does not take place, as this may lead to severe necrosis. The irritative effects of the drug can cause phlebitis. During infusion of antimony potassium tartrate, paroxysms of coughing and vomiting often occur. Epinepherine should be kept at hand in case hypotension occurs during the infusion. The antimonial drugs are primarily excreted by the kidneys, and their use is contraindicated in the presence of renal disease.

Antimony potassium tartrate frequently causes muscle and joint pain, bradycardia, and electrocardiographic changes. The drug can also cause rashes, pruritis, abdominal pain and diarrhea, weakness, dizziness, renal damage, and occasionally cardiac arrhythmias and circulatory collapse. Hepatocellular damage with jaundice and abnormal liver function is a rare side effect, and the drug is contraindicated in the presence of liver disease of non-schistosomal origin. The electrocardiographic changes eventually disappear but are sometimes observable for a time after cessation of drug therapy. The drug is contraindicated in the presence of cardiac disease. The other trivalent antimonials exhibit the same complex of adverse effects as antimony potassium tartrate, but the side effects occur less frequently and are less severe.

As with so many of the antiprotozoal and antiparasitic drugs, the antimonials are toxic compounds and are difficult to administer. Many people with schistosomiasis discontinue therapy, because they feel worse while taking the drug (therapy involves numerous intravenous injections) than they do with the disease alone.

Niridazole

Niridazole is used orally in the treatment of a number of helminthic diseases, including schistosomiasis, dracontiasis, (Dracunculus medinensis), and amebiasis. The biochemistry, pharmacology, toxicity, and the therapeutic trials conducted with this
new drug, were reviewed in a recent symposium.[40] The drug's
mechanism of action is not known. Although it clearly does not
inhibit glycolysis as the antimonials do, niridazole affects carbohydrate metabolism in schistosomes by increasing the rate of
breakdown of glycogen stores in the parasite.[41] This is a selective
effect, as it does not occur in the host.

Niridazole

Niridazole has a relatively slow onset of action; the worms do
not shift to the liver until four days after administration.[31] The
drug is extensively metabolized in the liver, but the period of time
required for metabolism does not account for the delay in schisto-
somicidal action. This was demonstrated by incubating schistomes
in vitro with plasma from untreated animals containing added
niridazole and with plasma from treated animals containing the
as yet unidentified metabolites but no niridazole. Only the niri-
dazole-containing plasma damaged the schistosomes.[42] The stage
of the disease process being treated is very important in niridazole
therapy. Relatively few side effects are seen in the treatment of
patients with the intestinal form of the disease. In patients who
have hepatosplenic damage the levels of both niridazole and its
metabolites in the blood are markedly elevated.[42] Treatment of
the hepatosplenic form of S. mansoni infestation produces severe
central nervous system disturbances in a high percentage of
patients.[43]

The use of niridazole is frequently accompanied by gastrointestinal disturbances (vomiting, diarrhea, and cramps), headache, and skin rashes. Slight electrocardiographic changes occur frequently. Niridazole inhibits spermatogenesis in laboratory animals, but it is not known if this occurs in man. This growth inhibitory effect suggests that the compound may be teratogenic, and it is prudent not to employ the drug during pregnancy. The most serious toxic effect is disturbance of central nervous system function with changes in the electroencephalogram, psychosis, and convulsions. Extreme care should be taken in administering the drug to patients who have a history of psychosis or convulsions. Niridazole has been shown to produce hemolysis in glucose-6-phosphate dehydrogenase-deficient erythrocytes.

Lucanthone

Lucanthone (Miracil D) and hycanthone are anthelminthic thioxanthone derivatives that inhibit the growth of bacteria and mammalian cells; S. Mansoni and S. haematobium appear to be about equally sensitive to lucanthone, but at doses which are therapeutic for them S. japonicum is unaffected. The receptor for lucanthone in the cell is DNA. The drug has been demonstrated to bind to DNA, thereby increasing its stability to thermal denaturation and the intrinsic viscosity of the DNA.[44] Lucanthone and hycanthone bind to DNA by intercalating between the base pairs of the double helix.[45] Lucanthone inhibits RNA synthesis in intact bacteria and reduces the priming activity of DNA for purified RNA polymerase.[46]

Lucanthone

Lucanthone is well absorbed from the gastrointestinal tract, extensively metabolized, and rapidly excreted. It is given every eight hours. The most frequent toxic effects of this drug are dizziness, vomiting, epigastric pain, headache, and depression.[47] A number of patients experience hallucinations while taking the drug. These psychiatric disturbances have been reported for adults, but they apparently do not occur in children.[48] Some experts feel that lucanthone should be used only in children under 16; however, this recommendation is not universally agreed upon. The drug is contraindicated in patients with severe hepatic or renal disease. The compound itself is yellow in color and it causes a benign, reversible discoloration of the skin and sclera.

It is surprising that leukopenia has not been reported as a frequent toxic effect of lucanthone. The drug is very much like actinomycin D with respect to its effects on mammalian cell growth. At low concentrations (about 10^{-5} M), it inhibits the growth of human cells in culture.[49] At this concentration the drug totally inhibits RNA synthesis in bacteria; it is also the therapeutic dose in man. The effect of lucanthone is readily reversible, whereas that of actinomycin D is not, and this might help explain the absence of side effects typical of cytotoxic drugs. It is also possible that schistosomes concentrate the drug and that circulating blood levels in the patient are relatively low in comparison with the concentration of drug in the parasite. It is known that actinomycin D enhances X-ray damage in mammalian cells by interfering with postradiation repair processes, and this effect has been exploited in the therapy of some tumors. Lucanthone also potentiates the radiation effect on HeLa cells,[50] and, as it is less toxic than actinomycin D, it may be useful in similar combined radiation and drug therapy of certain tumors.

Bithionol

Bithionol, like hexachlorophene, is a diphenolic compound. Both chemicals were shown to have antibacterial activity in the early part of this century. Bithionol given orally is now the drug of choice for infestation by the lung fluke *Paragonimus westermani*,[51] and it has also been used successfully in the treatment of liver fluke disease. The drug is not very effective in treating cerebral infestation with *P. westermani.* Vomiting, diarrhea, abdominal pain, rashes, and skin photosensitivity reactions are common side effects.

Tapeworm Infestation

Tapeworm infestation (cestodiasis) occurs when uncooked meat or fish containing the encysted larval forms of the organism are ingested. In the intestine of the host the head of the tapeworm, or scolex, attaches to the intestinal wall. The worm then grows by producing large numbers of egg-containing segments. Growth can continue until, in the fish tapeworm *(D. latum)*, for example, there are three to four thousand segments and the worm is 30 feet long. Tapeworms are hermaphroditic, and the fertilized eggs are excreted as the segments are passed with the feces. The eggs can then be ingested by the intermediate host in which the larval form develops, thus completing the cycle. In some cases the normal course of events is altered when man accidently ingests the eggs instead of the larvae. This happens with the pork tapeworm *(T. solium)* where man is the usual definitive host and the intermediate host is the pig. If tapeworm eggs are accidently ingested by man, the larvae can develop in human tissues.

The clinical symptoms of tapeworm infestation by adult forms growing in the intestine are surprisingly mild in the well nourished, otherwise healthy patient. There may be vague abdominal discomfort and pain, which is relieved by food, as well as weakness, weight loss, epigastric fullness, and anemia. Intestinal obstruction due to the mass of the worms is rare. Ingestion of eggs that produce migratory larvae can be very serious, as the larvae may develop in the orbit, brain, or other organs and become growing, space-occupying masses. There is no chemotherapeutic treatment for infestation by these intermediate stages of the life cycle of the tapeworm, but surgical removal of the mass is sometimes possible.

Quinacrine Hydrochloride

Quinacrine, an acridine derivative formerly used as an antimalarial agent, is very effective in the treatment of several

$$CH_3$$
$$NH-CH-(CH_2)_3-N(C_2H_5)_2$$
$$CH_3O$$
$$N$$
$$Cl$$

Quinacrine

tapeworm infestations[52] (Table 8-3). It is also the drug of choice for the treatment of infestation by *Giardia lamblia*, a flagellated protozoon that invades the bowel and is sometimes associated with *E. histolytica* infestation.

Quinacrine's mechanism of action as an inhibitor of growth in plasmodium is similar, if not identical, to that of chloroquine.[53] The drug is employed in an acute manner at much higher local concentrations for the eradication of tapeworms from the bowel. The mechanism of the drug effect under these conditions is not clear. Quinacrine is also used in the treatment of neoplastic effusions. Again the mechanism of the drug effect is unknown.

Quinacrine is taken orally. It commonly causes nausea and vomiting. For the treatment of tapeworm infestation quinacrine can be administered by duodenal tube directly into the upper small intestine. This results in less vomiting and a higher drug concentration in the intestinal lumen.[3] The patient should be fasting and should have been on a fluid diet the preceding day. When it is taken orally, the tendency to vomit can be reduced by the concomitant administration of sodium bicarbonate. Quinacrine frequently causes headache and dizziness and occasionally toxic psychosis, anemia, and exfoliative dermatitis (patients with psoriasis are especially prone to develop this last complication). Aplastic anemia and acute hepatic necrosis have been reported on rare occasion. One of the more annoying side effects to the patient is a yellowish discoloration of the skin due to binding of the drug in the tissues (see Chapter 7). When quinacrine was used for prolonged therapy of malaria, occasional blue discoloration of the nailbeds occurred. This resembled cyanosis and was due to deposition of blood pigment. Quinacrine is strongly bound in the liver and is slowly eliminated from the body. The metabolism of primaquine can be inhibited as long as ten to twelve weeks after the last dose of quinacrine. The free blood levels of primaquine are elevated in the presence of quinacrine, and, therefore, treatment with primaquine is a contraindication for quinacrine use.

Niclosamide and Dichlorophen

Niclosamide is very effective in the treatment of tapeworm infestations in man.[54] Its mechanism of action is probably inhibition of the anaerobic production of ATP. It has been reported that both niclosamide and desaspidin (the active principle of aspidium oleoresin) uncouple oxidative phosphorylation in mammalian mitochondria.[55] In addition, these drugs in low concentrations

Niclosamide

have been shown to inhibit the anaerobic incorporation of inorganic phosphate into ATP by the tapeworm *H. diminuta*.[56] Tapeworms, like the adult forms of many other helminths, derive their major source of energy from anaerobic rather than aerobic metabolism of carbohydrate.[31] This is consonant with their location in the lumen of the intestine, where oxygen tension is very low. Their heavy dependence on anaerobic metabolism of carbohydrate is probably the biochemical difference between the parasite and the host that provides the basis for selective drug action.

Niclosamide and the structurally similar drug dichlorophen are given orally. They are not absorbed from the gastrointestinal tract. Aspidium oleoresin, a plant extract that may act in the same manner, is absorbed from the gastrointestinal tract. This difference in absorption probably accounts for the lesser toxicity of niclosamide. Cure rates of 70 to 80 per cent are achieved with the use of niclosamide in *T. saginata* and *D. latum* infestation.[3] When niclosamide is employed in treatment, the segments of the tapeworm are destroyed, and large numbers of viable eggs are released into the intestine. In the case of the pork tapeworm (*T. solium*), where man can be an intermediate host, this may possibly result in the dissemination of the larval forms to the tissues (cysticercosis). Therefore, quinacrine, which acts to expel the intact worm segments, is used in *T. solium* infestation. There are two characteristics in addition to good cure rates that make niclosamide the drug of choice for other tapeworm infestations. First, its use is accompanied by few side effects (occasionally nausea and abdominal pain). Second, the drug can be given after an overnight fast without any other dietary restrictions.[57] Purgatives do not have to be given after therapy with this drug.

Aspidium Oleoresin

This drug is an extract of the male fern. The active component, desaspidine, may work like niclosamide. It is potentially toxic, for sometimes convulsions and respiratory or cardiac arrest occur after administration. An optic neuritis that can lead to blindness may also develop. The risk of toxic side effects can be lowered by keeping the patient on a fat-free diet for a few days (fat increases the absorption of the drug from the gastrointestinal tract) and administering a purgative (thus evacuating more of the unabsorbed drug) after therapy is terminated. This drug is unpleasant to take, and it should not be given to pregnant women, emaciated individuals, or people with ulcers or kidney, liver, or heart disease. It should be used only if less toxic drugs cannot be employed or if the clinical response to them is not satisfactory. In a few years this drug preparation, at least in its present crude form, will probably no longer be employed.

Paromomycin is currently receiving clinical trial in the treatment of tapeworm infestations, and it appears that it will be effective and less toxic than the agents presently in use.

Drugs Employed in the Treatment of Roundworm Infestation

Ascariasis

Ascaris lumbricoides is the most common human pathogen of all of the helminths. Infestation with *Ascaris* is more prevalent in tropical countries, but it occurs all over the world. The adult worm, which looks rather like an earthworm, lives in the lumen of the small intestine. Humans become infested by ingesting embryonated eggs. When the eggs reach the duodenum, the larvae hatch and begin a remarkable odyssey that eventually returns them to the intestinal lumen. The larvae penetrate the wall of the small intestine and are carried through the right heart to the lungs. They then penetrate the walls of the pulmonary capillaries, emerge into the air sacs, and migrate up the pulmonary tree to the epiglottis. This period of larval migration is often accompanied by cough, dyspnea, fever, bronchial rales, and dullness to percussion. Occasionally there is hemoptysis. Signs of hypersensitivity, like eosinophilia and urticaria, are also observed. Occasionally the larvae reach the general circulation and become lodged in tissues where they can provoke local reactions.

The larvae are swallowed after they reach the epiglottis, and upon their second arrival in the small intestine they develop into adult male and female worms. The patient at this stage of infection may be asymptomatic or may have vague symptoms of abdominal distress (epigastric pain, nausea, vomiting, and anorexia). More serious problems can arise as a result of migration of the adult worms into the pancreatic and bile ducts, gallbladder, and liver or from complete obstruction of the appendix or intestinal lumen. The by-products of living or dead worms can produce severe reactions in sensitized patients. It is interesting that migration of the adult worms, and the resulting complications, can be stimulated by drug therapy. A number of people who are infected with *Ascaris* are also infected with other parasites like hookworm. Treatment of hookworm infestation with tetrachlorethylene can provoke the migration of *Ascaris*. In this case the symptoms that arise as a side effect of tetrachlorethylene therefore are due to an effect of the drug on an entirely different parasite from that being treated. The drug of choice for the treatment of ascariasis is piperazine.

Piperazine

Piperazine citrate is a drug of choice for both roundworm *(Ascaris)* and pinworm *(Enterobius vermicularis)* infestation (Table 8-5). It acts by paralyzing the worm. The paralyzed worm, unable to maintain its position in the intestinal tract, is then passively expelled by the normal peristaltic action of the bowel; no purgative is required.

Piperazine

If piperazine citrate is added to a bath containing an *Ascaris* attached to a strain gauge, the irregular contraction of the worm ceases after a few minutes, and the worm remains in flaccid paralysis (Figure 8-6, A).[58] The delay may reflect the time required for the drug to reach its site of action. The time of onset of the paralysis in the intact worm preparation decreases with increasing doses of the drug. If a crudely dissected section from *Ascaris* is suspended in a similar bath, there is no spontaneous movement of the muscle. The muscle contracts readily upon addition of acetylcholine, and the response to acetylcholine is reversibly antagonized by piperazine (Figure 8-6, B).[58] Electrical stimulation of the muscle of the body wall causes a contraction that is not blocked by piperazine. These observations were felt to be consistent with the conclusion that piperazine paralyzes *Ascaris* by a blocking action at the myoneural junction. If this were true, one would then expect piperazine to be a toxic drug by

Table 8-5 Drugs used to treat nematode (roundworm) infestation
(A selected listing according to recommendations from *The Medical Letter.*[4])

Infesting organism	Drug of choice	Alternative
Roundworms		
Ascaris lumbricoides	Piperazine citrate	Thiabendazole
Trichuris trichiura (whipworm)	Hexylresorcinol (adult dose— 500 ml of a 0.3% solution by rectal retention enema for 1 hour)	Thiabendazole
Necator americanus (hookworm)	Tetrachloroethylene (adult dose—a single dose of 0.12 ml/kg to a maximum of 5 ml) or bephenium hydroxynaph-thoate (adult dose—one 5 gm packet b.i.d. for 3 days)	Thiabendazole
Ancylostoma duodenale (hookworm)	Bephenium hydroxynaph-thoate (adult dose—one 5 gm packet b.i.d. for 1 day)	Tetrachloroethylene (single dose as for *N. americanus*) or thiabendazole
Strongyloides stercoralis	Thiabendazole	Pyrvinium pamoate
Enterobius (Oxyuris) vermicularis (pinworm)	Piperazine citrate or pyrvinium pamoate	Thiabendazole
Filaria		
Wuchereria bancrofti		
Wuchereria (Brugia) malayi	Diethylcarbamazine	None
Loa loa		
Onchocerca volvulus	Diethylcarbamazine plus suramin	None
Dracunculus medinensis (guinea worm)	Niridazole	None

virtue of this effect, since it is readily absorbed from the intestinal tract of humans. This, however, is not the case; mammalian muscle is resistant to the effects of piperazine.

What then is the basis of the selective action of this nontoxic drug? Although the data are somewhat sketchy, it appears that contraction of *Ascaris* muscle is initiated by rhythmic spike

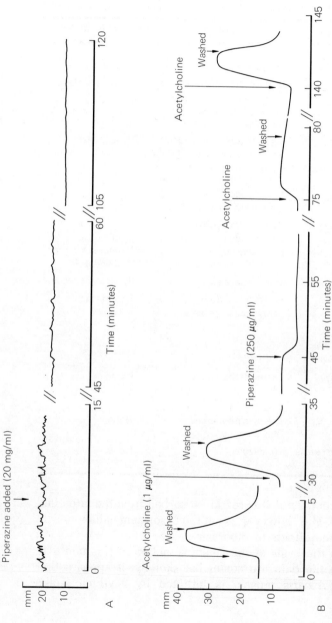

Figure 8-6 A. The effect of piperazine on the spontaneous contraction of a whole *Ascaris* attached to a strain gauge. When a whole *Ascaris* is exposed to piperazine there is a delay period followed by the development of flaccid paralysis. A 10-mm deflection on the record is equivalent to a 2 gm increase in tension. (The tracing is adapted from Norton and deBeer.[58] B. The effect of piperazine on the response of a crude nerve-muscle preparation of *Ascaris* to acetylcholine. The anterior portion of a worm (containing the main ganglia) was cut off, the worm was split, and the intestinal tract removed. The remainder was attached to a strain gauge and suspended in Ringer's solution. Piperazine decreases the response of the preparation in a reversible manner. (The tracing is adapted from Norton and deBeer.[58]

potentials generated by pacemakers in the muscle membrane itself.[59] Acetylcholine depolarizes the muscle cells, thereby increasing the frequency of the spike potentials and the degree of muscle contraction. Electrophysiological studies demonstrate that piperazine increases the resting potential of the muscle so that pacemaker activity is suppressed, and flaccid paralysis ensues.[60] Piperazine may therefore act as an inhibitory neurotransmitter. Indeed, it may be an analog of a natural inhibitory transmitter in *Ascaris*. The difference in the response of the host and the parasite to the drug would rest on the development of different control mechanisms at the muscle membrane in the more advanced species, man. That is, through differentiation the receptor has been lost or altered in higher life forms.

Piperazine is administered orally as a tablet or a liquid preparation for children. It is also prepared in a number of salt combinations. There is probably no difference between the citrate, the phosphate, the tartrate, etc. The drug generally is quite safe. Occasional rashes and dizziness are observed. Patients who are epileptic may have an exacerbation of seizures. Rarely, patients experience difficulty in focusing as a side effect of the drug. The lack of toxicity and ease of administration, in addition to the drug's high effectiveness in eradicating *Ascaris* and pinworm infestation,[52] make piperazine an excellent chemotherapeutic agent.

Thiabendazole

Thiabendazole is an oral drug that kills both the adult and larval forms of the many roundworm parasites of both humans and animals. The mechanism of its broad-spectrum anthelminthic effect is not known. The extensive literature on this drug has been reviewed by Cuckler and Mezey.[61]

Thiabendazole

Thiabendazole is highly effective in the treatment of infestation by *Strongyloides stercoralis*[62] and in cutaneous larva migrans. Cutaneous larva migrans, also called creeping eruption, is caused by larvae of canine and feline hookworms that penetrate and migrate under the skin. Their presence causes intense irritation and itching. Administered orally, thiabendazole produces a rapid and effective clinical response in this condition,[63] and it can also be effectively administered topically.

Because a number of different nematode infestations (e.g., *Ascaris*, hookworm) are sensitive in varying degrees to thiabendazole, this drug may provide a key to a means by which multiple intestinal parasitic worm infestations can be treated on a mass scale. A definitive program of research on its mechanism of action may very well turn up a biochemical process unique to the nematodes that can be exploited as a basis for rational drug design. The drug's efficacy does not extend to other helminths such as schistosomes or tapeworms.

It is interesting that thiabendazole has been reported to prevent the development of nematode eggs and larvae.[64] The drug may have a place in veterinary medicine in controlling the spread of helminthic disease in animal populations. This observation has led to the use of thiabendazole in the treatment of human disease by larval forms as in trichinosis and cutaneous larva migrans. The limited experience with thiabendazole in the treatment of trichinosis indicates that it produces a prompt clinical improvement with decreased temperature and muscle pain; however, not all the larvae in man are killed by the drug.[65]

Thiabendazole is rapidly absorbed after oral administration, and plasma levels reach their peak in one hour. The drug is excreted principally as its glucuronide and sulfate ester metabolites by the kidney within 24 to 48 hours.[61] Transient side effects, including anorexia, nausea, vomiting, and dizziness, are frequently encountered with thiabendazole. Less commonly, there may be leukopenia and crystalluria (both reversible), rashes, and xanthopsia, a disturbance of color vision in which objects appear yellow. Patients may notice a malodorous urine and sweat. Occasionally vomiting of live *Ascaris* occurs. In summary, thiabendazole is a reasonably safe and useful drug that, with more basic research concerning its mechanism of action, may provide a key to the development of still more potent broad-spectrum anti-nematodal compounds.

Pyrvinium Pamoate

Pyrvinium is one of the cyanine dyes. These are basic dyes characterized by a quaternary nitrogen linked to a tertiary nitrogen by a conjugated chain of an odd number of carbon atoms. Dithiazanine, another cyanine dye, was formerly used in the treatment of nematode infections; it has been withdrawn from the market because of its toxicity. The mechanism of action of pyrvin-

Pyrvinium (base)

ium is not known, but it has been demonstrated that cyanine dye compounds inhibit oxygen consumption by the adult filarial worm *Litomosoides carinii*,[30] whereas oxygen consumption by mammalian cells is not inhibited even at drug concentrations several orders of magnitude higher than those affecting the parasite.

Pyrvinium pamoate is effective in the treatment of pinworm infestation. A single oral dose yields high rates of cure (98 per cent in one study).[66] The drug is not absorbed from the intestinal tract, and it is well tolerated. Nausea, vomiting, cramping, and diarrhea occur occasionally, and patients should be warned that the stool is frequently red in color. Although pyrvinium pamoate and piperazine are able to effectively eradicate the pinworms, rein-festation is common, and patients should be examined for the presence of eggs at the anus several weeks after treatment.

Hexylresorcinol

Hexylresorcinol is a phenolic compound that was widely used for the oral treatment of parasitic infections in the past, but it has been replaced by newer, more effective drugs. This drug is principally used today in the treatment of whipworm (trichuriasis) infestation. It is reserved for heavily infected, hospitalized patients who are critically ill and is given by retention enema. This procedure results in a high cure rate (92 per cent in one study).[67] Patients who are asymptomatic are not treated.

There is systemic absorption of orally administered hexylresorcinol and presumably also of the rectally administered drug. The absorbed drug does not produce side effects at the levels reached therapeutically. Hexylresorcinol is a severe topical irritant, and for this reason the drug is not given to people with severe colonic disorders. On contact the drug produces painful burning and ulceration of the perianal skin, which can be reduced by coating the area liberally with petrolatum ointment.

Hookworm

The two types of hookworm infestation of major importance to man are by *Necator americanus* and *Ancylostoma duodenale*. Upon coming in contact with the skin, hookworm larvae actively burrow through the skin to the lymphatics or venules where they are carried via the blood through the right heart to the lungs. The larvae are unable to pass through the capillaries and they break through capillary walls to the alveoli. Then, like *Ascaris*, they migrate up the bronchi and the trachea and are swallowed, finally reaching the lumen of the intestine. By the time they reach the intestine the larvae have developed a buccal capsule by which they become attached to the intestinal mucosa. Ulcerations are created at the point of contact. The worms ingest blood from the mucosal vessels of the patient and lay eggs, which are passed with the feces. Definitive diagnosis depends upon finding eggs in the feces.

The penetration of the larvae into the skin produces localized erythema and severe itching, and the passage of large numbers of worms through the lungs may produce signs of penumonitis. The adult worms in the intestine can produce gastrointestinal symptoms such as abdominal fullness and epigastric pain; often, there are no acute symptoms. The symptoms of hookworm infestation are characteristic of a progressive, hypochromic microcytic anemia of the nutritional deficiency type. Anemia is secondary to chronic blood loss, which is superimposed on such contributing factors as malnutrition and an iron-deficient diet in many infested individuals. The result of heavy infestation in children is physical and mental retardation, which, when present on a mass scale, compromises the growth of whole communities and societies. There are two drugs of choice for the treatment of hookworm infestation, bephenium hydroxynaphthoate and tetrachloroethylene.

Bephenium Hydroxynaphthoate

Bephenium is a quaternary ammonium compound that is effective against both *N. americanus* and *A. duodenale*. It is also effective against *Ascaris* and *Trichuris* as well as a number of nematodes that infest livestock. The primary mechanism of action of the drug is not known. The gross physiological response of *Ascaris* skin muscle preparations to bephenium hydroxynaphthoate consists of a phase of excitation lasting for approximately 20 minutes followed by an inhibition of movement together with a loss of muscle sensitivity to acetylcholine.[68] The stimulatory effect of bephenium on *Ascaris* muscle, like that of acetylcholine, is blocked by piperazine and d-tubocurarine.[69] Both bephenium

Bephenium (base)

and acetylcholine contain a quarternary nitrogen, and it is possible that they act in a similar manner in the worms.

The cure rate following a single dose of bephenium hydroxynaphthoate is approximately 85 per cent in *A. duodenale* infestation.[70] This is to be compared to a cure rate of about 55 per cent and a 95 per cent reduction in the worm load with *N. americanus*.[71] The drug is given orally, and no pretreatment fasting or posttreatment purgation is required. Very little of the drug is absorbed from the gastrointestinal tract. Bephenium has a low toxicity. Vomiting and diarrhea are occasionally seen.

Tetrachloroethylene

Tetrachloroethylene (C_2Cl_4) is a colorless volatile liquid that is very effective in the treatment of *Necator americanus* infestation. The drug must be stored in a cool, dark place; if exposed to air at warm temperatures, it will oxidize to phosgene. How this drug eliminates hookworms from the intestine is not known. A single dose will cure 80 per cent of *N. americanus* infestations.[72] The cure rate in *A. duodenale* infestation is very low—approximately 25 per cent. The reason for the different sensitivities of these two organisms to the drug is unknown.

The absorption of tetrachloroethylene from the gastrointestinal tract is minimal in the absence of fat or alcohol. To reduce the absorption of the drug, fatty foods and alcohol should not be ingested before and for 24 hours after the drug is administered. The drug may cause nausea, vomiting, dizziness, and a burning sensation in the stomach. Rarely, tetrachloroethylene causes a loss of consciousness, so the patient should be kept at rest for four hours after it is administered. This drug is contraindicated if the patient is infested with *Ascaris* as well as hookworm. As mentioned previously, tetrachloroethylene stimulates the migration of *Ascaris*, thereby increasing the risk of serious complications due to organ invasion and obstruction by these worms. When *Ascaris* organisms are present, they must first be eliminated with piperazine. When *Ascaris* eggs are no longer found in the feces, the hookworm can then be treated with tetrachloroethylene. In these mixed infestations it is probably more sensible to use bephenium hydroxynaphthoate, which has some efficacy against both organisms. If this treatment fails, then the physician can turn to piperazine followed by tetrachloroethylene. Tetrachloroethylene is only available as a veterinary preparation in the United States, but it can be used effectively and safely in humans.

Diethycarbamazine in the Treatment of Filariasis

Filaria worms, a subgroup of nematodes, are transmitted to man by insects. The adult forms of filaria inhabit the tissues or body cavities of a vertebrate host. Some of the more important members of this family are *Wuchereria bancrofti*, *W. malayi*, *Loa loa*, *Onchocerca volvulus*, and *Dracunculus medinensis* (guinea worm).

Diethylcarbamazine is the drug of choice (Table 8-5) for the treatment of *W. bancrofti*, *W. malayi*, and *Loa loa*. It kills the microfilaria (the prelarval forms of the organism), which circulate in the blood and lymphatics, but whether or not the adult filaria, which reside statically in the lymphatics, are eliminated is not clear. Though the drug has been reported to kill the adult forms of *W. malayi* and *Loa loa*, definitive proof is not yet available.[73] Though diethylcarbamazine is a derivative of piperazine, unsubstituted piperazine has no filaricidal action. The mechanism of the filaricidal action of diethylcarbamazine is unknown.

Diethylcarbamazine

Diethylcarbamazine is absorbed well from the gastrointestinal tract. The drug is rapidly distributed in all the tissues except adipose tissue. All of the drug is excreted, both as the parent drug and metabolites, by the kidney within forty-eight hours. Reactions to the drug are of two types. Patients may experience headache, malaise, weakness, nausea, and vomiting as a direct effect of the drug. A second complex of side effects represents allergic reactions to substances released from the killed microfilariae. These reactions are usually mild in the case of *W. bancrofti*, but they are often severe when the drug is used to treat *O. volvulus*. Symptoms include swelling and edema of the skin, intense itching, enlargement and tenderness of the inguinal lymph nodes, rash, fever, tachycardia, and headache. Nodular swellings may develop along the course of the lymphatics. These symptoms persist for three to seven days and then subside; then, quite high doses can be tolerated without further reaction. For this reason the following schedule is used in treating *O. volvulus* infestation (adult dosages): 25 mg daily for three days; 50 mg daily for three days, 100 mg daily for three days, and 150 mg daily for twelve days. Caution must be exercised in the use of diethylcarbamazine in *Loa loa* because it can provoke an encephalopathy.

References

1. M. Farooq: Progress in Bilharziasis control: The situation in Egypt. *Wld. Hlth. Org. Chron.* 21:175 (1967).

2. R. S. Desowtiz: Antiparasite chemotherapy. *Ann. Rev. Pharmacol.* 11:351 (1971).

3. P. D. Marsden and M. G. Schultz: Intestinal parasites. *Gastroenterology* 57:724 (1969).

4. Editorial: Drugs for parasitic infections. *Med. Letter Reference Handbook* pp. 23–29 (1971).

5. F. Scott and M. J. Miller: Trials with metranidazole in amebic dysentery. *J.A.M.A.* 211:118 (1970).

6. M. W. Fisher and P. E. Thompson: "Antibiotics with specific affinities. Part 3: Paromomycin" in *Experimental Chemotherapy*, ed. by R. J. Schnitzer and F. Hawking. New York: Academic Press, 1964, pp. 329–345.

7. B. P. Phillips and P. A. Wolfe: The use of germfree guinea pigs in studies on the microbial interrelationships in amoebiasis. *Ann. N.Y. Acad. Sci.* 78:308 (1959).

8. S. J. Powell, I. MacLeod, A. J. Wilmot, and R. Elsdon-Dew: Metronidazole in amoebic dysentery and amoebic liver abscess. *Lancet* 2:1329 (1966).

9. S. J. Powell, A. J. Wilmot, and R. Elsdon-Dew: Further trials of metronidazole in amoebic dysentery and amoebic liver abscess. *Ann. Trop. Med. Parasit.* 61:511 (1969).

10. H. C. Hesseltine and G. Lefebvre: Treating vaginal trichomoniasis with metronidazole. *J.A.M.A.* 184:1011 (1963).

11. S. J. Powell, A. J. Wilmot, and R. Elsdon-Dew: Single and low dosage regimens of metronidazole in amoebic dysentery and amoebic liver abscess. *Ann. Trop. Med. Parasit.* 63:139 (1969).

12. P. O. Kane, J. A. McFadzean, and S. Squires: Absorption and excretion of metronidazole. *Br. J. Vener. Dis.* 37:276 (1961).

13. J. E. Stambaugh, L. G. Feo, and R. W. Manthei: The isolation and identification of the urinary oxidative metabolites of metronidazole in man. *J. Pharm. Exptl. Ther.* 161:373 (1968).

14. J. A. Edwards and J. Price: Metronidazole and human alcohol dehydrogenase. *Nature* 214:190 (1967).

15. S. Lal: Metronidazole in the treatment of alcoholism. A clinical trial and review of the literature. *Quart. J. Stud. Alc.* 28:544 (1969).

16. E. Rothstein and D. D. Clancy: Toxicity of disulfiram combined with metronidazole. *New Eng. J. Med.* 280:1006 (1969).

17. I. de Carneri, G. Achilli, G. Monti, and F. Trane: Induction of *in-vivo* resistance of *Trichomonas vaginalis* to metronidazole. *Lancet* 2:1308 (1969).

18. S. J. Powell, I. N. MacLeod, A. J. Wilmot, and R. Elsdon-Dew: The treatment of acute amebic dysentery. *Ann. Trop. Med. Parasit.* 59:205 (1965).

19. J. N. Scragg and S. J. Powell: Emetine hydrochloride and dehydroemetine combined with chloroquine in the treatment of children with amoebic liver abscess. *Arch. Dis. Child* 43:121 (1968).

20. A. P. Grollman: Structural basis for inhibition of protein synthesis by emetine and cycloheximide based on an analogy between ipecac alkaloids and glutarimide antibiotics. *Proc. Natl. Acad. Sci.* 56:1867 (1966).

21. J. M. Clark and A. Y. Chang: Inhibitors of the transfer of amino acids from aminoacyl soluble ribonucleic acid to proteins. *J. Biol. Chem.* 240:4734 (1965).

22. A. P. Grollman: Inhibitors of protein synthesis: Effects of emetine on protein and nucleic acid biosynthesis in HeLa cells. *J. Biol. Chem.* 243:4089 (1968).

23. B. M. Beller: Observations on the mechanism of emetine poisoning of myocardial tissue. *Circulation Res.* 22:501 (1968).

24. G. Klatskin and H. Friedman: Emetine toxicity in man; studies on the nature of early toxic manifestations, their relation to dose level, and their significance in determining safe dosage. *Ann. Int. Med.* 28:892 (1948)

25. A. I. Gimble, C. Davison, and P. K. Smith: Studies on the toxicity, distribution and excretion of emetine. *J. Pharmacol. Exptl. Ther.* 94:431 (1948).

26. K. K. F. Ng: A new pharmacological action of emetine. *Brit. Med. J.* 1:1278 (1966).

27. S. J. Powell, I. MacLeod, A. J. Wilmot, and R. Elsdon-Dew: Ambilhar in amoebic dysentery and amoebic liver abscess. *Lancet* 2:20 (1966).

28. K. A. Western, D. R. Perera, and M. G. Schultz: Pentamidine isethionate in the treatment of Pneumocystis carinii pneumonia. Ann. Int. Med. 73:695 (1970).

29. T. P. Waalkes, C. Denham, and V. T. DeVita: Pentamidine: Clinical pharmacologic correlations in man and mice. Clin. Pharm. Ther. 11:505 (1970).

30. H. J. Saz and E. Bueding: Relationships between anthelmintic effects and biochemical and physiological mechanisms. Pharm. Rev. 18:871 (1966).

31. E. Bueding: Some biochemical effects of anthelmintic drugs. Biochem. Pharmacol. 18:1541 (1969).

32. G. Chen and E. M. K. Geiling: The determination of antitrypanosome effect of antimonials in vitro. J. Infect. Dis. 77:139 (1945).

33. J. D. Fulton and L. P. Joyner: Studies on protozoa. Part I. The metabolism of Leishman-Donovan bodies and flagellates of Leishmania donovani. Trans. Roy. Soc. Trop. Med. Hyg. 43:273 (1949).

34. T. E. Mansour and L. Peters: "Chemotherapy of infections by flagellates and flukes" in Drill's Pharmacology in Medicine, ed. by J. R. DiPalma. New York: McGraw-Hill, 1971, pp. 1813.

35. L. G. Goodwin and J. E. Page: A study of the excretion of organic antimonials using a polarographic procedure. Biochem. J. 37:198 (1943).

36. E. Bueding: Carbohydrate metabolism of Schistosoma mansoni. J. Gen. Physiol. 33:475 (1950).

37. T. E. Mansour and E. Bueding: The actions of antimonials on glycolytic enzymes of Schistosoma mansoni. Brit. J. Pharmacol. 9:459 (1954).

38. E. Bueding and J. M. Mansour: The relationship between inhibition of phosphofructokinase activity and the mode of action of trivalent organic antimonials on Schistosoma mansoni. Brit. J. Pharmacol. 12:159 (1957).

39. G. A. H. Buttle and M. T. Khayyal: Rapid hepatic shift of worms in mice infected with Schistosoma mansoni after a single injection of tartar emetic. Nature 194:780 (1962).

40. Symposium: The pharmacological and chemotherapeutic properties of niridazole and other antischistosomal compounds. Ann. N.Y. Acad. Sci. 160:423–946 (1969).

41. E. Bueding and J. Fisher: Biochemical effects of schistosomicides. Ann. N.Y. Acad. Sci. 160:536 (1969).

42. J. W. Faigle and H. Keberle: Metabolism of niridazole in various species, including man. Ann. N.Y. Acad. Sci. 160:544 (1969).

43. A. Coutinho and F. T. Barreto: Treatment of hepatosplenic schistosomiasis mansoni with niridazole: Relationships among liver function, effective dose and side effects. Ann. N.Y. Acad. Sci. 160:612 (1969).

44. R. A. Carchman, E. Hirschberg, and I. B. Weinstein: Miracil D: Effect on the viscosity of DNA: Biochim. Biophys. Acta 179:158 (1969).

45. M. Waring: Variation of the supercoils in closed circular DNA by binding of antibiotics and drugs: Evidence for molecular models involving intercalation. J. Mol. Biol. 54:247 (1970).

46. B. Weinstein, R. Carshman, E. Marner, and E. Hirshberg: Miracil D: Effects on nucleic acid synthesis, protein synthesis, and enzyme induction in *Escherichia coli*. *Biochim. Biophys. Acta.* 142:440 (1967).

47. D. M. Blair: Lucanthone hydrochloride. *Bull. World Health Org.* 18:989 (1958).

48. A. Einhorn, A. Fritsch, K. G. Dwork, and H. B. Schookhoff: *Schistosoma mansoni* infection in children. *Am. J. Dis. Children.* 104:30 (1962).

49. R. Bases and F. Mendez: Reversible inhibition of ribosomal RNA synthesis in HeLa by lucanthone (Miracil D) with continued synthesis of DNA-like RNA. *J. Cell. Physiol.* 74:283 (1969).

50. R. Bases: Enhancement of X-ray damage in HeLa cells by exposure to lucanthone (Miracil D) following radiation. *Canc. Res.* 30:2007 (1970).

51. S. Yang and C. Lin: Treatment of paragonimiasis with bithionol and bithionol sulfoxide. *Dis. Chest* 52:220 (1967).

52. O. D. Standen: "Chemotherapy of helminthic infections" in *Experimental Chemotherapy*, ed. by R. J. Schnitzer and F. Hawking. New York: Academic Press 1963, pp. 701–892.

53. F. E. Hahn, R. L. Obrien, J. Ciak, J. L. Allison, and J. G. Olenick: Studies on modes of action of chloroquine, quinacrine, and quinine and on chloroquine resistance. *Military Med.* 131:1071 (1966).

54. J. E. D. Keeling: "The chemotherapy of Cestode infections" in *Advances in Chemotherapy*, ed. by A. Goldin, F. Hawking, and R. J. Schnitzer. New York: Academic Press, 1968, pp. 109–152.

55. L. Runeberg: Uncoupling of oxidative phosphorylation in rat liver mitochondria with desaspidin and related phlorobutyrophenone derivatives. *Biochem. Pharmacol.* 11:237 (1962).

56. L. W. Scheibel, H. J. Saz, and E. Bueding: The anaerobic incorporation of ^{32}P into adenosine triphosphate by *Hymenolepis diminuta*. *J. Biol. Chem.* 243:2229 (1968).

57. G. J. Abrams, H. C. Seftel, and H. J. Heinz: The treatment of human tapeworm infections with "Yomesan." *S. Afr. Med. J.* 37:6 (1963).

58. S. Norton and E. J. deBeer: Investigations on the action of piperazine on *Ascaris lumbricoides*. *Am. J. Trop. Med. Hyg.* 6:898 (1957).

59. J. T. DeBell, J. Del Castillo, and V. Sanchez: Electrophysiology of the somatic muscle cells of *Ascaris lumbricoides*. *J. Cell Comp. Physiol.* 62:159 (1963).

60. J. Del Castillo, W. C. De Mello, and T. Morales: Mechanism of the paralyzing action of piperazine on *Ascaris* muscle. *Brit. J. Pharmacol.* 22:463 (1964).

61. A. C. Cuckler and K. C. Mezey: The therapeutic efficacy of thiabendazole for helminthic infections in man. *Arzneim.-Forsch.* 16:411 (1966).

62. K. H. Franz, W. J. Schneider, and M. H. Pohlman: Clinical trials with thiabendazole against intestinal nematodes infecting humans. *Am. J. Trop. Med. Hyg.* 14:383 (1965).

63. O. J. Stone and J. F. Mullins: Thiabendazole effectiveness in creeping eruption. *Arch. Dermatol.* 91:427 (1965).

64. H. D. Brown, A. R. Matzuk, I. R. Ilves, L. H. Peterson, S. A. Harris, L. H. Sarett, J. R. Egerton, J. J. Yakstis, W. C. Campbell, and A. C. Cuckler: Antiparasitic drugs. IV. 2-(4'-thiazolyl)-benzimidazole, a new anthelmintic. *J. Am. Chem. Soc.* 83:1764 (1961).

65. B. H. Kean and D. W. Hoskins: Treatment of trichinosis. *J.A.M.A.* 190:852 (1964).

66. J. W. Beck: Treatment of pinworm infections with reduced single dose of pyrvinium pamoate. *J.A.M.A.* 189:511 (1964).

67. R. C. Jung: Use of a hexylresorcinol tablet in the enema treatment of whipworm infection. *Am. J. Trop. Med. Hyg.* 3:918 (1954).

68. A. I. Krotov and S. N. Federova: Effect of bephenium hydroxynaphthoate on ascarids. *Fed. Proc.* (Translation supplement) 23:T55 (1964).

69. A. W. J. Broome: "Mechanisms of anthelminthic action with particular reference to drugs affecting neuromuscular activity" in *Drugs, Parasites and Hosts,* ed by L. G. Goodwin and R. H. Nimmo-Smith, Boston: Little, Brown, 1962, pp. 43–61.

70. H. H. Salem, W. M. Morcos, and H. M. El-Ninny: Clinical trials with bephenium hydroxynaphthoate against *A. duodenale* and other intestinal helminths. *J. Trop. Med.* 68:21 (1965).

71. M. D. Young, G. M. Jeffery, W. G. Morehouse, J. E. Freed, and R. S. Johnson: The comparative efficacy of bephenium hydroxynaphthoate and tetrachlorethylene against hookworm and other parasites of man. *Am. J. Trop. Med. Hyg.* 9:488 (1960).

72. R. C. Jung and J. E. McCroan: Efficacy of bephenium and tetrachloroethylene in mass treatment of hookworm infection. *Am. J. Trop. Med. Hyg.* 9:492 (1960).

73. F. Hawking: "Chemotherapy of filariasis" in *Experimental Chemotherapy,* Vol. I, ed. by R. J. Schnitzer and F. Hawking. New York: Academic Press, 1963, pp. 893–912.

Part III
Drugs Employed in the Treatment of Viral Infection

Medical efforts to combat viral infection include a variety of approaches. As with the parasitic diseases, vector control is helpful in limiting those viral infections transmitted by insects (e.g. yellow fever transmitted by mosquitos) and animals (e.g. rabies transmitted by dogs). In some cases, isolation of infected patients will limit the spread of a virus in the community. Other efforts to control viral infection have been directed at active stimulation of the immune response by eliciting specific antibody production (immunization) or at passive assistance to the patient's defense mechanism by the use of human gamma globulin, equine antiserums, and, more recently, antiserum from successfully vaccinated humans. In addition to these approaches, there are several new drugs for the treatment and prevention of selected viral infections. The role of each of these forms of treatment in the control of virus infections in man has been concisely discussed by Stevens and Merigan[1] and by Hilleman.[2]

Prophylaxis by immunization has been the most effective form of control for many viral infections. Mass immunization with live, attenuated virus vaccines is currently effectively employed to prevent diseases like polio, mumps, measles, and yellow fever. The use of vaccinia virus immunization to prevent smallpox has been so successful that the disease has been virtually eradicated in many areas of the world. In fact, in the United States the mortality associated with smallpox vaccination is greater than that associated with the disease itself. The use of killed virus vaccines against influenza provides partial protection against serious infection. Influenza vaccines are currently used during epidemics to protect the elderly, the young, and people debilitated because of chronic disease (these are the groups that suffer the greatest morbidity and mortality during influena epidemics).

In addition to effecting production of antibodies, viruses stimulate production of interferon by host cells. This substance in turn induces production of a translation inhibitory protein that acts to prevent the synthesis of viral proteins. Two methods have been employed experimentally to increase the amount of interferon in the body. The first is the administration of exogenous interferon and the second is the use of compounds that induce production of interferon by the host. This second method holds the promise of providing a new class of effective antiviral drugs, and it will be discussed in the following chapter. The action of interferon and interferon inducers has been reviewed in a series of papers entitled "Symposium on Interferon and Host Response to Viral Infection."[3]

Three groups of drugs are currently marketed in the United States for antiviral chemotherapy: the pyrimidine analogs, amantadine, and the isatin-β-thiosemicarbazones. There is no broad-spectrum antiviral drug available for clinical use, and the application of each of these drug groups is severely restricted to the treatment of only a few viral infections. The chemotherapy of virus disease has been reviewed by Eggers and Tamm[4] and by Prusoff.[5] A comparison of the three approaches to antiviral therapy (immunization, interferon production, and chemotherapy) is presented in Table III-1.

Table III-1 Approaches to specific control of viral infections
(From Hilleman,[2] Table I.)

| Approach | Characteristics: | | |
	Level of effectiveness	Antiviral spectrum	Duration of effect
Immunological	Usually high	Very narrow	Relatively long to lifetime
Host resistance (interferon)	Moderate to high	Very broad	Relatively short term
Chemical	Low to moderate	Narrow	Short term

References

1. D. A. Stevens and T. C. Merrigan: Approaches to the control of viral infections in man. *Rational Drug Ther.* 5 (Issue No. 9): pp. 1–5 (1971).

2. M. R. Hilleman: Toward control of viral infections of man. *Science* 164:506 (1969).

3. T. C. Merrigan (Ed.): Symposium on interferon and host response to virus infection. *Arch. Int. Med.* 126: pp. 49–157 (1970).

4. H. J. Eggers and I. Tamm: Antiviral chemotherapy. *Ann. Rev. Pharmacol.* 6:231 (1966).

5. W. H. Prussoff: Recent advances in chemotherapy of viral diseases. *Pharm. Rev.* 19:209 (1967).

Chapter 9
Chemotherapy of Viral Infections

Introduction

Definition and Classification of Viruses

Viruses are organisms composed of a nucleic acid core (the genome may be either DNA or RNA) surrounded by a protein-containing shell; they reproduce only inside living cells. They derive their energy supply and their substrates from the parasitized cell; they use its synthetic machinery to produce the virus-specific protein required for production of the mature viral particle. Mature virus particles possess only one type of nucleic acid, and they lose their organized form during replication of the genome in the host cell. These characteristics distinguish the viruses from intracellular parasites like the chlamydiae (psittacosis-lymphogranuloma venerum-trachoma group of organisms), which possess two types of nucleic acid in their infectious particles and retain their organized form in the intracellular phase, dividing by binary fission.[1] Still more complex intracellular parasites like the plasmodia, the leprosy bacillus, and the rickettsiae have even higher levels of cellular organization, possessing protein-synthesizing and energy-generating systems of their own.

The animal viruses are classified according to various characteristics such as nucleic acid content (RNA viruses, DNA viruses), gross morphology, location of viral multiplication (in the cytoplasm or nucleus of the parasitized cell), composition of the virus shell (enveloped or non-enveloped), and serological typing. A selected list of the viruses that infect man is presented in Table 9-1.

The Biology of Viral Reproduction

It is impossible in this text to provide a background review of the molecular biology of animal viruses. But by presenting examples of some of the biochemical events that take place during viral infection, we can provide a basis for understanding some

Table 9-1   Classification of some viruses infecting man
(Adapted from Luria and Darnell,[2] Table 1-1.)

Group	Agent	Characteristics
RNA VIRUSES		
Small RNA viruses		Cubic symmetry, no envelope, multiply in cytoplasm, RNA about 2×10^6 daltons
Enteroviruses	Polio Coxsackie A Coxsackie B ECHO	
Rhinoviruses		
Reoviruses		Cubic symmetry, no envelope, double-stranded RNA, multiply in cytoplasm
Myxoviruses		Enveloped virions
Subgroup I		Nuclear phase in replication cycle
	Influenza	Three serotypes (A,B,C,); type A most frequent, causes large epidemics
Subgroup II		Multiplies in cytoplasm; very large RNA (6 to 8×10^6 daltons)
	Parainfluenza Mumps Measles	
Arboviruses		Small, enveloped virions with central RNA-containing core; transmitted by arthropods, cause encephalitis
Subgroup A		Includes Western and Eastern equine encephalomyelitis
Subgroup B		Includes yellow fever and denge
DNA VIRUSES		
Poxviruses		Large, brick-shaped enveloped virions containing at least 10 proteins and a large DNA

(Table continued on p. 234)

Table 9-1 (continued)

Group	Agent	Characteristics
		molecule; multiply in cytoplasm
	Variola	Causes smallpox
	Vaccinia	Used for vaccination against smallpox
Herpesvirus		Large, enveloped virions with well-defined icosahedral capsid
	Herpes simplex	Causes fever blisters
	Varicella	Causes chickenpox
	Cytomegalovirus	Infection leads to giant cell formation
Adenovirus		Icosahedral, non-enveloped virions
	Human subgroup	Cause upper respiratory disease and conjunctivitis
Small DNA viruses		Icosahedral, non-enveloped virions containing circular DNA molecules
	Human papilloma	Causes warts
	SV-40	Can transform cultured human cells

of the possible sites where the process of viral infection can be selectively inhibited by drugs. For comprehensive discussions of the biology of viral reproduction, the reader is referred to the appropriate chapters in three general texts on this subject.[2,3,4] The process of viral infection can be conveniently considered in three stages: (I) entry of the virus into the host cell and release of nucleic acid; (II) replication of the genome and synthesis of viral proteins; (III) assembly of the virion and release from the cell. A schematic summary[5] of the replication cycle of poliovirus, a non-enveloped RNA virus, is presented in Figure 9-1 for reference during the following discussion.

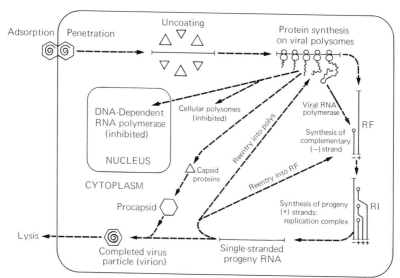

Figure 9-1 The replication cycle of poliovirus. RF, replicative form; RI, replicative intermediate. (From Pearson.[5])

Stage I—Adsorption, Penetration, and Uncoating

The initial attachment of viruses to mammalian cells appears to be mediated by an electrostatic interaction between the virus capsid or outer envelope and the cell membrane. In some cases specific receptors for a virus have been demonstrated on the surface of mammalian cells. Polio, for example, a virus that possesses a protein capsid composed of 60 repeating units, (four separate proteins per unit) becomes attached to receptors found only in membranes of susceptible cells.

After attachment, a variety of mechanisms operate to introduce the virus into the cell. Certain bacterial viruses (the T-even bacteriophages, for example) have developed elaborate mechanisms for injecting their nucleic acid through the cell wall and membrane into the cytoplasm, but this does not occur with animal viruses. Viruses may often penetrate animal cells by a process of pinocytosis, but in general their entry mechanisms are not well defined. Certain viruses (e.g. influenza viruses and other myxo-viruses) are surrounded by an envelope containing carbohydrate, lipid, and protein. One of the proteins is a neuraminadase, which may facilitate cell penetration by digesting components of the cell membrane.

Some poxviruses have developed elaborate mechanisms of becoming uncoated and releasing their nucleic acid after they have entered the cell. For example, the vaccinia virus, a large DNA virus with an envelope, undergoes a two-stage uncoating process in the cell.[6] In the first stage the virion is attacked by host cell enzymes that partially degrade the virus particle, which loses some of its protein and all of its phospholipid. This particle, called a core, is composed of DNA surrounded by protein. Pox-virus cores contain a DNA-dependent RNA polymerase,[7] and they can synthesize mRNA.[8] The second stage of the uncoating process proceeds only after a delay, releasing the viral DNA into the cell cytoplasm. This second uncoating process is prevented by inhibitors of protein synthesis.[6] The most plausible model of this sequence of events is that the virus is attacked by host cell enzymes, which partially uncoat the virus; the resulting virus core synthesizes a mRNA for a virus-specific protein synthesized in the cell cytoplasm that degrades the core, releasing naked vaccinia DNA. The delay between the first and second stage of the uncoating process represents the time required for synthesis of the virus-specific uncoating protein.

These examples of viral penetration and uncoating point up the complicated interaction between the virus and the host cell required for the initiation of a viral infection. The infective pro-cess can be interrupted here at the first stage of the virus-cell interaction. Antiviral antibodies, for example, can prevent attach-ment of the virus to the cell by reacting with the coat protein of the virion; when added shortly after adsorption of the virus to the cell surface, they can prevent initiation of infection. Amanta-dine, one of the clinically useful antiviral drugs, acts at this first stage of the infection process. This drug does not prevent adsorp-tion of the virus to the cell surface, but apparently blocks pene-tration of the cell by the virus. As has just been demonstrated, drugs that inhibit animal cell protein synthesis may in some cases inhibit the uncoating process; however, such drugs are not useful in therapy because they have no selective toxicity.

Stage II—Synthesis of Viral Components

In the second stage of viral infection the genome of the virus is duplicated, and the viral proteins are synthesized in the appropriate sequence. The events that take place in the second stage involve a variety of control mechanisms that direct the energy-producing and synthetic functions of the cell to serve in the synthesis of viral nucleic acid and protein. When some DNA viruses infect a population of growing cells, for example, they may inhibit the synthesis of host DNA, thus reserving the pools of nucleic acid precursors for their own use. This inhibition of host cell DNA synthesis is apparently mediated by a virus-specific protein.

Although viruses use cellular enzymes in the synthesis of viral components, they also produce their own enzymes for specialized functions. For example, enzymes produced after infection with RNA viruses are necessary for replicating the RNA genome. As far as is known at present, RNA does not serve a template function in mammalian cells, and specific enzymes, coded in the viral genome, must be produced so that the genetic information of the RNA virus can be replicated. One of these enzymes, produced after virus infection (e.g. by poliovirus or mengovirus), is RNA synthetase; it requires a single-stranded RNA for a template and directs the synthesis of a second strand of RNA. This second strand (−) is complementary to the first strand (+), which contains the genetic information of the virus, and it can in turn serve as a template upon which multiple viral RNA genomes, (+) strands, are synthesized. This enzyme is completely different from the RNA polymerase of the host cell, which uses double-stranded DNA as a template. It is also different from another viral polymerase, the RNA-dependent DNA polymerase (or reverse transcriptase), which synthesizes DNA from single-stranded viral RNA template.[9]

The production and function of key virus-specific enzymes like

RNA synthetase stand out as logical points for selective attack by chemotherapeutic agents. There are two compounds, guanidine and 2-(α-hydroxybenzyl)-benzimidazole, which block the formation of active viral RNA synthetase in certain small RNA viruses (e.g. poliovirus, Coxsackie B virus, and most ECHOviruses). They do not inhibit the activity of the enzyme *in vitro,* and they have not proved useful in chemotherapy because of the rapid emergence of resistance and limited activity *in vivo.*

The detailed study of the viral enzymes responsible for nucleic acid synthesis may yield new viral-inhibitory drugs. The substrate site of the viral enzyme, for example, may "accept" nucleotide analogs not accommodated by the mammalian polymerases. Such nucleotide analogs could then have an antiviral effect either by blocking the function of the viral enzyme or by being incorporated into viral nucleic acid, producing a faulty inactive RNA or DNA. In either case a selective toxicity would obtain. Iododeoxyuridine (IUdR) is a clinically useful antiviral drug which is incorporated into DNA in place of thymidine. The abnormal DNA thus formed is more susceptible to breakage and apparently is unable to direct the synthesis of mRNA's that produce functional viral proteins. The incorporation of IUdR into DNA is not a very selective event, as the drug is incorporated into the DNA of the patient's cells as well as into that of the virus.

The production of viral proteins in all DNA viruses requires the synthesis of mRNA's, which are then translated by the protein synthesizing machinery (ribosomes, tRNAs, amino acids, activating enzymes, etc.) of the host cell. In the case of single-stranded RNA viruses (e.g. polio, Coxsackie, ECHO, mumps, measles), the ($+$) RNA is unique in that it serves both as a messenger for protein synthesis and as a template for ($-$) RNA synthesis. In general the mRNA's for proteins involved in the replication of the viral genome and in the direction of host cell synthesis of viral-specific components are produced earlier in the infection process than the mRNA for proteins like the capsid proteins which are not required until the end, when assembly of the virion takes place. This statement is certainly an oversimplification, but it points out the fact that production of the various components of the virus is not just a random process in which all of the viral genes are turned on at the same time.

The synthesis of viral-specific proteins is another potential mechanism for selective inhibition by chemotherapeutic drugs. Indeed, one of the clinically useful antiviral compounds, N-methyl-isatin-β-thiosemicarbazone, appears to inhibit the multiplication of poxviruses by selectively inhibiting the synthesis of late viral structural proteins. Translation inhibitory protein, a substance produced by cells exposed to interferon, apparently acts at the ribosome to prevent translation of viral mRNA, thus preventing synthesis of protein necessary for viral replication. This effect is specific; translation of cell mRNA is unaffected.

Stage III—Assembly and Release of the Virus

In the final stage of the infection process the viral components are assembled into a mature virion. During replication, the viral nucleic acid is not associated with viral structural protein. The capsid proteins accumulate in the cell late in the infection. The viral genome then becomes enveloped by capsid proteins and, once associated with them, is no longer able to replicate. In the case of nonenveloped viruses (e.g. poliovirus, adenovirus) the virion is now complete and is released from the cell. With other viruses, however, the capsid is enveloped by a membrane, the lipid portion of which is derived from host cell membranes. The poxviruses are even more complex. They contain a large DNA molecule surrounded by many viral proteins and more than one membrane. These complex viruses are synthesized in cytoplasmic factories, and they possess a higher degree of organization than the other viruses.

The release of mature virions from the cell may be rapid and may be accompanied by cell death and lysis; this is often the case with the simpler non-enveloped viruses like polio. In contrast to this method of release, some enveloped viruses are released (often over a long period of time) by a process of budding at the cell membrane. In this case the cytoplasmic membrane remains intact during the release of the viruses, and the cell may survive.

No drugs are known that inhibit the release of mature virions from animal cells; however, there is one drug that seems to block the assembly of viral DNA and protein into mature virus particles. Rifampicin, a drug used in the treatment of tuberculosis (see Chapter 1), also inhibits the replication of poxviruses. [10, 11] Comprehensive studies (discussed in detail in Chapter 1) have demonstrated that the antibacterial effect of rifampicin is due to its ability to selectively inhibit bacterial RNA polymerases. The mechanism of the drug's antiviral action, however, may be quite different. Concentrations of rifampicin that completely inhibit viral growth do not inhibit RNA polymerase activity associated with the mature vaccinia virus particle or the virus core. [12] Further experiments have demonstrated that viral DNA, RNA, and protein synthesis continues in the presence of rifampicin, but that assembly into mature virus particles is prevented. [13] This drug effect is reversible. If rifampicin is removed, the virus particles are assembled into mature virions even in the absence of new protein synthesis. It is entirely possible that the receptor for rifampicin in both bacteria and viruses is RNA polymerase. In bacteria the association of the drug with the receptor inhibits enzyme activity, and in the virus the rifampicin-RNA polymerase complex, although enzymatically active, may be structurally altered so that it is unable to interact with other parts of the virus as a necessary component of the virus core.

Because viruses parasitize many of the functions of their host cells, there are many biochemical mechanisms common to both the infecting agent and the animal cell. This of course limits the number of functions that may be selectively interrupted by chemical agents.

It is hoped that this introduction has served to underscore the fact that fundamental research into the molecular biology of viral replication is providing a basis for the rational development of antiviral drugs. One of the problems in chemotherapy of viral infection is that the clinical symptoms of infection are often not evident until there has already been extensive viral replication, and the immune responses of the host are already building an effective deterrent to the virus. For many infections, therefore, antiviral chemotherapy may be more useful as prophylaxis than as therapy for the well-developed clinical case.

Interferon

Interferons are small-molecular-weight, carbohydrate-containing proteins produced by animal cells infected with viruses. They are released from the cells in which they are produced, and they inhibit the multiplication of viruses in other cells. The principal source of the circulating interferon in the body appears to be the cells of the lymphoreticular system. Both DNA and RNA viruses are interferon inducers. In addition, a wide variety of other intracellular parasites (including trachoma agent, several bacteria, and at least three protozoa), microbial extracts, and several synthetic polymers can elicit the production of interferon (see Table 9-2). The interferons produced by different animals are quite species specific.[14] That is, they inhibit viral multiplication only in cells of the same animal species (or closely related ones) in which they were produced. In contrast, the antiviral action of the interferons is very broad. They are active in a wide variety of viral infections, and they have been reported to inhibit higher organisms, including some protozoa. The literature in this field has been reviewed by De Clercq and Merrigan[15] and by Hilleman.[16]

Studies on the Mechanism of Induction of Interferon

Some indirect evidence suggests that interferon is produced as a result of the induction of new host cell protein synthesis by viral components. Double-stranded RNA's of both synthetic and viral origin are good interferon inducers, and it may be that this viral component is the active inducing moiety. The production of virus-induced and synthetic RNA-induced interferon is blocked by actinomycin D, an inhibitor of RNA synthesis (see Chapter 10).[17] In addition puromycin, an inhibitor of protein synthesis, inhibits the production of virus-induced interferon.[17, 18, 19] These observations are consistent with (but do not prove) the hypothesis that interferon-inducing substances cause the mammalian cell

Table 9-2　List of interferon inducers
(From DeClercq and Merigan,[15] Table 1.)

Microorganisms
　Viruses (both DNA and RNA)
　Chlamydia (trachoma, inclusion conjunctivitis)
　Rickettsiae
　Bacteria (e.g. *E. coli, S. typhimurium, B. abortus, H. influenzae*)
　Protozoa (e.g. *Toxoplasma gondii, Plasmodium berghei, Trypanosoma cruzi*)
Microbial extracts
　Viral extracts (double-stranded RNAs from several viruses)
　Bacterial extracts [endotoxins, toxoids, tuberculo-protein, exotoxins (strepto-lysin O)]
　Fungal extracts
　　Statolon (a double-stranded RNA from *Penicillium stoloniferum*—of probable viral origin)
　　Helenine (a double-stranded RNA from *Penicillium funiculosum*—of probable viral origin)
　Plant extracts.
　　Phytohemagglutinin (from the kidney bean)
Synthetic polymers
　Polycarboxylates (maleic anhydride copolymers, polyacrylic and polymethyl-acrylic acids)
　Polysulfates (polyvinylsulfate)
　Polyphosphates
　　Polyribonucleotide homopolymer pairs (e.g. poly rI:rC and poly rA:rU)
　　Alternating polyribonucleotides
　　Phosphorylated polysaccharides (e.g. dextran phosphate)
　Polythiophosphate (thiophosphate analogs of polyribonucleotides)

---

to transcribe a specific cellular gene into mRNA to produce inter-feron. It is, however, possible that cellular RNA and protein syn-thesis are required for release of preformed interferon in the active form as a soluble molecule. If this is the case, the produc-tion of interferon would be blocked by inhibitors of RNA and pro-tein synthesis, but the mechanism would not represent a specif-ic gene derepression by the interferon-inducing agent. The fact that interferon is specific for the cell in which it was synthesized rather than for the inducer supports the concept that interferons are cellular gene products.

Studies on the Mechanism of Action of Interferon

Interferon does not interact directly with viruses or affect their adsorption or penetration into the cell. Studies with actinomycin D and puromycin indicate that both cellular RNA and protein synthesis are necessary for the development of antiviral activity in interferon-treated cells.[20,21] This has been interpreted as an indication that interferon itself is an inducer molecule that derepresses the host cell genome, producing a protein that inhibits virus multiplication. The specific viral process inhibited is the synthesis of viral protein,[22,23,24] but the reason for this inhibition is not yet clear. Some experiments indicate that viral RNA cannot combine with ribosomes to form functional polysomes in interferon-treated cells.[23,24] Other studies indicate that ribosome-viral RNA complexes can be formed, but that protein synthesis is inhibited.[25,26] At any rate, the translation of viral RNA into protein is inhibited in interferon-treated cells, and the protein produced by the host cell in response to interferon is called translation inhibitory protein.

Interferon Inducers as Antiviral Drugs

Of the three approaches to the specific control of viral infections, immunization provides the longest lasting protection, but its usefulness is restricted to those infections in which there are only a few serotypes. In the case of viruses causing the common cold, for example, there are so many different serotypes, and immunity is so short lived, that control by immunization is not a practical prospect for the future. The chemotherapeutic agents developed to date have a very narrow spectrum of action, and their effects are transient. Interferon has a broad spectrum of activity, and it does not have the delay period inherent to the development of the antibody response in immunization. Exploitation of the antiviral effect of interferon would thus seem to be a promising therapeutic approach. This can be done in two ways: the administration of purified interferon or the administration of compounds that stimulate the production of interferon by the cells of the host. The administration of interferon itself has several drawbacks. Because of its species specificity, interferon prepared for use in humans must be purified from human or perhaps primate cells. This would be a costly and laborious procedure, and it would yield only limited amounts of the compound. Animal experiments have shown that intravenously injected interferon has a serum half-life of only about ten minutes.[27] This short half-life appears to result from interferon's rapid distribution throughout all of the body compartments, rapid inactivation, and excretion.[15] Large quantities of the active, highly purified compound would thus be required for therapy. These difficulties may be circumvented by the use of interferon inducers.

Some microbial extracts and synthetic polymers that induce the production of interferon are listed in Table 9-2. The ideal interferon inducer would be a non-pyrogenic, non-antigenic, non-toxic compound, it would not be rapidly inactivated or excreted, and it would induce high levels of interferon. There is no compound that satisfies these criteria. The most promising of the interferon inducers developed to date is poly I:C, a double-stranded homopolymer of inosine and cytosine. This compound has been shown to protect cells in culture from a variety of viruses, including the production of resistance to many common respiratory viruses in cultured human cells.[28,29] It also elicits antiviral activity in animals.[28] Poly I:C has a number of side effects,[30] including endotoxin-like effects,[31] pyrogenicity,[32] and embryotoxicity[33] (at high concentrations). Poly I:C is also immunogenic in some strains of mice that spontaneously develop an autoimmune disorder resembling human systemic lupus erythematosus,[34] a condition in which anti-nucleic acid antibodies are commonly found. This compound and the other synthetic interferon-inducing polymers, in their present form, are clearly not going to create a revolution in the clinical treatment of viral infection. But the study of these agents may very well provide the basis for new, effective, clinically practical therapy of virus-caused disease.

Amantadine

Structure and Mechanism of Action

Amantadine hydrochloride is a water-soluble amine with a unique structure that prevents infection of cultured cells by influenza viruses. The mechanism of action of amantadine has not been completely elucidated. The drug inhibits penetration of

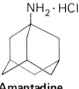

$NH_2 \cdot HCl$

Amantadine

viruses into the cell; there is no effect on either viral multiplication or assembly and release.[35] Amantadine is more effective if given prior to infection and has little *in vitro* effect if it is introduced after viral multiplication has begun. Amantadine does not interact with the virus directly or prevent the adsorption of the virus to the cell membrane. The virus adsorbed to cells in the presence of amantadine is susceptible to inactivation by antiviral antibody several hours after infection (Figure 9-2).[35,36] These observations strongly suggest that amantadine inhibits penetration of the virus into the cell, leaving it attached to the cell surface in a form that can react with antibodies. The drug is active against only a few viruses *in vitro*; these include influenza A, A_1, and A_2[37], parainfluenza 1 (Sendai),[37] and rubella.[38] The possibility that these few viruses employ a common mechanism of membrane penetration may explain the drug's limited spectrum of action. Further understanding of the mechanism of action of amantadine will probably depend upon the elucidation of the various mechanisms of viral penetration.

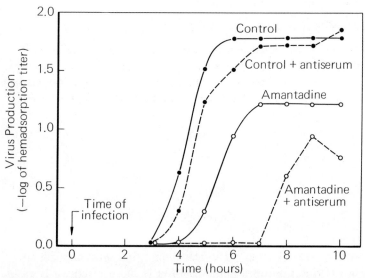

Figure 9-2 Effect of amantadine, antibody, and the combination of both on virus production in chick embryo fibroblasts infected with influenza A2/AA/2/60. Control (●-●); control, plus antiserum (●--●); amantadine (o-o); amantadine plus antiserum (o--o). Monolayer cultures and chick embryo fibroblasts were infected with influenza A_2, and, after 15 minutes of incubation, the unadsorbed virus was removed by washing the cells. Amantadine ($20\mu g/ml$) was present from 15 minutes before to 2 hours after infection. Antibody-treated cultures were exposed to specific virus rabbit antiserum for a 15-minute period between 1.75 and 2 hours postinfection. The amount of virus produced was determined by a hemadsorption test. It is clear that the antiserum had no effect on the production of virus when added to the control cultures during the indicated period. Amantadine alone produced a delay in the initial appearance of virus as well as a reduction in the total amount of virus. Amantadine plus antiserum resulted in a long delay in the appearance of virus as well as a reduction in the total amount of virus produced. This experiment provides evidence for the concept that in the presence of amantadine virus remains adsorbed at the cell surface. (Redrawn from Hoffmann et al.[35])

The Clinical Use of Amantadine

Despite the *in vitro* sensitivity of influenza A and A_1, Sendai virus, and rubella, amantadine is clinically useful only in the treatment of influenza A_2 infection. It is currently recommended that the use of amantadine be restricted to prophylaxis against influenza A_2 (Asian) and that it should not be used in the treatment of patients with established A_2 influenza. This recommendation is based on the results of clinical trials comparing the incidence and severity of infection in subjects treated with the drug or a placebo. The interpretation of the results of several of the early clinical trials has been questioned because of a number of deficiences in their design, including an inadequate number of patients, an occasional failure to confirm the infection serologically, inappropriate matching of control and drug-treated groups, and lack of double-blind procedures of administration and patient evaluation.[39]

It is easy to understand the difficulty in determining the effectiveness of an antiviral drug in reducing the incidence of naturally acquired infection during an influenza epidemic. The experimental protocol has to be prepared and the participating investigators organized before the epidemic has developed. Otherwise, it is difficult to assure uniformity of methods and adequate sample sizes. Consistent and accurate methods of identifying index cases, defining the presence of infection, and quantitating its severity and duration must be employed. Appropriate serological identification of the infection must be carried out, and antibody titers should be followed in all controls and treated patients to determine possible effects of the drug on subclinical infection and to control for those patients suffering from virus infection other than influenza A_2. The population studied must be assigned to drug-treated or control groups by an appropriate random process, and the groups must be compared, at the end, to assure that they are matched according to age and sex. Finally, the drug or placebo should be administered and the patient response assessed according to double-blind procedure.

Several studies have been carried out that take these considerations into account; they demonstrate that amantadine, given before the onset of clinical symptoms, decreases the occurrence of Asian influenza in humans when the infection is experimentally induced[40,41] and when it is naturally acquired.[42] The results of one of these studies are presented in Table 9-3. They demonstrate that

Table 9-3 **The effect of amantadine on the incidence of infection in contacts of serologically confirmed, active cases of influenza A_2**

Index cases were identified during an influenza A_2 epidemic, and their families were divided at random into drug-treated and placebo groups. All members of one family except the index case received the same treatment (drug or placebo). Index cases received only the placebo, so as not to reduce the possible spread of influenza virus among contacts. Treatment consisted of 100 mg of amantadine (adult dose) every twelve hours for ten days from the time the index case was first seen. The drug, or placebo, was given on a double-blind basis. Blood samples were taken from everybody on the first visit and again two to three weeks later. During the ten days, the family members were visited regularly with daily recording of temperature and the presence of a cough. A cough accompanied by a temperature of $100°F$ or higher was accepted as the criterion for a diagnosis of clinical influenza. Subclinical infection was identified by a fourfold or greater rise in antibody titer to A_2/England/10/67 virus without cough and temperature elevation. The data presented in the table refer only to family members of index cases in which there was serological confirmation of influenza A_2 infection (Data taken from Galbraith et al.[42] Tables II and III.)

Contacts who developed clinical influenza within ten days of entering the study:

Treatment	All cases			Confirmed serologically		
	Number	Per cent	Probability	Number	Per cent	Probability
Amantadine	2/55	3.6		0/48	0	
			0.07			0.05–0.01
Placebo	12/85	14.1		10/69	14.5	

Contacts with serological evidence of influenza infection:

Treatment	Clinical and subclinical infections			Subclinical infections only	
Amantadine	7/48	14.6		7/48	14.6
			<0.01		0.2
Placebo	27/69	39.1		17/69	24.6

amantadine treatment of contacts (people living in the same household) of active cases of influenza A_2 results in both a decreased incidence of clinical influenza and a significant reduction in subclinical infection (i.e., where there is only serological evidence). The sample size in this study is not large but the results are representative. Amantadine certainly does not provide complete protection, but the results have been encouraging enough to warrant its use with high risk patients.

Since amantadine prevents the virus from entering the cell, it seems reasonable to assume that the drug is effective if it is given to a person before he is infected. There is also some indication, however, that the clinical course of the viral infection may be altered by the administration of amantadine after the appearance of symptoms. Several double-blind, placebo-controlled studies with serologically confirmed cases of naturally occurring A2 influenza demonstrate that amantadine treatment results in more rapid defervesence and a milder clinical course.[43,44,45] The clinical improvement is probably due to a reduction in the number of additional cells infected by the virus. Thus this drug may be of some use in the treatment, as well as the prophylaxis, of influenza A2 infection. At present, the prophylactic effect of amantadine justifies its administration on a continuous basis for up to 90 days to reduce the likelihood of infection in high risk patients during A2 influenza epidemics. The drug may be used with or without vaccine.

Amantadine is well absorbed when taken orally; maximum blood levels are reached in two to four hours. There is no evidence of metabolism of the drug in man, and the primary route of excretion is renal.[46] Amantadine has not been found to be toxic to any organ, and in animal tests it is essentially free of pharmacodynamic actions in the dose ranges used for viral chemotherapy.[47] Patients sometimes complain of subjective central nervous system side effects, including feelings of depression, drowsiness, detachment, lethargy, nervousness, and dizziness. Occasionally some patients experience tremors; however, exactly the opposite response was noted in one Parkinsonian patient who experienced a remission of her symptoms of rigidity, tremor, and akinesia while being treated with amantadine for the flu.[48] This serendipitous observation has been followed up by clinical trials that demonstrate that amantadine is of significant and persistent benefit for the patient with mild Parkinson's disease.[48,49] The mechanism of this effect is not known.

Methisazone

Structure and Mechanism of Action

   Methisazone (N-methylisatin-β-thiosemicarbazone) is one of a group of derivatives of isatin-β-thiosemicarbazone that possess antiviral activity. The mechanism of action of this compound is not well defined. Studies on the parent compound, isatin-β-thiosemicarbazone, demonstrate that the drug affects the ability of late

Methisazone

vaccinia virus mRNA to express itself normally.[50, 51] The viral mRNA, which is synthesized in cells during the first three hours of infection, is normal in size and fully functional in the presence of the drug. The late viral mRNA (produced after three hours) is apparently of normal size when synthesized, and it can enter polysomes; however, within a very short period, the RNA decreases in size, and protein synthesis is drastically reduced. As a result, few if any viral progeny are formed.

   Viruses, like bacteria, can become drug resistant. Resistance to all of the antiviral drugs in clinical use (amantadine,[52] the pyrimidine analogs,[53] and the isatin-β-thiosemicarbazones[54]) has been demonstrated. A strain of virus made resistant to isatin-β-thiosemicarbazone was also resistant to methisazone, and this suggests that the mechanism of action of the two drugs may be similar (i.e. inhibition of "late" viral protein synthesis). Another interesting observation made with this resistant subline was that the resistant viruses were much less resistant to the drug when they were replicating in cells that were also infected with the sensitive strain. One interpretation of this phenomenon is that the resistant virus is still sensitive to the action of an intermediate inhibitor produced by the sensitive virus but cannot itself produce the inhibitor. A second interpretation is that the sensitive virus produces a viral component affected by the drug, whereas the resistant virus produces a modified form of the component not affected by the drug, and the resistant virus responds to the drug-bound product of the sensitive virus.

The basis for the antiviral activity of some analogs of isatin-β-thiosemicarbazone may not be the inhibition of "late" viral protein synthesis. A study of the effects of busatin (a dibutyl-derivative of isatin-β-thiosemicarbazone) on poliovirus replication demonstrates that this analog inhibits viral RNA synthesis and, to some extent, cellular DNA synthesis, but not cellular RNA synthesis.[55] As this effect could be demonstrated in a cell-free poliovirus RNA polymerase reaction, it seems to be entirely different from the inhibition of "late" viral protein synthesis. Methisazone, the clinically useful thiosemicarbazone, does not inhibit poliovirus and clearly does not act in the same manner as busatin.

Methisazone inhibits the reproduction of poxviruses and several adenoviruses. This drug is used clinically for the prophylaxis of smallpox in people exposed to the infection. It has the advantage of being active during the incubation period of the virus at a time when vaccination would be too late to prevent the development of infection. Preliminary trials indicate that methisazone may also be useful in the treatment of eczema vaccinatum and vaccinia gangrenosa.[56]

A trial of the prophylactic effect of methisazone against smallpox was carried out in Madras, India in 1963.[57] Drug treatment of close contacts was begun 1 to 2 days after hospital admission of the patient with active smallpox. Of 2610 contacts treated, there were 18 cases of smallpox (0.69%), and 4 cases died. In the control sample of 2710 contacts, 113 cases developed active smallpox (4.17%), and 21 cases died. Methisazone has also been found to reduce the incidence of variola minor (alastrim) in contacts of active cases.[58] Although it exhibits a clinically mild course, this disease is caused by a virus that is closely related to variola major, the causative agent of smallpox. Methisazone is taken orally; the principal side effect is vomiting, which occurs in the majority of patients.

Pyrimidine Analogs

Structures and Mechanism of Action

A wide variety of pyrimidine analogs have been synthesized and tested as antiviral and anticancer drugs. The most important of these compounds in clinical antiviral therapy are 5-iodo-2'-deoxyuridine (IUdR, idoxuridine) and cytosine arabinoside. Cytosine arabinoside and another pyrimidine analog, 5-fluorouracil, are employed in the chemotherapy of cancer, and their structures and mechanisms of action are discussed in Chapter 10. IUdR is a halogenated derivative of deoxyuridine. The iodine atom has a van der Waals radius of 2.15 Å. This is approximately the size of a methyl group (2.00 Å); therefore, IUdR is able to function in many ways as an analog of thymidine (5-methyl-deoxyuridine).

IUdR   Thymidine

IUdR inhibits the replication of several DNA viruses such as herpes simplex, vaccinia, pseudorabies, adenovirus, and polyoma. With very few exceptions RNA viruses are not inhibited. One of these exceptions is the inhibition of Rous sarcoma virus,[60] which replicates its RNA genome by first synthesizing a DNA to serve as a template for further RNA synthesis.[9] The studies on the mechanism of the antiviral action of IUdR have been reviewed by Prusoff.[59] There are two levels at which IUdR could affect the biochemistry of the DNA-containing viruses. First, the drug or the phosphorylated derivatives could inhibit the formation of DNA by blocking the production of the required precursor molecules or their polymerization into DNA. Second, the incorporation of IUdR into the DNA could prevent it from functioning normally. In cells IUdR is converted to the triphosphorylated derivative, which can become incorporated into viral DNA. The drug itself competitively inhibits the thymidine kinase reaction, and IUdR monophosphate competitively inhibits the thymidylate kinase step.[61] In addition, 5-iodo-2'-deoxyuridine triphosphate may function, like the natural compound deoxythymidine triphosphate, as a feedback inhibitor of some of the reactions involved in the synthesis of pyrimidine nucleotides. These effects do not contribute in a significant way to the antiviral activity of the drug, although a feedback inhibition of pyrimidine biosynthesis may be important in explaining the toxicity of IUdR to animal cells. The triphosphate of IUdR also competes with thymidine triphosphate in a cell-free reaction directed by a DNA polymerase preparation from mammalian cells, but in the reaction the utilization of the other nucleotides is not inhibited by IUdR triphosphate in the absence of thymidine triphosphate.[59]

At present, it seems that the incorporation of the drug into viral DNA is primarily responsible for the antiviral effect. The DNA containing the halogenated compound may be altered in a number of ways. The drug-containing viral DNA, for example, is more susceptible to strand breakage,[62] an effect that could conceivably modify the ability of the altered molecule to function properly. IUdR is mutagenic in E. coli,[63] and this suggests that its presence in viral DNA could result in abnormal base-pairing to produce altered or non-functional viral proteins. Studies of the effect of IUdR on pseudorabies virus multiplication suggest that non-functional viral proteins are produced.[64] Both viral DNA and proteins are synthesized and accumulate in IUdR-treated cells; however, there is little or no assembly of these viral components into viral particles. If thymidine is added for a short period of time, the IUdR-containing DNA can enter into virus particles, demonstrating that the inability to form virus particles is not the result of a structural distortion of the DNA. This inhibition must, therefore, be the result of malfunction of some of the proteins that are coded by IUdR-containing progeny viral DNA. In addition to inhibition of viral assembly, the production of viral DNA and protein is reduced as a result of the synthesis of inactive viral protein. The selectivity of action of IUdR for the DNA virus compared to the host cell is low. When IUdR is employed topically to treat viral infections in the eye, some selective toxicity is achieved. The replication of viruses in the cell requires the rapid, sustained synthesis of DNA, whereas normal mammalian cells in the conjunctiva of the eye are not synthesizing DNA at a high rate. The drug is probably selectively toxic to the virus in this instance because the virus is synthesizing DNA at a very rapid rate and because, although the local concentration of IUdR is high, the systemic levels are too low to be toxic. Even under these conditions the rate of local wound healing may be inhibited as a result of the toxic effect on the cells of the conjunctiva.[65]

Resistance to IUdR has been demonstrated in vitro[53] and has developed during clinical treatment of herpetic keratitis.[66] The resistant cells are still sensitive to cytosine arabinoside (cytarabine), and this drug can be used to treat conjunctival lesions that develop a resistance to IUdR.

The principal use of IUdR in clinical medicine is in the treatment of herpes simplex keratitis.[67] It is applied to the eye locally in drops or as an ointment. IUdR has also been used topically for the treatment of herpes simplex infection of the skin, and for this purpose it is given in dimethylsulfoxide (DMSO), a compound that increases the absorption of the drug. The effect of IUdR on the clinical course of cutaneous herpes simplex is not dramatic; DMSO alone can shorten the process somewhat; however, recurrence of lesions at the same site is much less frequent with the drug.[68] Given as a constant intravenous infusion, IUdR has proved useful for the treatment of herpes simplex encephalitis.[69,70] The drug should be given systemically only when there is a life-threatening situation such as viral encephalitis. Varicella zoster virus is a DNA virus closely related to herpes simplex. IUdR in DMSO applied topically limits pain and accelerates healing in the disease.[71]

The topical application of IUdR results in high local concentrations of the drug, but systemic levels remain low and severe toxic effects are avoided. Toxic reactions including inflammation, itching and edema of the eyelids, and photophobia are observed with local application to the conjunctiva. Systemic administration of IUdR produces stomatitis, leukopenia, thrombocytopenia, and alopecia.[72] This complex of symptoms is seen with many drugs that are cytotoxic to mammalian cells, and they are discussed in the introduction to Chapter 10. The toxic effects of IUdR are reversible. IUdR has been reported to produce liver damage and to be teratogenic in animals. In addition to its being toxic, the systemic use of the drug is compromised by its rapid metabolism.[73]

IUdR-containing DNA is especially sensitive to the effects of radiation (strand breakage occurs, as well as cross-linking of thymidine residues, resulting in covalent linkage between the two strands in the DNA helix). For this reason the halogenated pyrimidines are being studied as possible adjuncts to X-irradiation of cancer. The IUdR-containing DNA is sensitive to ultraviolet irradiation, an effect that may contribute to the therapeutic action of the drug in the treatment of superficial infection of the conjunctiva which is exposed to some solar ultraviolet radiation.

References

1. J. W. Moulder: The Psittacosis Group as Bacteria, New York: John Wiley, 1964.

2. S. E. Luria and J. E. Darnell: General Virology (second ed.), New York: John Wiley, 1967.

3. J. D. Watson: Molecular Biology of the Gene (second edition), New York: W. A. Benjamin, 1970.

4. B. D. Davis, R. Dulbecco, H. N. Eisen, H. S. Ginsberg, and W. B. Wood: Microbiology, New York: Harper and Row, 1969.

5. G. D. Pearson: The Inhibition of Poliovirus Replication by N-Methyl-isatin-β-4':4'-dibutylthiosemicarbazone. Ph.D. Thesis, Stanford University, 1968.

6. W. K. Joklik: The intracellular uncoating of poxvirus DNA, II. The molecular basis of the uncoating process. J. Mol. Biol. 8:277 (1964).

7. J. R. Kates and B. R. McAuslan: Poxvirus DNA-dependent RNA polymerase. Proc. Natl. Acad. Sci. U.S. 58:134 (1967).

8. J. R. Kates and B. R. McAuslan: Messenger RNA synthesis by a "coated" viral genome. Proc. Natl. Acad. Sci. U.S. 57:314 (1967).

9. H. M. Temin and S. Mizutani: RNA-dependent DNA polymerase in virions of Rous sarcoma virus. 226:1211 (1970).

10. J. H. Subak-Sharpe, M. C. Timbury, and J. F. Williams: Rifampicin inhibits the growth of some mammalian viruses. *Nature* 222:341 (1969).

11. E. Heller, M. Argaman, H. Levy, and N. Goldblum: Selective inhibition of vaccinia virus by the antibiotic rifampicin. *Nature* 222:273 (1969).

12. B. Moss, E. Katz, and E. N. Rosenblum: Vaccinia virus directed RNA and protein synthesis in the presence of rifampicin. *Biochem. Biophys. Res. Commun.* 36:858 (1969).

13. B. Moss, E. N. Rosenblum, E. Katz, and P. M. Grimley: Rifampicin: a specific inhibitor of vaccinia virus assembly. *Nature* 229:1280 (1969).

14. R. Z. Lockart: "Biological properties of interferons; criteria for acceptance of a viral inhibitor as an interferon." in *Interferons*, ed. by N. B. Finter, Philadelphia: W. B. Saunders, 1966, pp. 1–20.

15. E. DeClercq and T. Merigan: Current concepts of interferon and interferon induction. *Ann. Rev. Med.* 21:17 (1970).

16. M. R. Hilleman: Interferon induction and utilization. *J. Cell, Physiol.* 71:43 (1968).

17. M. S. Finkelstein, G. H. Bausek, and T. C. Merigan: Interferon inducers *in vitro*: Difference in sensitivity to inhibitors of RNA and protein synthesis. *Science* 161:465 (1968).

18. A. Buchan and D. C. Burke: Interferon production in chick-embryo cells. The effect of puromycin and p-fluorophenylalanine. *Biochem. J.* 98:530 (1966).

19. R. R. Wagner and A. S. Huang: Reversible inhibition of interferon synthesis by puromycin: Evidence for an interferon-specific messenger RNA. *Proc. Natl. Acad. Sci. U.S.* 54:1112 (1965).

20. J. Taylor: Studies on the mechanism of action of interferon. I. Interferon action and RNA synthesis in chick embryo fibroblasts infected with Semliki Forest virus. *Virology* 25:340 (1965).

21. S. Levine: Effect of actinomycin D and puromycin dehydrochloride on action of interferon. *Virology* 24:586 (1964).

22. R. M. Friedman: Inhibition of arbovirus protein synthesis by interferon. *J. Virol.* 2:1081 (1968).

23. H. B. Levy and W. A. Carter: Molecular basis of the action of interferon. *J. Mol. Biol.* 31:561 (1968).

24. W. K. Joklik and T. C. Merigan: Concerning the mechanism of action of interferon. *Proc. Natl. Acad. Sci.* 56:558 (1966).

25. W. A. Carter and H. B. Levy: The recognition of viral RNA by mammalian ribosomes. An effect of interferon. *Biochim. Biophys. Acta* 155:437 (1968).

26. P. I. Marcus and J. M. Salb: Molecular basis of interferon action: Inhibition of viral RNA translation. *Virology* 30:502 (1966).

27. S. Baron, C. E. Buckler, R. V. McCloskey, and R. L. Kirschstein: Role of interferon during viremia. I. Production of circulating interferon. *J. Immunol.* 96:12 (1966).

28. M. R. Hilleman: Double-stranded RNA's (poly I:C) in the prevention of viral infections. *Arch. Int. Med.* 126:109 (1970).

29. D. A. Hill, S. Baron, and R. M. Chanock: Sensitivity of common respiratory viruses to an interferon inducer in human cells. *Lancet* 2:187 (1969).

30. E. DeClercq and T. Merigan: Induction of interferon by nonviral agents. *Arch. Int. Med.* 126:94 (1970).

31. M. Absher and W. R. Stinebring: Toxic properties of a synthetic double-stranded RNA. *Nature* 223:715 (1969).

32. H. L. Lindsay, P. W. Trown, J. Brandt, and M. Forbes: Pyrogenicity of poly I: poly C in rabbits. *Nature* 223:717 (1969).

33. R. H. Adamson and S. Fabro: Embryotoxic effect of poly I. poly C. *Nature* 223: 718 (1969).

34. A. D. Steinberg, S. Baron, and N. Talal: The pathogenesis of autoimmunity in New Zealand mice, I. Induction of antinucleic acid antibodies by polyinosinic polycytidylic acid. *Proc. Natl. Acad. Sci. U.S.* 63:1103 (1969).

35. C. E. Hoffmann, E. M. Neumayer, R. F. Haff, and R. A. Goldsby: Mode of action of the antiviral activity of amantadine in tissue culture. *J. Bacteriol.* 90:623 (1965).

36. W. L. Davies, R. R. Grunert, R. F. Haff, J. W. McGahen, E. M. Neumayer, M. Paulshock, J. C. Watts, T. R. Wood, E. C. Hermann, and C. E. Hoffman: Antitiviral activity of 1-adamantanamine (Amantadine). *Science* 144:862 (1964).

37. E. M. Neumayer, R. F. Haff, and C. E. Hoffman: Antiviral activity of amantadine hydrochloride in tissue culture and *in ovo. Proc. Soc. Exptl. Biol. Med.* 119:393 (1965).

38. H. F. Maassab and K. W. Cochran: Rubella virus: Inhibition *in vitro* by amantadine hydrochloride. *Science* 145:3639 (1964).

39. A. B. Sabin: Amantadine hydrochloride. *J. Am. Med. Assoc.* 200:135 (1967).

40. Y. Togo, R. B. Hornick, and A. T. Dawkins: Studies on induced influenza in man. I. Double-blind studies designed to assess prophylactic efficacy of amantadine hydrochloride against A2/Rockville/1/65 strain. *J. Am. Med. Assoc.* 203:1089 (1968).

41. A. T. Dawkins, L. R. Gallager, Y. Togo, R. B. Hornick, and B. A. Harris: Studies on induced influenza in man. II. Double-blind study designed to assess the prophylactic efficacy of an analogue of amantadine hydrochloride. *J. Am. Med. Assoc.* 203:1095 (1968).

42. A. W. Galbraith, J. S. Oxford, G. C. Schild, and G. I. Watson: Protective effect of 1-adamantanamine hydrochloride on influenza A2 infections in the family environment, *Lancet* 2:1026 (1969).

43. W. L. Wingfield, D. Pollack, and R. R. Grunert: Therapeutic efficacy of amantadine HCl and rimantidine HCl in naturally occurring influenza A2 respiratory illness in man. *New Eng. J. Med.* 281:579: (1969).

44. Y. Togo, R. B. Hornick, V. J. Felitti, M. L. Kaufman, A. T. Dawkins, V. E. Kilpe, and J. L. Claghorn: Evaluation of therapeutic efficacy of amantadine in patients with naturally occurring A_2 influenza. *J. Am. Med. Assoc.* 211:1149 (1970).

45. A. W. Galbraith, J. S. Oxford, G. C. Schild, C. W. Potter, and G. I. Watson: Therapeutic effect of 1-adamantanamine hydrochloride in naturally occurring influenza A_2/Hong Kong infection. A controlled double-blind study. *Lancet* 2:113 (1971).

46. W. E. Bleidner, J. B. Harmon, W. E. Hewes, T. E. Lynes, and E. C. Hermann: Absorption, distribution and excretion of amantadine hydrochloride. *J. Pharm. Exptl. Ther.* 150:484 (1965).

47. V. G. Vernier, J. B. Harmon, J. M. Stump, T. E. Lynes, J. P. Marvel, and D. H. Smith: The toxicologic and pharmacologic properties of amantadine hydrochloride. *Toxic. Appl. Pharmacol.* 15:642 (1969).

48. R. S. Schwab, A. C. England, D. C. Poskanzer, and R. R. Young: Amantadine in the treatment of Parkinson's disease. *J. Am. Med. Assoc.* 208:1168 (1969).

49. J. D. Parkes, R. C. H. Baxter, G. Curzon, R. P. Knill-Jones, P. J. Knott, C. D. Marsden, R. Tattersall, and D. Vollum: Treatment of Parkinson's disease with amantadine and levodopa. A one year study. 1:1083 (1971).

50. W. K. Joklik: "Studies on the mode of action of two antiviral agents: Isatin-β-thiosemicarbazone and interferon" in *Medical and Applied Virology*. ed. by M. Sanders and E. H. Lennette, St. Louis: Warren H. Green, 1968, pp. 299–326.

51. B. Woodson and W. K. Joklik: The inhibition of vaccinia virus multiplication by isatin-β-thiosemicarbazone. *Proc. Natl. Acad. Sci. U.S.* 54:946 (1965).

52. J. S. Oxford, I. S. Logan, and C. W. Potter: *In vivo* selection of an influenza A_2 strain resistant to amantadine. *Nature* 226:82 (1970).

53. H. E. Renis and D. A. Buthala: Development of resistance to antiviral drugs. *Ann. N.Y. Acad Sci.* 130:343 (1965).

54. G. Appleyand and H. J. Way: Thiosemicarbazone-resistant rabbitpox virus. *Brit. J. Exptl. Path.* 47:144 (1966).

55. G. D. Pearson and E. F. Zimmerman: Inhibition of poliovirus replication by N-methylisatin-β-4':4'-dibutylthiosemicarbazone. *Virology* 38:641 (1969).

56. D. J. Bauer: Clinical experience with the antiviral drug Marboran ® (1-methylisatin 3-thiosemicarbazone). *Ann. N.Y. Acad. Sci.* 130:110 (1965).

57. D. J. Bauer, L. St. Vincent, C. H. Kempe, P. A. Young, and A. W. Downie: Prophylaxis of smallpox with methisazone. *Am. J. Epidemiol.* 90:130 (1969).

58. L. A. R. de Valle, P. R. de Melo, L. F. De Salles Gomez, and L. M. Proenca: Methisazone in prevention of variola minor among contacts. *Lancet* 2:976 (1965).

59. W. H. Prussoff: Recent advances in the chemotherapy of viral diseases. *Pharm. Rev.* 19:209 (1967).

60. E. E. Force and R. C. Stewart: Effect of 5-iodo-2'-deoxyuridine on the multiplication of Rous sarcoma virus *in vitro. Proc. Soc. Exp. Biol. Med.* 116:803 (1964).

61. W. H. Prusoff, Y. S. Bakhle, and L. Sekely: Cellular and antiviral effects of halogenated deoxyribonucleosides. *Ann. N.Y. Acad. Sci.* 130:135 (1965).

62. J. F. McCrea and M. B. Lipman: Strand-length measurements of normal and 5-iodo-2'-deoxyuridine-treated vaccinia virus deoxyribonucleic acid released by the Kleinschmidt method. *J. Virol.* 1:1037 (1967).

63. Z. Lorkiewicz: Effects of incorporation of iododeoxyuridine on *Escherichia coli. Nature* 197:314 (1963).

64. A. S. Kaplan and T. Ben-Porat: Mode of antiviral action of 5-iodouracil deoxyriboside. *J. Mol. Biol.* 19:320 (1966).

65. P. Payrau and C. H. Dohlman: IDU in corneal wound healing. *Am. J. Ophthal.* 57:999 (1964).

66. P. R. Laibson, T. W. Sery, and I. H. Leopold: The treatment of herpetic keratitis with 5-iodo-2'-deoxyuridine (IDU). *Arch. Ophthal.* 70:52 (1963).

67. H. E. Kaufman: Problems in virus chemotherapy. *Progr. Med. Virol.* 7:116 (1965).

68. F. O. MacCallum and B. E. Juel-Jensen: Herpes simplex virus infection in man treated with idoxuridine in dimethyl sulfoxide. Results of double-blind control trial. *Br. Med. J.* 2:805 (1966).

69. D. C. Nolan, M. M. Carruthers, and A. M. Lerner: Herpesvirus hominis encephalitis in Michigan: Report of thirteen cases, including six treated with idoxuridine. *New Eng. J. Med.* 282:10 (1970).

70. H. Ashton, E. Frenk and C. J. Stevenson: Herpes simplex virus infections and idoxuridine. *Br. J. Derm.* 84:496 (1971).

71. B. E. Juel-Jensen, F. O. MacCallum, A. M. R. Mackenzie, and M. C. Pike: Treatment of zoster with idoxuridine in dimethyl sulfoxide. Results of two double-blind controlled trials. *Br. Med. J.* 4:776 (1970).

72. P. Calabresi: Current status of clinical investigations with 6-azauridine, 5-iodo-2'-deoxyuridine, and related derivatives. *Cancer Res.* 23:1260 (1963).

73. A. D. Welch and W. H. Prusoff: A synopsis of recent investigations of 5-iodo-2'-deoxyuridine. *Cancer Chem. Rep.* 6:29 (1960).

There are many differences between the drug treatment of infectious or parasitic disease and of cancer. The rationale underlying treatment of infectious or parasitic disease is epitomized by the concept of selective toxicity. The biochemistry of the pathogenic organism is in many ways qualitatively different from that of the host, thereby providing specific points where growth of the organism can be selectively inhibited. On the other hand, the differences that have been defined between cancer cells and normal cells are largely quantitative (differences in the rate of cell division or in properties related to invasiveness), and treatment with the cytotoxic drugs is for the most part based on a nonselective interference in cell growth.

Normal cell populations are kept within certain size limits by a number of mechanisms (most of them undefined) controlling the rates of cell division and degradation that set their steady state level. In cancer cells the mechanisms controlling the rate of cell growth are either less responsive or nonexistent. The most pernicious aspect of this change is that cancer cells often develop the capacity to invade neighboring tissue areas and to grow at distant sites after being transported in the blood or the lymphatics. These capacities for invasion and transplantability account for the malignancy of many tumors, which so often compromises the possibility of completely eradicating the tumor process by local surgical excision or radiotherapy.

Rapidly growing neoplastic cells become dedifferentiated. That is, they lose the ability to express certain enzymatic functions of the differentiated cells from which they arise. This loss of function differs greatly from one type of tumor to another. Asparagine synthetase activity, for instance, is lost in some human leukemia cells and some animal tumors that cannot synthesize the amino acid asparagine. The former observation has led to the use of asparaginase (an enzyme that degrades the free amino acid in the blood) in the treatment of acute leukemias. Normal cells, which can synthesize asparagine intracellularly, survive, but the neoplastic cells are selectively starved for the amino acid. In addition to quantitative differences in enzyme levels between normal cells and cancer cells, there are morphological differences by which pathologists can diagnose tumor processes. Rapidly growing tumor cells often exhibit gross karyotypic abnormalities, including excessive and abnormal chromosomes. In general, however, it can be stated that no common factor distinguishing cancer cells from normal cells has yet been identified; thus there is no focus for specific chemotherapeutic attack to destroy cancer cells without also adversely affecting normal cells.

Certain therapeutically useful properties of the normal cell type are sometimes retained by tumor cells. For example, tumors of hormone-sensitive cells often retain their ability to respond to steroid hormones, and this response has been exploited. The use of sex steroid hormones in the treatment of carcinoma of the prostate, breast, and endometrium and of glucocorticoid steroids in lymphocytic leukemias are examples of this type of drug therapy.

The treatment of infection by drug administration is potentiated by the body's immune response to foreign substances. This is not generally the case in chemotherapy of neoplastic disease. Until recently it was felt that tumor cells could not elicit an antibody response in the host, but recent evidence casts doubt on this belief. The studies of Gold,[1,2] for example, suggest that certain tumors of the gastrointestinal tract may produce substances that initiate the production of specific antibodies in the patient. These antigens are similar or identical to substances present in embryonic and fetal gut, pancreas, and liver during the first two trimesters of gestation (they have been called carcinoembryonic antigens). The possibility that antigenic substances present in the embryo are re-expressed in certain carcinomas may lead to an immunological approach to the treatment of these tumors in the future.

Two tumors respond remarkably well to chemotherapy: choriocarcinoma in the female and Burkitt's lymphoma. The basis for the relatively high rate of cure in these tumors is probably related to the patient's ability to develop antibodies to the tumor cells. The choriocarcinoma is unique in that it develops from fetal tissue (epithelial cells covering the chorionic villi) and not from maternal tissue. In Burkitt's lymphoma, there is a good deal of evidence suggesting that a virus is associated with the lymphoma[3] and that tumor-specific immune reactions are elicited in patients with the disease.[4] It has been demonstrated that patients with

Burkitt's tumor who benefit the most from chemotherapy have a higher titer of antibodies than those who do not respond well. These two tumors are major exceptions, and there is no measurable immune response to most tumors. In order to eliminate a tumor by means of chemotherapy, at the present time, it is thus probably necessary to kill *all* the tumor cells by drug action alone.

The possibility of eliciting an immune response, or augmenting low level responses, is nevertheless one of the most promising approaches to cancer therapy being investigated today. It has been proved that a number of experimental tumors are caused by viruses, and there is a reasonable possibility that some human cancers are of viral origin. If this proves to be the case, then immunotherapy may well become a more important clinical tool in advanced cancer than chemotherapy. In contrast to most drugs used in the treatment of infectious disease, many of the drugs employed in cancer chemotherapy suppress the immune response. In addition to suppressing the patient's ability to fight infection (which is most often the immediate cause of death in malignancies), this effect may be counter productive in some tumors where low level immune responses might possibly be elicited.

In most cases the criteria for success in the treatment of infectious or parasitic disease are the patient's return to well being and the elimination of the organism. An analogous goal, complete tumor regression without recurrence, is not a useful way for the physician to judge the effectiveness of his treatment of neoplastic disease. Complete cures of localized cancers may be achieved by surgical resection and in some cases by radiotherapy or a combination of the two methods. In the two cases already mentioned, Burkitt's lymphoma and choriocarcinoma, the achievement of tumor regression through chemotherapy has been successful enough to make complete cure a realistic goal. With other tumors, however, clinical success is measured in terms of the patient's survival for a longer period than with other treatment regimens. In a number of tumor types chemotherapy may be palliative without prolonging life. In these cases a favorable response to therapy is gauged by alleviation of the patient's symptoms, improvement in cellular functions as determined by laboratory assessment, and regression in tumor size (or the extent of tumor-associated pathology such as effusions) as determined by palpation and radiological measurement. In some cancers, such as melanoma or carcinoma of the bladder, chemotherapy is rarely palliative, or the patient's symptomatic relief is only transient. With the exception of steroid hormones, the drugs used in cancer chemotherapy are extremely toxic and give the patient a great deal of distress. Chemotherapy must be considered only after surgery and/or radiotherapy are judged inappropriate. In the advanced stages of some cancers, which respond poorly to the anticancer drugs, there is a very real decision to be made regarding the use of chemotherapy directed against the disease process itself or merely symtomatic therapy to minimize the patient's suffering. As Hiatt has pointed out, this is a positive clincal decision, it is not a decision ". . . to neglect or to abandon the patient and his family . . .".[5]

It would go beyond the limits of this text to present a discussion of the drug therapy of neoplastic disease from the clinical standpoint of indications for drug use and specific management of different tumors. The reader is referred here to three concisely written books that deal with this aspect of the subject.[6,7,8] It is also beyond our scope to delve deeply into the research in molecular biology, immunology, and virology that is changing our concept of the chemotherapy of cancer. For a view of this research the reader is referred to the symposium, *A Critical Evaluation of Cancer Chemotherapy.*[9] The next chapter describes the mechanisms of action and the pharmacology of some of the drugs most widely used in the therapy of neoplastic disease. The mechanisms are in many cases well worked out and often quite different from the mechanisms of action of any of the drugs employed in the treatment of infectious or parasitic disease. It is encouraging that several of the anticancer drugs were developed, by logical design of a molecule, to interfere with well-defined biochemical processes for the treatment of a specific disease. This is the opposite of discovering that a natural plant product inhibits cell growth and then determining the mechanism of inhibition. With the extension of our knowledge of the molecular biology of the cell in lower life forms and man, logical drug design will become the basis for developing new agents in the treatment of both infectious and neoplastic disease.

References

1. P. Gold and S. O. Freedman: Demonstration of tumor-specific antigens in human colonic carcinomata by immunological tolerance and absorption techniques. *J. Exptl. Med.* 121:439 (1965).
2. P. Gold and S. O. Freedman: Specific carcinoembryonic antigens of the human digestive system. *J. Exptl. Med.* 122: 467 (1965).
3. M. A. Epstein, B. G. Achong and Y. M. Barr: Virus particles in cultured lymphoblasts from Burkitt's lymphoma. *Lancet* 1:702 (1964).
4. G. Klein, P. Clifford, E. Klein, and J. Stjernsward: "Search for tumor specific immune reactions in Burkitt lymphoma patients by the membrane immunofluorescence reaction" in *Treatment of Burkitt's Tumor,* ed. by J. H. Burchenal and D. P. Burkitt. Berlin: Springer-Verlag. 1967, pp. 209–232.
5. H. H. Hiatt: Cancer chemotherapy—Present status and prospects. *New Eng. J. Med.* 276:157 (1967).
6. W. H. Cole, ed.: *Chemotherapy of Cancer.* Philadelphia; Lea and Febisher, 1970.
7. E. Boesen and W. Davis: *Cytotoxic Drugs in the Treatment of Cancer.* London. Edward Arnold. 1969.
8. M. J. Cline: *Cancer Chemotherapy.* Philadelphia. W. B. Saunders. 1971.
9. Symposium (Various authors): A Critical Evaluation of Cancer Chemotherapy *Cancer Res.* 29:2261–2485 (1969).

Chapter 10

The Anticancer Drugs

Introduction

General Features of the Toxicity of Cytotoxic Drugs

Certain types of cells in the adult human replicate very rapidly under normal growth conditions. This rapid growth is seen, for example, in the cells of the bone marrow that are responsible for continually supplying the body with leukocytes, lymphocytes, erythrocytes, and platelets. The cells of the mucosa of the gastro-intestinal tract are constantly sloughed off and regenerated. The cells of the hair follicles, the germinal epithelium in the testis, and extra-marrow sites of lymphocyte synthesis like the thymus normally turn over at a rapid rate. Indeed, the normal generation rate of these cells is higher than that observed for most neoplastic cells. The action of cytotoxic drugs, such as alkylating agents and anti-metabolites, is non-selective with respect to normal and neoplastic cells. When these drugs are employed in doses sufficient to inhibit the rate of growth of tumor cells, they will also have an effect on normal cells possessing a high turnover rate. Most of the anti-cancer drugs possess a therapeutic index that is virtually unity— that is, at an effective therapeutic level, toxic effects are also observed.

Depression of the growth rate of rapidly dividing cells accounts for a complex of toxic symptoms that is observed with high doses of almost all the anticancer drugs. Depression of bone-marrow and lymphoid cells results in leukocytopenia, lymphocytopenia, and thrombocytopenia. Thus, many patients who are receiving a course of chemotherapy with a cytotoxic drug will have an increased tendency to hemorrhage and a decreased ability to fight infection. Anemia also occurs, but the depression in erythrocyte count develops at a slower rate than the depression in leukocyte and platelet counts. The cytotoxic effect on the cells of the hair follicles results in alopecia. Ulceration of the oral and intestinal mucosa also occurs, with symptoms of gastrointestinal distress like vomiting and diarrhea. The cell destruction that results from the drug action is sometimes responsible for releasing large amounts of nucleic acid degradation products into the system. For this reason, high levels of serum uric acid are seen during therapy of certain cancers, and renal function may be impaired. These general toxic effects are extremely distressing to the patient. In addition to the common cytotoxic properties, the individual drugs produce a variety of specific toxic effects that will be discussed later in this chapter.

Anticancer Drugs and the Cell Cycle

In considering the inhibition of mammalian cell growth by drugs, it is helpful to relate drug action to the ordered cycle of events that occurs during the course of a cell generation. As presented in Figure 10-1, the division cycle of animal cells consists of four phases. G_1 is the interval following cell division to the point where DNA synthesis begins. In general the variability in the length of the cell cycle between rapidly replicating cells and slowly replicating cells is accounted for by differences in the length of the G_1 interval.[1] Dormant cells, that is cells not in the process of preparing for cell division, are considered to be in a subphase of G_1 called G_0. The S phase is that portion of the cell cycle during which DNA synthesis takes place; it lasts most often six to eight hours.[2] G_2 is the premitotic interval or postsynthetic phase, and it is shorter than the S phase. During the G_2 period, RNA and protein synthesis, but not DNA synthesis, take place. During mitosis, the M phase, synthetic activity of the cell is low, and the chromosomes separate into two daughter cells—a process that has been divided on morphological grounds into the subphases prophase, metaphase, anaphase, and telophase.

Some cytotoxic drugs are effective in inhibiting cell replication during only one phase of the division cycle. These drugs are characterized as cell cycle-dependent. For example, vinblastine and vincristine act in mitosis, while methotrexate, arabinosylcytosine, and fluorouracil, all inhibiting DNA synthesis, act in the S phase. The alkylating agents are cytotoxic for cells at any point in the division cycle and are therefore called cell cycle-independent agents. It is important to realize that neoplastic cells are not

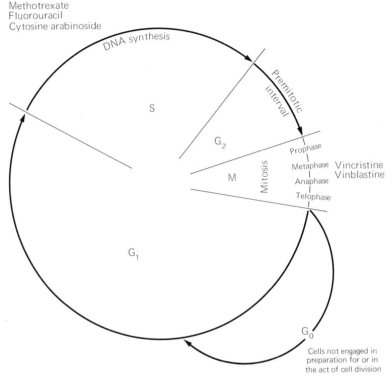

Figure 10-1   The cell cycle. G_1 is the period between mitosis and the beginning of DNA synthesis. In G_0 cells are dormant. S is the period of DNA synthesis; G_2 is the premitotic interval; and M is the period of mitosis. Examples of cell cycle-dependent anticancer drugs are listed next to the phase at which they act.

always in a state of rapid division. A significant proportion of the cells in a tumor may be in G_0, and cell cycle-dependent drugs will have little or no effect on cells in G_1 or G_0. Some evidence indicates that a course of cell cycle-independent therapy resulting in reduction of the number of neoplastic cells will be followed by a recruitment of the resting cells into active replication, at which point they will be sensitive to cell cycle-dependent drugs. For example, after X-irradiation (a cell cycle-independent modality) of rat rhabdomyosarcomas, the cells that are still able to proliferate have a shorter average cell cycle time than the tumor cells had before x-irradiation.[4]

The Alkylating Drugs

The alkylating drugs were developed from the sulfur mustard gases used during World War I. It was observed on autopsy of soldiers who were killed in gas attacks that the mustard gas caused bone-marrow aplasia, leukopenia, dissolution of lymphoid tissue, and ulcerations of the mucosa of the gastrointestinal tract.[5] Research conducted between the wars led to the development of the nitrogen mustards. Because of their antilymphocytic properties the effect of nitrogen mustards on lymphosarcoma in mice was studied. The first human application of these drugs in the treatment of cancer was carried out in 1942 on a patient with far advanced lymphosarcoma.[6] A number of alkylating agents have been developed for clinical use since then. There are three major chemical classes of these drugs: the nitrogen mustards, the ethylenimines, and the methanesulfonic acid esters. The structure of important members of each class is presented in Figure 10-2.

The Mechanism of Action of the Alkylating Drugs

The Chemical Reaction

The alkylating drugs are highly reactive compounds that form covalent bonds with a variety of nucleophilic groups. The proposed reaction mechanism for the nitrogen mustards is presented in Figure 10-3. Under neutral or alkaline conditions, one of the chlorethyl side chains undergoes a cyclization, releasing chloride ion and forming an immonium ion intermediate. This intermediate is highly reactive; strained ring scission yields the electrophilic carbonium ion that reacts with water or with nucleophilic groups like amino, carboxyl, phosphate, or sulfhydryl groups of proteins and nucleic acids. One favored reaction of great importance in producing the cytotoxic effect is the formation of a covalent bond between the drug and the 7-nitrogen group of guanine. After forming a covalent bond with one molecule, the bifunctional alkylating agents (those containing two reactive chloroethyl side chains) can then undergo a similar cyclization of the second side chain and form a covalent bond with a second nucleophilic group. This second reaction could involve the 7-nitrogen group of another

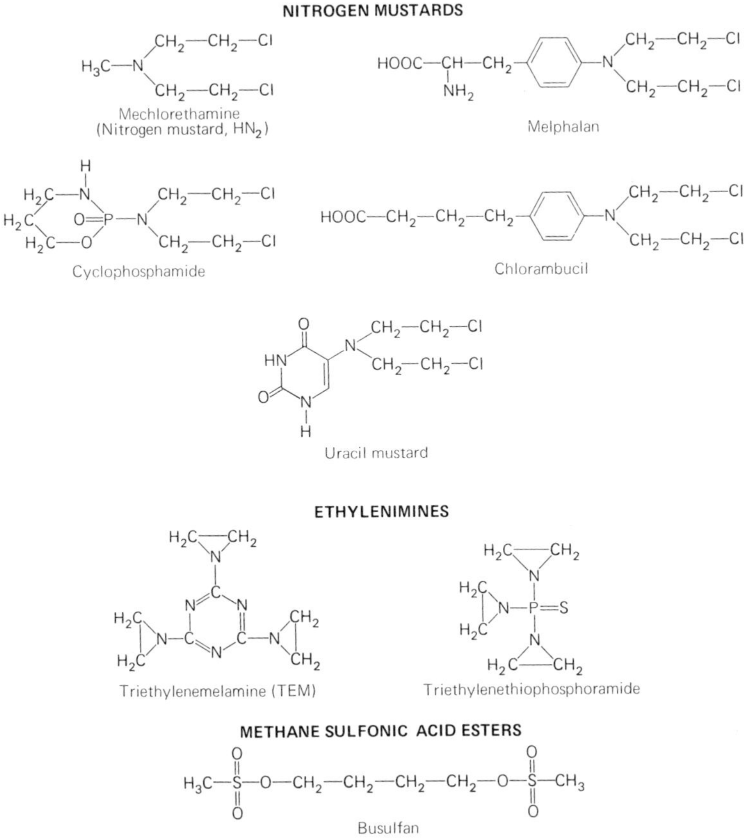

Figure 10-2 Structures of some of the major alkylating drugs.

guanine or some other nucleophilic moiety. This sequence of reactions can have a number of results. For example, adjacent DNA strands may become cross-linked, a DNA strand may be cross-linked to proteins, protein-protein linkages can occur.

The alkylating agents are potent mutagens. Experiments with monofunctional alkylating agents have demonstrated that a guanine with the drug covalently bonded to the 7-nitrogen can form anomalous base pairs with thymine. The major mutagenic effect of the alkylating drugs seems to result from the subsequent transi-

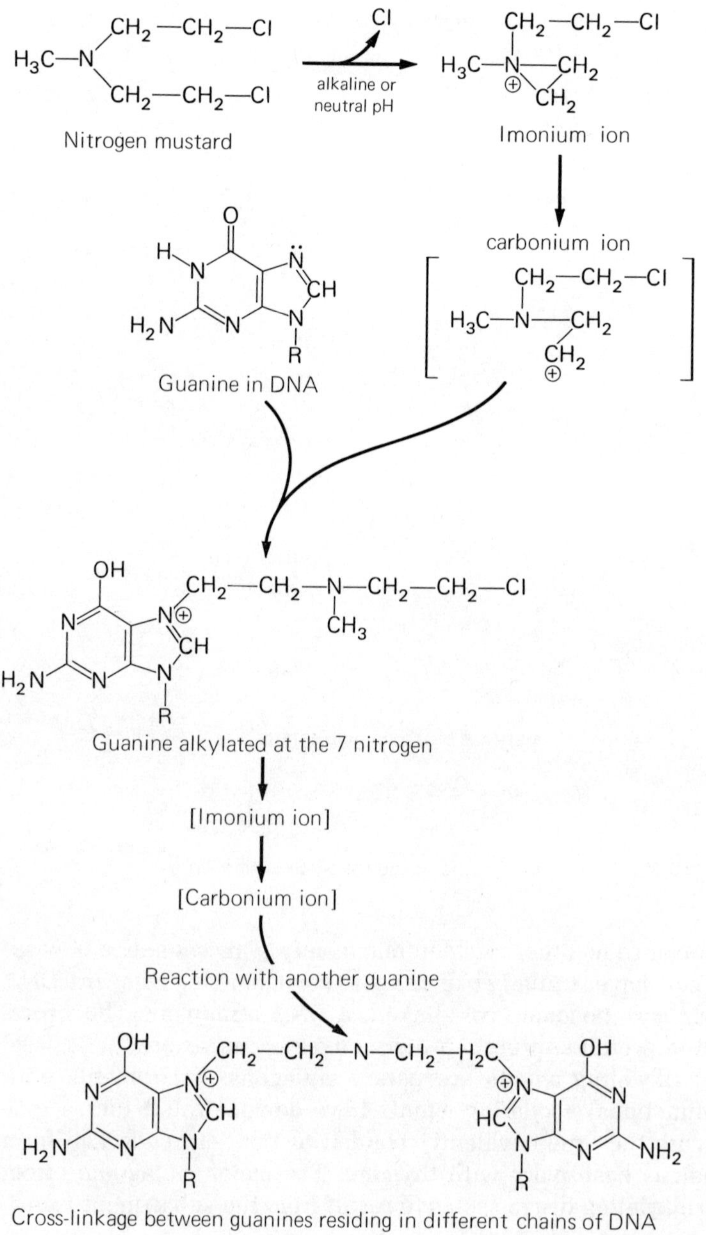

H₃C—N with CH₂—CH₂—Cl and CH₂—CH₂—Cl

Nitrogen mustard

alkaline or neutral pH

Imonium ion

carbonium ion

Guanine in DNA

Guanine alkylated at the 7 nitrogen

[Imonium ion]

[Carbonium ion]

Reaction with another guanine

Cross-linkage between guanines residing in different chains of DNA

tions from guanine-cytosine base pairs to adenine-thymine.[7] Depurination of the DNA and splitting of the imidazole ring can also occur as a result of the alkylation of the 7-nitrogen group of guanine.

The Cross-Linking of DNA

The alkylating agents in high enough concentrations affect a wide variety of biochemical events in the cell.[8] The best evidence available indicates that the cytotoxicity of the drug at therapeutic levels is mainly due to inhibition of DNA synthesis. It has been demonstrated that nitrogen mustard in low doses inhibits the synthesis of DNA by mammalian cells in culture more rapidly and to a greater extent than it inhibits RNA or protein synthesis.[9] Studies with other difunctional alkylating agents have demonstrated that DNA synthesis is preferentially inhibited in sarcoma 180 cells *in vivo*[10] and in *E. coli.*[11]

Although alkylating agents in high enough doses will inhibit a number of reactions necessary for the synthesis of DNA by mammalian cells and bacteria, it is the interaction between the drug and DNA itself that promises to be the most meaningful with respect to the major cytotoxic effect. The possibility that alkylating agents may form cross-links between the two DNA strands in the double helix was suggested by the observation that DNA treated with nitrogen mustard is converted to a reversibly denaturable form.[12] The type of experiment that suggests this (Figure 10-4) and the interpretation of the data are as follows: DNA purified from *Bacillus subtilis* is treated with various concentrations of nitrogen mustard; the solution of treated DNA is adjusted to alkaline pH for 1.5 minutes, neutralized, and dialyzed against a buffer. When normal double-stranded, helical DNA is made

Figure 10-3 The mechanism by which nitrogen mustard becomes covalently bonded to the 7 nitrogens of two guanines. In solution the drug forms a reactive cyclic intermediate that reacts with the 7 nitrogen of a guanine residue in DNA to form a covalent linkage. The second arm can then cyclize and react with nucleophilic groups such as a second guanine moiety in an opposite DNA strand or in the same strand. Reactions between DNA and RNA and between DNA and protein also occur.

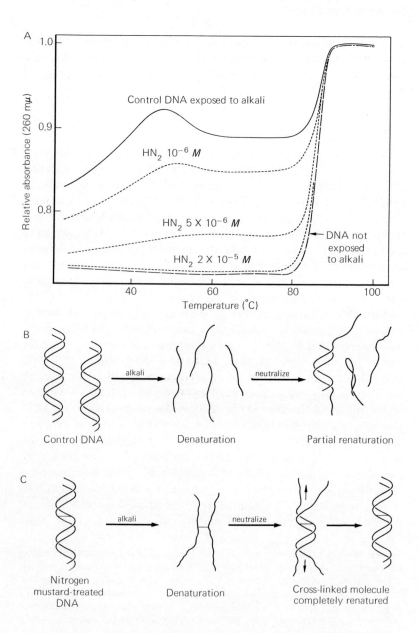

A

B

Control DNA   Denaturation   Partial renaturation

C

Nitrogen
mustard-treated
DNA   Denaturation   Cross-linked molecule
completely renatured

alkaline, the DNA denatures to yield two separated strands. When the solution is neutralized, portions of the DNA strands containing appropriate hydrogen-bonding sequences come into opposition on a random basis, and partial renaturation takes place (Figure 10-4, B). The partially renatured DNA solution contains a large amount of single-stranded DNA. Single-stranded DNA absorbs more light at 260 mμ than the native, double-stranded DNA. This can be seen in the melting curve profile of the treated DNA (Figure 10-4, A) as an elevated baseline of absorbance at temperatures lower than that at which thermal transition from double-stranded to single-stranded DNA takes place. This baseline is much lower in samples exposed to nitrogen mustard prior to denaturation in alkali and subsequent neutralization. The drug effect is outlined in Figure 10-4, C. Nitrogen mustard has formed a cross-link between the two strands of DNA. In the alkali hydrogen bonding is disrupted, and strand separation takes place. Strands which are cross-linked by the drug, however, are oriented so that renaturation is more complete than with the control DNA where appropriate sequences for hydrogen bonding must come into apposition on a purely random basis.

Figure 10-4 The effect of interstrand cross linkage on the ability of DNA to renature. A. Purified *B. subtilis* DNA or samples of the same DNA treated with various concentrations of nitrogen mustard were made alkaline for 1.5 minutes, neutralized, and dialyzed against buffer. Melting curves were then carried out on each DNA sample. The graph presents the absorbance of each sample at 260 mμ, expressed as a fraction of the absorbance of fully denatured DNA, versus temperature. Solid line, control DNA which was treated with alkali and neutralized; dotted lines, DNA treated with various concentrations of nitrogen mustard then alkali and neutralized; dashed line, untreated DNA (i.e., not exposed to either drug or alkali treatment). (From Kohn, Spears and Doty.[13]) B. A schematic presentation of the response of normal double-stranded DNA to alkali treatment and neutralization. In alkali the native DNA denatures; upon neutralization partial renaturation takes place as possible hydrogen-bonding sequences on the single strands become opposed to one another in a random fashion. C. A schematic presentation of the response to denaturation and renaturation of DNA that has been cross-linked by nitrogen mustard. Under alkaline conditions the hydrogen bonding of the double-stranded DNA is dissolved, but the strands are held together by the drug. On neutralization, complete renaturation takes place ("zipping up" process indicated by the vertical arrows) because the complementary DNA strands are able to reassume the "correct" hydrogen-bonding sequence.

In other words the two drug-linked strands are able to "zip up" in their normal base-pairing relationships.

Other experiments designed to demonstrate that the bi-functional alkylating agents form cross-links between the two strands of the DNA helix have confirmed this hypothesis. Interstrand cross-linking is certainly not the only reaction of biological importance between the drug and DNA. Actually, about five times more monoalkylation products than dialkylation products form.[14] Not all of the diguaninyl derivative formed on reaction of sulfur mustard with DNA can be accounted for as interstrand cross-linkages.[14, 15] Some of the diguaninyl-drug products are formed by reaction of the nitrogen mustard with two guanines in the same DNA strand. The monofunctional alkylating agents can form only one covalent bond with DNA. Of course, they cannot cross-alkylate two DNA strands, and they are considerably less potent cytotoxic agents than their bifunctional analogs.

Resistance to the Alkylating Drugs

There is evidence to support the concept that formation of the diguaninyl-drug product is the major lethal event that accounts for the cytotoxicity of the alkylating agents. The most convincing evidence has been derived from studies on bacterial cells that have become resistant to concentrations of the alkylating agents lethal to the sensitive parent strains. There are a number of ways in which cells can become resistant to the action of the alkylating agents. Many of these resistance mechanisms are not particularly helpful in elucidating the mechanism of action of the drug. For example, it has been demonstrated that resistant Ehrlich ascites tumor cells have a decreased ability to take up the drug.[16] This mechanism, although interesting, does not provide any insight into the mechanism of the drug's cytotoxic action. However, experiments with a strain of E. coli resistant to both alkylating drugs and ultraviolet irradiation (ultraviolet radiation produces covalent interstrand cross-linking between thymidine residues) have demonstrated that the drug-DNA interaction is crucial for the cytotoxic effect in bacteria. The drug resistance of these cells is due to an increased ability of the resistant cells to excise the cross-

linked residues in the DNA and repair the defect. The existence of
a mechanism for excision and repair of thymidine dimers in DNA
is well established.[17] In the experiment presented in Figure 10-5
drug-resistant (*E. coli* B/r) and drug-sensitive (*E.coli* B/s) bacteria
are exposed to a submaximal concentration of radioactive-labeled
sulfur mustard (10^{-4} M); they are then diluted into a growth
medium, and growth is allowed to proceed.[11] The amount of radio-

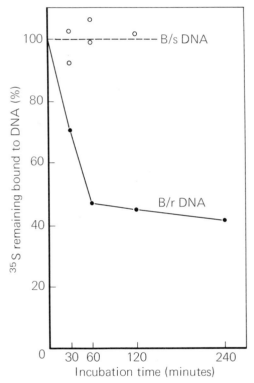

Figure 10-5 Excision of radioactive-labeled sulfur mustard from the DNA
of drug-resistant *E. coli*. Drug-resistant (B/r) and drug-sensitive (B/s) *E. coli*
were exposed to 25 µg/m1 of ^{35}S-mustard gas and diluted into growth medium.
The amount of ^{35}S remaining bound to the DNA of sensitive and resistant cells
was measured at various times of growth after dilution into drug-free medium.
(From Lawley and Brookes.[11])

active drug associated with the DNA is assayed at various times after dilution into growth medium. The resistant bacteria remove the radioactive alkylated groups from the DNA, while the drug remains attached to the DNA of the sensitive organism. Furthermore hydrolysis of the DNA of the resistant and sensitive cells and subsequent chromatography of the hydrolysis products demonstrates that the resistant cell had excised from the DNA all of the cross-linked guanine moieties and some of the monofunctionally alkylated guanines. It has also been demonstrated that mammalian cells (e.g., mouse fibroblasts and lymphoma cells) can excise the guanine-drug complexes from DNA.[18, 19] In bacteria with an unusual sensitivity to the effects of ultraviolet irradiation, there is also an increased sensitivity to nitrogen mustard.[20] These unusually sensitive bacteria have deficient repair mechanisms and cannot excise the drug-induced cross-links. Experiments with drug-resistant cells do not rule out the possibility that reactions of alkylating drugs with cellular components other than DNA contribute to their cytotoxic effect. However, the ability of an organism to become resistant by acquiring an enhanced capacity to correct the drug-induced defect on DNA is potent support for the hypothesis that this interaction is the major factor behind the cytotoxic effect.

BCNU

BCNU, 1,3-bis(2-chloroethyl)-1-nitrosourea, is one of a group of nitrosurea compounds found to be useful in the treatment of intracerebral leukemia.

$$Cl-CH_2-CH_2-NH-\overset{\overset{O}{\|}}{C}-\underset{\underset{NO}{|}}{N}-CH_2-CH_2-Cl$$

BCNU

At low concentrations BCNU inhibits the synthesis of DNA; at higher concentrations there is inhibition of de novo synthesis of purine ribonucleotides.[21] The drug is an alkylating agent,[22] and it has been demonstrated that plasmacytomas that are resistant to alkylating agents like nitrogen mustard and cyclophosphamide are also resistant to BCNU.[23] It would therefore seem that the cytotoxic effect of this drug is basically the same as that of other alkylating agents.

Other Effects of the Alkylating Drugs

The apparent parallelism between the effects of the alkylating agents and X-irradiation on biological systems has been studied. For example, both alkylating agents and X-irradiation are carcinogenic, mutagenic, teratogenic, and immunosuppressive. The biological effects of both can be diminished by cysteine, and they produce many similar toxic effects such as destruction of lymphoid tissue and bone marrow. These similarities have been reviewed extensively.[8] The various alkylating drugs differ from one another in the extent to which they produce these effects, and it is probably of little value to retain the "catch-all" concept that the alkylating drugs are radiomimetic.

The Pharmacology of the Alkylating Drugs

Administration

The principal routes of administration of the major alkylating drugs are listed in Table 10-1. Administration of these drugs is modified by their aqueous solubility, vesicant (blister-producing) properties, and the rapid rate at which chemical transformation to the active intermediate takes place. Mechlorethamine (nitrogen mustard) is soluble in water, it is rapidly activated, and it has a potent vesicant effect. The drug is provided as a sterile powder. The powder must be dissolved in sterile distilled water and immediately injected into the patient. Because the drug is a potent vesicant care should be exercised to avoid contact with the skin of the physician and the patient. Great care should also be exercised in avoiding extravasation of the drug into the tissues at the injection site. The safest way to administer the drug is to inject the fresh solution directly into the tubing of a rapidly flowing intravenous infusion. The drug is given at a dose of 0.4 mg/kg, usually

Table 10-1 **The alkylating agents**
Route of administration and some distinguishing characteristics of a selected list of alkylating agents. At high to excessive doses all of these drugs will cause severe depression of the bone marrow, gastrointestinal disturbances, alopecia, hyperuricemia, etc.

Drug	Principal route of administration	Characteristics
Mechlorethamine (nitrogen mustard, HN_2)	Intravenous	Nausea and vomiting on administration, severe vesicant effect, very rapid acting
Chlorambucil	Oral	Slow rate of conversion to carbonium ion
Melphalan	Oral	
Cyclophosphamide	Intravenous or oral	Nausea and vomiting on administration, must be metabolized by liver before it is active, produces alopecia more frequently, metabolites can produce hemorrhagic cystitis
Busulfan	Oral	Selectively myelosuppressive, used in chronic granulocytic leukemia
BCNU	Intravenous	Penetrates into the central nervous system, bone marrow depression is delayed for up to a month after administration

in a single injection. It stands to reason that this agent, which rapidly reacts with the tissue components and is not cell cycle-dependent will produce a chemical effect immediately. Therefore, a single injection can constitute a course of treatment with mechlorethamine. Evidence of cytotoxicity, however, will develop over a period of the next several days. In comparison with mechlorethamine, other more fat-soluble mustards, like chlorambucil and melphalan, can be given orally in tablet form with good absorption from the gastrointestinal tract.

Distribution and Metabolism

The distribution, metabolism, and excretion of the alkylating agents as well as many of the other anticancer drugs has been reviewed by Mandel.[24] Experiments using small animals have shown that over 90 per cent of the radioactive-labeled mechlorethamine disappears from the blood within 30 seconds following intravenous injection. Tissues near the injection site in the direction of blood flow have a somewhat higher concentration of the drug than those at a greater distance. This is not the case with agents like chlorambucil or melphalan where the electron-withdrawing action of the aromatic ring results in a slower rate of formation of the reactive carbonium ion. These drugs are distributed to distant sites before they become reactive. In some unusual cases the rapid reactivity of mechlorethamine has been exploited therapeutically by delivering the drug directly into the arteries supplying the tumor-bearing area. In the case of a tumor localized in an extremity, high local concentrations can be achieved by limb perfusion.

Heroic attempts have occasionally been made to achieve high concentrations of drug in one area of the body while sparing the bone marrow in others. For example, the blood supply to marrow-bearing areas in the lower body has been limited by means of an abdominal tourniquet during the time the chemical reaction is taking place. There is rarely a real advantage to these efforts, but they offer a unique example of a drug effect so rapid that physicians have sought to modify its toxicity by physically altering the drug's distribution. These attempts to limit marrow suppression were based on the demonstration in animals that temporary occlusion of the blood supply to tissues could prevent local cytotoxic effects.[25] One routine application of this principle is the use of a scalp tourniquet with vincristine administration. The blood supply to the scalp is occluded while the drug rapidly becomes fixed in the other tissues, thus sparing the patient embarrassing hair loss.

The cells in the center of many tumors are often poorly vascularized and not exposed to high concentrations of drugs. This situation parallels the experiment just cited, and alkylating agents would not be expected to greatly affect these cells. The problem of poor drug response in poorly vascularized tissue areas applies to all the antineoplastic drugs with the possible exception of the steroid hormones, which are sufficiently lipid soluble and have a biological half-life long enough to allow good equilibrium distribution.

A number of alkylating agents have been synthesized in an attempt to obtain a preferred localization in a particular type of tumor (e.g. melanoma) or in particular organ sites, but these efforts have not been successful. Phenylalanine mustard, for instance, was designed on the basis of the entirely rational concept that melanomas would be particularly sensitive to phenylalanine analogs, since phenylalanine is a precursor of melanin. Agents such as phenylalanine mustard have been referred to as "site-directed inhibitors." Unfortunately clinical trials have not yet shown any promise for this type of anticancer drug.

The nitrosurea compound BCNU is very lipid soluble and has been found to pass through the blood-brain barrier into cerebrospinal fluid. Experiments in mice have demonstrated that BCNU given orally is active against intracerebral L 1210 leukemia.[26] Meningeal leukemia is currently treated with radiation and intrathecal methotrexate; however, it may be that BCNU will provide an avenue for the development of cytotoxic drugs that readily distribute into the cerebrospinal fluid and do not have to be given by the intrathecal route.

One of the mustards, cyclophosphamide, is not active in the form in which it is administered; it is metabolized by the liver to one or more active alkylating agents. Cyclophosphamide is not cytotoxic to cells in culture, but serum from animals that have been given the drug and liver homogenates that have been incubated with the drug are cytotoxic.[27] There is no evidence that cyclophosphamide is less effective in patients with compromised liver function. This points out one of the interesting, although as yet unsuccessful, avenues of research in the attempt to develop an antineoplastic drug with some specificity of action. Although no great qualitative differences between neoplastic cells and normal cells exist, there are often differences in the levels of some enzyme activities. It is hoped that drugs may be developed, which, like cyclophosphamide, are not active in the administered form but may be metabolized more rapidly by neoplastic cells that have high levels of activity of enzymes capable of converting the drugs to an active form. In this way a selective killing effect would be produced.

Toxicities and Clinical Uses

The administration of mechlorethamine and cyclophosphamide is frequently accompanied by nausea and vomiting. Vomiting is apparently due to central nervous system stimulation. Administration of a phenothiazine and a barbiturate help alleviate these symptoms. As with all of the alkylating agents, severe bone-marrow depression can occur. It reaches a maximum in one to two weeks, and then function returns. A second course of mechlorethamine is not usually begun until marrow function has returned to normal. The rapid breakdown of neoplastic tissue that may occur during treatment of leukemias and some other tumors can cause hyperuricemia. In this case patients should be given allopurinol to prevent renal damage from uric acid. The use of alkylating agents is sometimes followed by amenorrhea. All the nitrogen mustards can produce central nervous system stimulation with convulsions when amounts in excess of the therapeutic doses are employed.

Therapeutic indications for the use of anticancer drugs are presented in Tables 10-2 and 10-3.[28] It is reasonable to presume from their mechanism of action that the alkylating drugs as a group would have a wide spectrum of action, and it is clear from the recommendations presented in the two tables that this is the case. The choice of one alkylating drug over another in single-drug therapy rests largely on clinical experience and is generally not subject to rational application of clear principles.

Chlorambucil produces remissions in a large percentage of lymphomas and is particularly useful in chronic lymphocytic leukemia. The cells of the lymphoid series are particularly sensi-

Table 10-2 Choice of anti-cancer drugs in disseminated or non-resectable cancers where more than 50 per cent of patients treated are responsive to therapy

(A selected list based on recommendations from *The Medical Letter.* [28])

Disease	Drugs	Per cent remissions	Prolongation of life
Leukemias			
Acute lymphoblastic	Induction: Prednisone usually combined with vincristine or 6-MP or daunorubicin or methotrextate or cyclophosphamide, cytarabine, L-asparaginase Maintenance: 6-MP, methotrexate, BCNU	90	Definite
Chronic granulocytic	Busulfan, 6-MP, melphalan, hydroxyurea, thioguanine	90	Uncertain
Chronic lymphocytic	Chlorambucil, cyclophosphamide, prednisone, cytarabine	50	Probable
Lymphomas			
Hodgkin's disease	Vinblastine, mechlorethamine, thiotepa, chlorambucil, cyclophosphamide, procarbazine, BCNU, prednisone	80	Uncertain
Lymphosarcoma	Chlorambucil, thiotepa, cyclophosphamide, prednisone, vinblastine, vincristine, BCNU	50	Uncertain
Polycythemia vera	Busulfan, chlorambucil, pipobroman	80	Uncertain
Waldenstrom's macroglobulinemia	Chlorambucil, melphalan, cyclophosphamide	60	Uncertain
Carcinomas			
Gestational choriocarcinoma	Dactinomycin, methotrexate, 6-MP, vincristine, vinblastine	75	Definite
Prostate	Estrogens, progestins, adrenal steroids	70	Definite

Table 10-3 **Choice of anticancer drugs in disseminated or non-resectable cancers where less than 50 per cent of patients are responsive to therapy**
(A selected list based on recommendations from *The Medical Letter.* [28])

Disease	Drugs	Per cent remissions	Prolongation of life
Acute myeloblastic leukemia	Induction: Cytarabine, thioguanine, vincristine, daunorubicin, 6-MP, L-asparaginase, methotrexate, prednisone, cyclophosphamide Maintenance: 6-MP	20–30	Probable
Reticulum cell sarcoma	Cyclophosphamide, vincristine, prednisone, chlorambucil, mechlorethamine	30	Uncertain
Multiple myeloma	Melphalan, cyclophosphamide, chlorambucil, prednisone	35	Uncertain
Carcinomas			
Breast			
Pre-menopausal, post-castration, or early post-menopause	5-FU; cyclophosphamide; androgens; chlorambucil; thiotepa; methotrexate; prednisone, azaribine; vincristine, vinblastine, or melphalan with or without methotrexate and progestins	20–50	Uncertain
Late post-menopause	Estrogens, 5-FU, androgens, cyclophosphamide, chlorambucil, thiotepa, prednisone, vincristine	30–40	Uncertain
Ovary	Thiotepa with melphalan; chlorambucil; cyclophosphamide; 5-FU; methotrexate	25–40	Uncertain
Uterus			
Body	Progestins, 5-FU, cyclophosphamide	25	Uncertain
Cervix	Thiotepa, methotrexate, 5-FU, vinblastine	5	Uncertain
Testis	Dactinomycin with methotrexate and chlorambucil; vincristine; mithramycin	30–40	Uncertain

(Table 10-3 continued on p. 286)

Table 10-3 (continued)

Disease	Drugs	Per cent remissions	Prolongation of life
Carcinomas			
Adrenal cortex	Mitotane	25	Uncertain
Lung	Mechlorethamine, cyclo-phosphamide, chlorambucil, methotrexate, 5-FU, vin-cristine	5	Uncertain
Stomach	5-FU, thiotepa	10	Uncertain
Large bowel	5-FU	20	Uncertain
Pancreas	5-FU	10	Uncertain
Head and neck	Mechlorethamine, metho-trexate, vinblastine, cyclophosphamide	15	Uncertain
Melanoma	Imidazole carboxamide, vin-blastine, vincristine, BCNU, thiotepa, chlorambucil, melphalan, hydroxyurea	5–15	Uncertain
Sarcomas			
Wilms' tumor	Dactinomycin, vincristine, an alkylating agent	30-40	Definite
Neuroblastoma	Cyclophosphamide, dauno-rubicin, vincristine, prednisone	40	Probable
Rhabdomyo-sarcoma	Thiotepa, dactinomycin, cyclophosphamide, vin-cristine, methotrexate	5–30	Uncertain

tive to chlorambucil in comparison with most of the other alkylating agents. The drug is taken orally and causes nausea and vomiting in only a few patients.

Cyclophosphamide is said to produce less thrombocytopenia than other alkylating agents, but it produces alopecia more frequently.[29] The metabolites of cyclophosphamide are excreted into the urine and can cause a hemorrhagic cystitis.[30] Patients receiving this drug should be kept on a high fluid output. Nausea and vomiting frequently occur regardless of whether the drug is administered orally or intravenously. It is not a vesicant, and local thrombophlebitis does not occur. Cyclophosphamide is used in the treatment of a wide variety of neoplastic diseases and is particularly helpful in treating the leukemias and lymphomas, a group of neoplasms that generally respond better to chemotherapy than do other tumors.

Busulfan (a methane sulfonic acid ester) preferentially depresses cells of the granulocyte series over lymphocytes. For this reason it is used in the treatment of chronic granulocytic leukemia. The fact that it spares lymphocyte function is of special value, since patients with chronic granulocytic leukemia are often treated on a continuous basis for several years. The drug increases pigmentation of the skin, and in some patients a diffuse interstitial pulmonary fibrosis has been reported. The cause of this is not clear. Amenorrhoea is frequently seen.

As previously mentioned, BCNU has the advantage over other alkylating agents of passing into the central nervous system. It is thus of value in treating central nervous system involvement in leukemia and may prove useful with tumors of central nervous system origin. This drug is quite toxic to the hematopoietic system, the liver, and the kidneys. The suppression of peripheral leukocyte count occurs after a delay of three to four weeks, and the leukopenia lasts an additional two to three weeks.[31] The delay occurs regardless of the dose.

The Antimetabolites (Folic Acid Analogs)

Mechanism of Action

Methotrexate (amethopterin) is a structural analog of folic acid. The chemistry, mechanism of action, and pharmacology of the folate antagonists have been discussed in a symposium entitled *Folate Antagonists as Chemotherapeutic Agents*.[32] The cell receptor for methotrexate is the enzyme folate reductase. This enzyme directs the conversion of folic acid (FA) to dihydrofolic acid (FH_2) and tetrahydrofolic acid (FH_4). Only the tetrahydrofolic acid can be converted into the coenzymes necessary for one-carbon transfer reactions in the cell (Figure 10-6). The drug binds very tightly to folate reductase. Apparently the binding causes a considerable conformational change in the enzyme, as the drug-bound enzyme

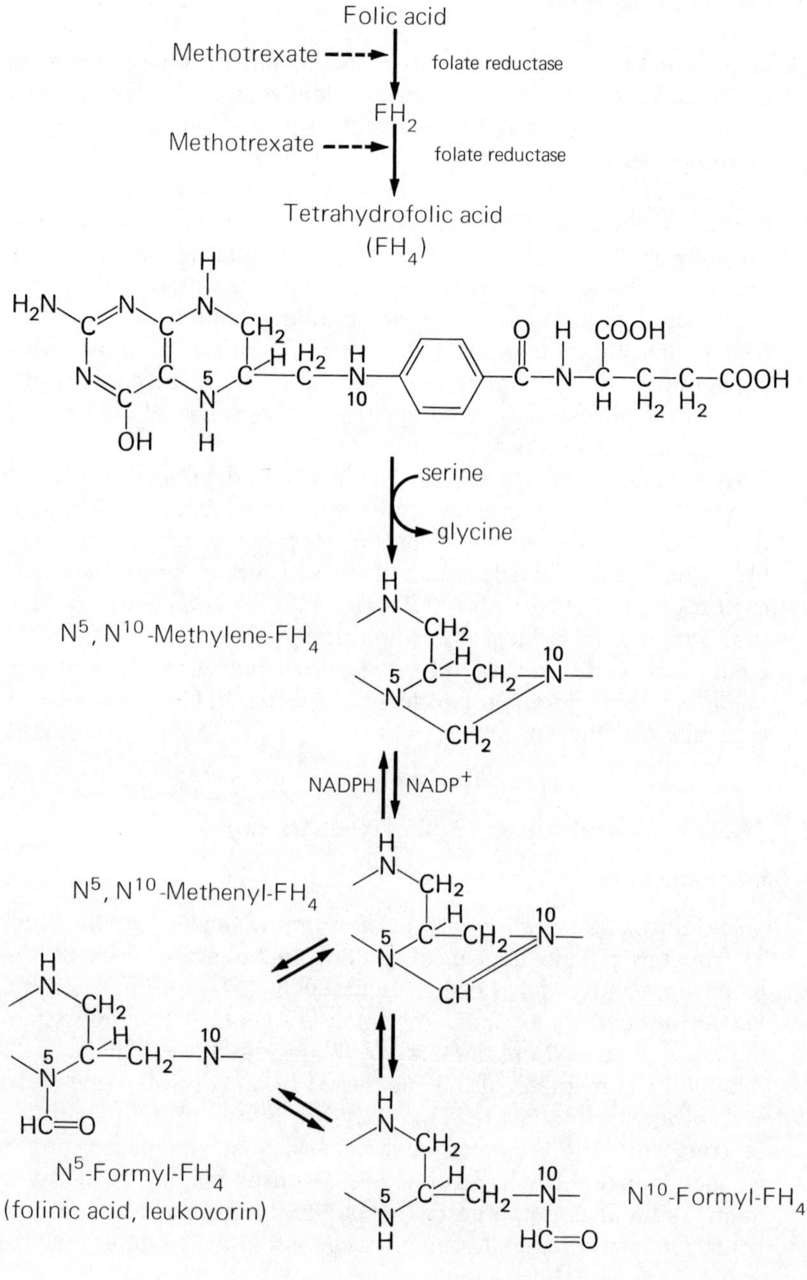

Folic acid

Methotrexate ----→ | folate reductase

FH_2

Methotrexate ----→ | folate reductase

Tetrahydrofolic acid
(FH_4)

serine

glycine

N^5, N^{10}-Methylene-FH_4

NADPH ⇅ $NADP^+$

N^5, N^{10}-Methenyl-FH_4

N^5-Formyl-FH_4
(folinic acid, leukovorin)

N^{10}-Formyl-FH_4

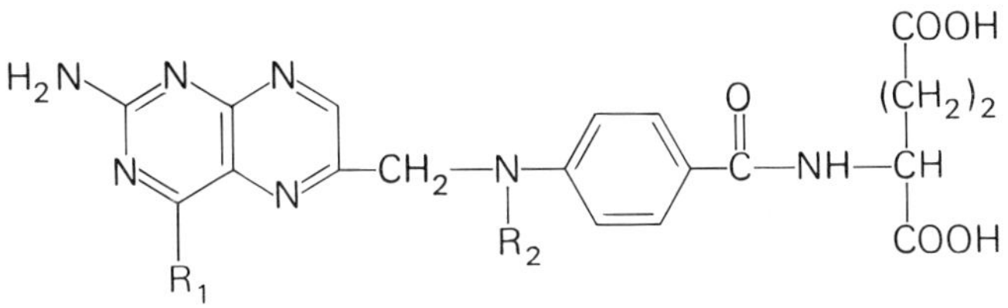

	R_1	R_2
Folic acid	OH	H
Methotrexate	NH_2	CH_3

is stabilized to digestion by proteolytic enzymes.[33] The binding is not covalent, but the dissociation constant for the drug-enzyme complex is several orders of magnitude lower than that for the folic acid-enzyme complex.[34] This means that the drug effect cannot be reversed by folic acid, and, as dissociation of the drug from its receptor does not readily take place, the drug has a long period of action. It has been shown, for example, that methotrexate remains in the liver and kidney of man for weeks.[35]

Inhibition of the conversion of folic acid to FH_4 inhibits the synthesis of thymidine and the purines, both of which are required for the synthesis of DNA. As diagrammed in Figure 10-10, thymidine monophosphate is synthesized by transfer of a methyl group from N^5,N^{10}-methylene FH_4 to deoxyuridine monophosphate under the direction of the enzyme thymidylate synthetase. In addition, carbon atoms 2 and 8 of the purine structure also are derived from reduced forms of the coenzyme. The reactions involved in the synthesis of the purines and the sites of inhibition by the antimetabolites are shown in Figure 10-8. In addition to the inhibition of synthesis nucleic acid precursors, the biosynthesis of serine is also inhibited and the drug effect can be reversed in cell culture by adding serine, thymidine, and hypoxanthine. A number of studies suggest that the primary effect that leads to cell death after treatment with methotrexate is inhibition of thymidylate synthesis.[36,37] This effect may be analogous to

Figure 10-6 The tetrahydrofolic acid coenzymes. The dashed arrows indicate reactions inhibited by methotrexate.

the well-known phenomenon of thymineless death in bacteria. Why mammalian cells die after blockade of thymidylate synthesis is not known.

There are two ways thymidylate synthesis could be blocked by methotrexate. The first is indirect—by inhibiting the synthesis of the necessary tetrahydrofolate coenzyme. This is clearly the most important mechanism. There is also some evidence that the drug may inhibit thymidylate synthetase directly by competing for the folate-coenzyme site on the enzyme.[38]

Because the binding between methotrexate and folate reductase is so tight, folic acid cannot reverse the effect of the drug; but if folic acid is given with the drug both will compete for the site, and the effect of the drug will be diminished. If cells are exposed to methotrexate and folinic acid (N^5-formyl FH_4), a compound that is able to participate in one-carbon transfer (Figure 10-6), then a much better competitive protection from the effects of the drug can be obtained. This observation has received some clinical application. If mice with experimental leukemia are exposed to high doses of methotrexate and then are given folinic acid 12 hours later, the 60-day survival rates are better than with the drug alone.[39] This delayed use of folinic acid is called "rescue." The theory behind the procedure is the following. As the leukemia cells are replicating rapidly, a large number pass into S phase during the 12-hour treatment, and a good drug effect is seen in the short exposure time at high dose levels. Some marrow cells are not replicating as rapidly as the neoplastic cells and will not pass through S phase during the period of therapy. If these cells are provided with folinic acid after a short period of time, they will survive. In essence the technique takes advantage of the different generation times and the different proportions of a cell population in the cell cycle between the neoplastic cells and the marrow cells. Thus by administering a compound that bypasses the drug-blocked reaction a short time after methotrexate administration, the therapeutic index is improved. In other words, for each course of treatment the ratio of neoplastic cell kill to normal cell kill is increased. Surprisingly, this procedure seems to work in some cases not only with experimental animal tumors but also in the treatment of some neoplasms in humans.[40]

Drug Resistance

Resistance to cytotoxic drugs develops in certain transplanted tumors in experimental animals by a process of mutation and selection as in bacteria.[41] A number of different mechanisms of resistance to methotrexate have been described. One such mechanism is selection of cells possessing an altered dihydrofolate reductase with a decreased affinity for amethopterin.[42] Folate compounds are actively transported into a number of cell types, and there is preliminary evidence that drug-sensitive human leukemia cells actively take up more methotrexate than do cells isolated from some patients who have had a poor clinical response to the drug.[43] It has been shown that two methotrexate-resistant sublines of sarcoma 180 cells have a high level of folate reductase activity.[44] One subline is 67-fold resistant and the other 174-fold resistant; they were found to contain 65 times and 155 times more folic acid reductase than the sensitive strains. As the kinetic characteristics of the sensitive and resistant enzymes were identical, it is clear that resistance to the drug arose as a result of the production of an increased amount of the drug receptor, folic acid reductase.

An increase in the amount of enzyme protein may result from an increased rate of synthesis or a decreased rate of degradation. In this respect it is interesting to note that in cultured cells exposed to submaximal concentrations of methotrexate, the total amount of enzyme protein increases with time.[45] This increase is secondary to the fact that the drug-bound enzyme is stabilized from degradation. The increase in amount of enzyme protein is not accompanied by an increase of enzyme activity, as the drug-bound enzyme is not functional at physiological pH.

Pharmacology

Methotrexate is given by the oral, intravenous, intra-arterial, or intrathecal route. The plasma levels achieved after administration of the drug at 0.1 mg/kg, a dose routinely employed in clinical practice, are equivalent regardless of whether the drug is given orally or intravenously. At higher doses, however, the efficiency of oral absorption diminishes.[46] The drug is probably absorbed from the small intestine in the same manner as folate. At low doses uptake of folate appears to be by active transport, but at high doses the transport mechanism becomes saturated, and absorption becomes diffusion limited. The drug is 50 per cent bound to plasma proteins. Methotrexate penetrates the blood-brain barrier very poorly, and it must be given by the intrathecal route for neoplastic involvement of the central nervous system. From 54 to 88 per cent of an intravenous or a small oral dose is excreted unchanged in the urine during the first 24 hours.[46] Accordingly, great caution must be exercised when the drug is given to patients with impaired renal function. As the drug is bound strongly by the folic acid reductase enzyme in tissue, it will persist for weeks in tissues like the liver and kidney. This results in a pattern of excretion that has two phases: a period of immediate rapid excretion of the unmetabolized free drug and then a period during which 1 to 2 per cent of the retained drug is excreted per day, largely in the form of metabolites.[47]

The toxic effects of methotrexate are primarily those expected with cytotoxic drugs. Bone-marrow depression must be carefully followed. To obtain the best therapeutic response in leukemia it is often necessary to give the drug at levels that greatly depress bone-marrow function. Ulceration of the mucous membrane of the mouth and gastrointestinal tract occur frequently. This is accompanied by vomiting, diarrhea, and abdominal pain. Alopecia, changes in skin pigmentation, and photosensitivity occur as well as impairment of liver function (occasionally hepatic fibrosis in children).

Methotrexate is particularly useful in the treatment of choriocarcinoma and of acute lymphoblastic leukemia in children. In addition to its use in neoplastic disease, the drug has been used to treat severe psoriasis (a condition in which there is a rapid proliferation of the cells of the skin).[48] Methotrexate is an immunosuppressive agent. It is not yet clear if it is of value in the treatment of immune diseases such as systemic lupus erythematosis.[49]

Purine Analogs

Structures and "Lethal Synthesis"

6-Mercaptopurine (6-MP) and 6-thioguanine are sulfhydryl-substituted analogs of purine bases. They are converted in the cell to nucleotides, in which form they are active as inhibitors of purine synthesis. The conversion of the inactive drug to the active nucleotide is called "lethal synthesis." There are two mechanisms

6-Mercaptopurine   **6-Thioquanine**
(6-MP)

Azathioprine

by which lethal synthesis can take place. The first mechanism (Type 1, Figure 10-7) involves the direct conversion of purine analogs to nucleotides by a nucleotide pyrophosphorylase.[50] This is called the salvage pathway. The second mechanism (Type 2, Figure 10-7) applies to pyrimidine analogs, which will be discussed in the next section of this chapter.

If a drug must be converted to an active form in the cell, then one might predict that resistance to the drug could arise by a mutation which decreases or abolishes the activity of the converting enzyme system, provided, of course, that such a change was compatible with continued cell viability. This has proved to

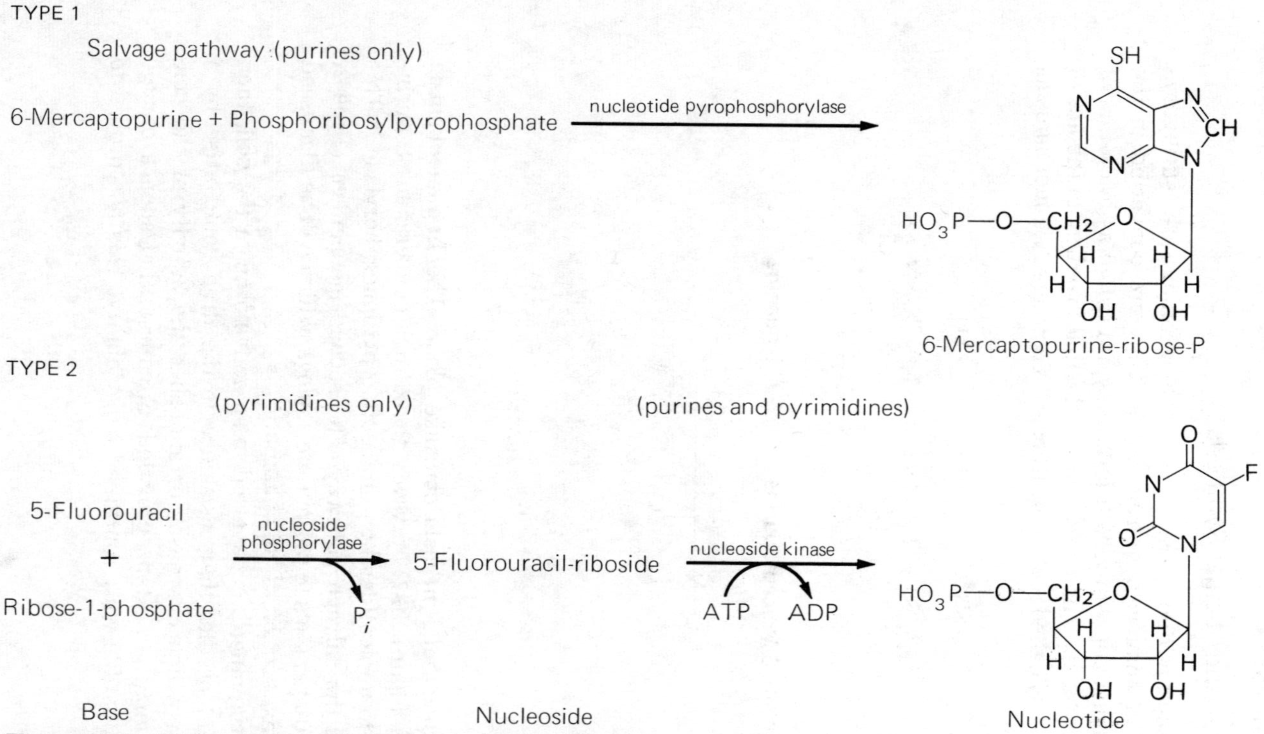

Figure 10-7 Lethal synthesis in animal cells—the conversion of purine and pyrimidine analogs to nucleotides. The purines are converted directly to their nucleotides by a reaction directed by a nucleotide pyrophosphorylase (Type 1). The pyrimidines cannot utilize this pathway, and they are converted to their nucleotides by a two-step mechanism (Type 2) in which the pentose is added first and the nucleoside is phosphorylated. There is no purine nucleoside phosphorylase in mammalian cells, but there are purine nucleoside kinases, so some purine nucleosides, like methylmercaptopurine riboside, can be phosphorylated by the second reaction in Type 2.

be the case with some cell lines and tumors that are resistant to 6-mercaptopurine.[51,52] The loss of this enzyme function is not lethal since the principal route of purine biosynthesis de novo involves an entirely different pathway (see Figure 10-8) and the salvage pathway can be eliminated without injuring the cell. The compound 6-methylmercaptopurine ribonucleoside (6-MMPR) is taken into mammalian cells and phosphorylated by a kinase, probably adenosine kinase, as in the second mechanism (Type 2, Figure 10-7).[53] The resulting nucleotide is a potent inhibitor of purine synthesis. Resistance to 6-MP resulting from a deficiency of nucleotide pyrophosphorylase can thus be circumvented with 6-MMPR, a drug analog which utilizes a different type of lethal synthesis.

Mechanism of Action

6-Mercaptopurine-riboside-phosphate (6-MPRP, thioinosine monophosphate) is a structural analog of inosine monophosphate, the common precursor of both adenylic acid and guanylic acid (Figure 10-9). It interacts with a number of enzymes active in purine metabolism, it inhibits NAD synthesis, and it interferes with coeyzyme A function.[54] Inhibition of three reactions is responsible for reducing the production of purines in the cell and the consequent inhibition of nucleic acid synthesis. 6-MPRP inhibits the conversions of inosinic acid to adenylosuccinic acid[55] and xanthylic acid,[56] thus preventing the synthesis of adenylic acid and guanylic acid (Figure 10-9). Studies with partially purified inosinate dehydrogenase demonstrate that inhibition occurs at the substrate site of the enzyme, and these studies also support the hypothesis that the drug reacts covalently at the IMP site.[57] A third site of inhibition of purine synthesis occurs at the first reaction presented in Figure 10-8. The amidotransferase that catalyzes the transfer of an amino group to 5-phosphoribosyl-1-pyrophosphate is a regulatory enzyme that is inhibited by the products of the purine synthetic pathway. Thus, when the concentration of the adenosine and guanosine phosphates rise in the cell they interact with a regulatory site on the enzyme and thereby decrease the rate of purine synthesis. 6-

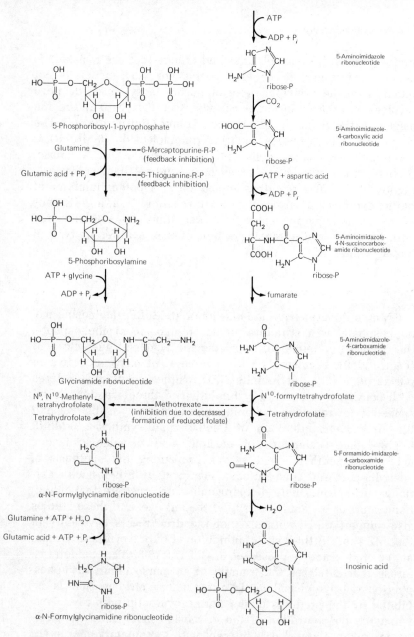

Figure 10-8 Purine synthesis. The dashed arrows indicate reactions inhibited by 6-mercaptopurine ribose-P and 6-thioguanine ribose-P and reactions inhibited as a result of methotrexate blockade of reduced folate production.

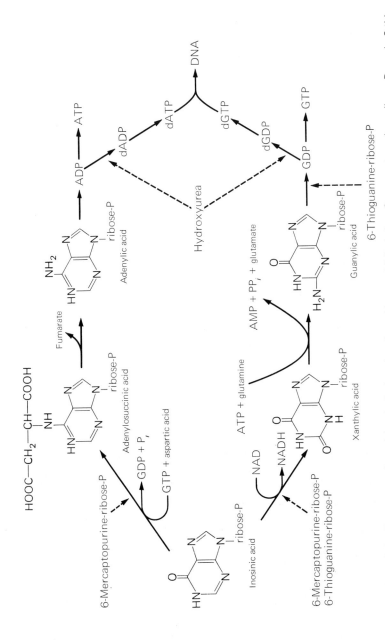

Figure 10-9 The conversion of inosinate to adenylic acid and guanylic acid. The dashed arrows indicate reactions inhibited by 6-mercaptopurine ribose-P and 6-thioguanine ribose-P.

MPRP is able to bind to this regulatory site and function as a "pseudo-feedback inhibitor" of purine biosynthesis.[58] The most potent pseudo-feedback inhibitor of the amidotransferase is 6-methyl-mercaptopurine nucleotide, the analog of 6-MP that follows a different pathway of lethal synthesis and is cytotoxic for certain 6-MP–resistant tumors.[59]

The ribonucleotide derivative of 6-thioguanine, another purine analog used in cancer chemotherapy, also inhibits inosinate dehydrogenase[56] and acts as a pseudo-feedback inhibitor of the amidotransferase.[58] In addition, 6-thioGMP competitively inhibits guanylate kinase, the enzyme that phosphorylates GMP to GDP.[60] Although small amounts of 6-thioguanine become incorporated into DNA, this does not appear to contribute significantly to the cytotoxic effect. 6-MP apparently is not incorporated into DNA.

A number of studies have demonstrated differences in the levels of anabolic and catabolic enzymes of purine metabolism between different tumor types and between tumor cells and normal cells. The differences observed may explain why 6-MP is selectively toxic to some types of tumors. For example, sarcoma 180 cells are quite sensitive to 6-MP. It has been demonstrated that the livers of host mice have twice the capacity for conversion of inosinic acid to adenylic acid (Figure 10-9) than 6-MP sensitive sarcoma 180 cells in the same animal.[61] The drug's inhibition of this conversion in the tumor could reduce the tumor's enzymatic activity below the level required for growth, while a similar reduction in the liver might not cause serious deficiency because of the organ's greater capacity to produce adenine derivatives. This hypothesis brings up the general concept that quantitative differences in the composition of tumor cells and normal cells may occasionally facilitate the selective toxicity of cytotoxic drugs.

Differences in levels of drug catabolizing activity between tumors and host cells may also on occasion contribute to the selective toxicity. For example, a number of tumors have low levels of activity of xanthine oxidase, an enzyme that catabolizes 6-MP to biologically inactive compounds.[54] Cells lacking this activity might be more sensitive to 6-MP, as indicated by the fact that the antitumor activity of 6-MP is potentiated by allopurinol, a purine analog that inhibits xanthine oxidase.[62] It has already been mentioned that allopurinol is used to lower serum uric acid levels resulting from degradation of tumor nucleic acids and release of purines following cytotoxic drug therapy. Allopurinol prevents the conversion of xanthine, which is quite soluble, to uric acid, which is less soluble and tends to precipitate in the kidney tubules. The administration of allopurinol will increase not only the antitumor effect of 6-MP but its systemic toxicity as well. Thus when allopurinol and 6-MP are given concomitantly to patients with leukemia, the dose of 6-MP must be greatly reduced.

Pharmacology

6-Mercaptopurine is usually given orally. About 50 per cent of the drug is absorbed from the gastrointestinal tract.[63] 6-MP is distributed widely in the body tissues, and studies with the radioactive-labeled drug demonstrate that it penetrates the blood-brain barrier. The level achieved in the spinal fluid is about one-twentieth of that in the blood, and about one-third of the amount in the spinal fluid is in the unchanged form.[64] Among several routes of drug metabolism, the chief one is by the enzyme xanthine oxidase to 6-thiouric acid. The principal route of drug excretion is by glomerular filtration in the kidney. The excreted forms include the unchanged drug, thiouric acid, and methylated and desulfurated metabolites. After intravenous administration the half-life of 6-MP in the blood is about ninety minutes. The half-life is considerably longer when the drug is given orally.

The principal toxic effect of 6-MP is bone-marrow depression. Gastrointestinal disturbances and oral ulceration are uncommon. Reports indicate that some people receiving 6-MP may develop jaundice and other evidence of liver damage. As this complication has been seen in patients without leukemia who have received the drug,[65] it seems reasonable to presume that it is drug related. The mechanism is unknown. 6-Mercaptotopurine is used alone to maintain remissions in both acute lymphoblastic and acute myeloblastic leukemia and in combination with other drugs to induce remissions. In addition, it is of value in the treatment of chronic myelocytic leukemia that is refractory to busulfan. The purine analogs depress the immune response. Azathioprine (Imuran ®), a somewhat less toxic drug than 6-MP, is being used to prevent transplant rejection and to treat immune diseases like rheumatoid arthritis and lupus erythematosis.

Pyrimidine Analogs

Fluorouracil

5-Fluorouracil (FU) is a fluorine-substituted analog of uracil, which was synthesized for the specific purpose of inhibiting the enzyme thymidylate synthetase and thereby stopping the cellular synthesis of thymidine. The van der Waals radius of the fluorine substituent (1.35 Å) is close to that of the hydrogen (1.20 Å) in uracil so that FU is a close structural analog of the natural base. The chemical reactivity of the molecule is altered as the carbon-fluorine bond is less susceptible to enzymatic cleavage.

Uracil   **5-Fluorouracil**

FU is not active as a cytotoxic agent until it has been changed in the cell to fluorouracil-ribose-phosphate (Figure 10-7) and subsequently reduced to 5-fluoro-2'-deoxyuridine-5'-monophosphate (FUdRP). The investigational drug 5-fluorouracil-2'-deoxyuridine (FUdR), which has a generally greater antitumor effect than FU, needs only to be phosphorylated before becoming an effective growth inhibitor. The mechanism of action of the pyrimidine analogs has been reviewed by Heidelberger, whose laboratory provided this example of the rational development of a cytotoxic drug.[66]

The addition of FUdR to cells in culture results in an inhibition of DNA synthesis with no immediate effect on RNA synthesis.[67] The inhibition of growth and DNA synthesis is prevented by thymidine. The principal receptor for the drug is thymidylate synthetase

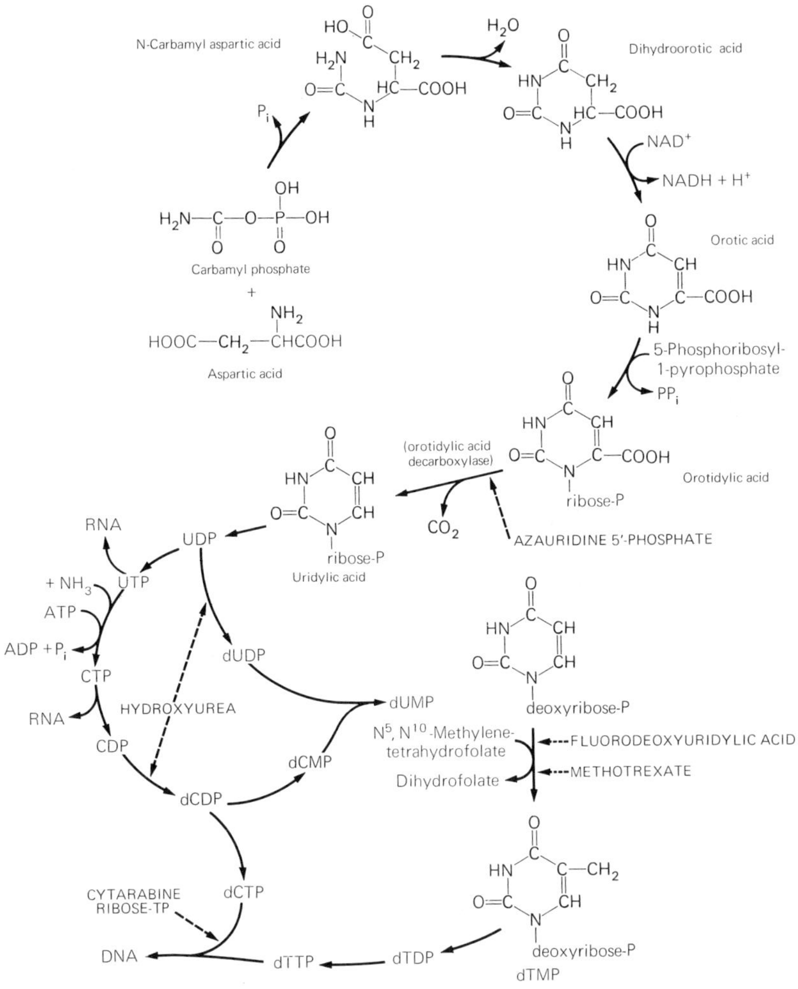

Figure 10-10 Pyrimidine synthesis. The dashed arrows indicate sites of drug inhibition.

(Figure 10-10), the enzyme that directs the transfer and reduction of a methylene group from reduced folic acid to deoxyuridine monophosphate to form thymidylic acid and FAH_2 [68] FUdRP inhibits the reaction in a manner that is reversible and competitive with the substrate deoxyuridine monophosphate. FUdRP is not itself a substrate for the enzyme. The enzyme's affinity for the drug is much greater than its affinity for the normal substrate.

The inhibition of thymidylate synthetase is clearly the major event responsible for the cytotoxic effect of FU and FUdR. It has been demonstrated that in some drug-resistant tumor cells the enzyme is altered; it readily converts uridylic acid to thymidylic acid and is inhibited only by high concentrations of FUdRP.[69] FU is incorporated into cellular RNA but not into DNA. The incorporation of the halogenated base into RNA may contribute to the toxicity of this compound.

Fluorouracil is given intravenously, as its absorption from the gastrointestinal tract is irregular and incomplete. The same amount of drug is less toxic when given by slow intravenous infusion than by a single intravenous injection. FU is distributed in the total body water. It is degraded by most tissues in man, but the liver is probably the main site of degradation. FU is converted to the dihydro-derivative, and the ring is split to form α-fluoro-β-guanidopropionic acid and α-fluoro-β-ureidopropionic acid, which in turn are catabolized to α-fluoro-β-alanine, urea, and CO_2.[70] The metabolites are excreted in the urine and as respiratory CO_2. Some mouse tumors, like sarcoma 180, do not readily degrade FU, a fact that may explain the selectivity of the drug action against these tumors.[71] When given directly to cells in culture, FUdR is much more potent than FU, probably because it is a more immediate precursor of FUdRP, the active form of the drug. When administered to man, however, FU and FUdR are essentially equipotent, because FUdR is rapidly degraded to FU in the body.

Fluorouracil is a very toxic drug. The usual earliest signs of toxicity are nausea, vomiting, stomatitis, and diarrhea. The drug can cause severe bone-marrow depression. Alopecia and hyperpigmentation are seen in about 10 per cent of patients. Great caution is necessary in patients with compromised hepatic function since the liver is a major site of metabolism. The administration of this drug, as with so many of the cytotoxic agents, is a difficult procedure requiring specialized experience on the part of the physician and close patient supervision.

Fluorouracil has produced clinical responses in a wide variety of solid tumors. It is most useful in the treatment of advanced carcinomas of the breast, ovary, uterus, and gastrointestinal tract. Remissions are achieved in from 5 to 50 per cent of patients, depending on the tumor type (Table 10-3).

6-Azauridine

6-Azauridine is an analog of uridine with a nitrogen subsituted for a carbon atom at position 6 of the ring. In the cell azauridine is phosphorylated to azauridine-5'-monophosphate a compound that competitively inhibits the enzyme orotidylic acid decarboxylase

Uridine   6-Azauridine

and thus blocks pyrimidine synthesis.[72] The site of action in the pathway of pyrimidine synthesis is shown in Figure 10-10.

When azauridine is given orally to man it is partly converted by microorganisms in the gut to azauracil, which is neurotoxic (its main toxic effects are lethargy and electroencephalographic changes). Accordingly, it is administered orally as the triacetyl derivative, azaribine, which is well absorbed and is converted to azauridine in the body. Azauridine does not pass into the central nervous system as azauracil does. The drug is distributed rapidly into most of the body water and is excreted by tubular secretion. This drug is surprisingly nontoxic in man. The most important toxic effect is anemia without severe leukopenia or thrombocytopenia. The anemia is readily reversible on cessation of therapy. Except for the treatment of mycosis fungoides, a condition often classified

as one of the lymphoma group of diseases, azaribine is not particularly useful in cancer chemotherapy. Although there is a high
incidence of malignant lymphoma associated with mycosis fungoides, it is probably not a cancer. Severe psoriasis also responds
well to treatment with azaribine.[73]

Cytarabine

Cytarabine (cytosine arabinoside) is a pyrimidine in which the
orientation of the hydroxyl group on the 2 carbon of the sugar is
reversed from that of cytidine; thus it becomes an analog of 2'-
deoxycytidine. In cell culture cytarabine inhibits DNA virus replication (see Chapter 9) as well as the growth of a variety of mammalian cells. It inhibits DNA synthesis while permitting RNA and
protein synthesis to continue for long periods. This effect is competed for, and at an early point it is reversed by, deoxycytidine.

Cytidine   **Cytarabine**

Cytarabine's precise mechanism of action is not yet completely
clear. It was first hypothesized that the phosphorylated form
of the drug inhibited the reduction of ribonucleosides to deoxyribonucleosides.[74] Nucleotides of arabinosylcytosine, however,
were found to be only weak inhibitors of the reduction reaction,
and this effect probably does not contribute greatly to the observed inhibition of DNA synthesis.[75] The triphosphorylated drug,
ara-CTP, is incorporated to a slight extent into DNA,[76] but there is
no correlation between the extent of incorporation and the degree

of lethality.[77] Ara-CTP competitively inhibits the polymerization of the natural nucleotide (deoxycytidine triphosphate) into DNA by mammalian DNA polymerase preparations.[77,78] At present this competitive inhibition of DNA synthesis at the polymerase level is the most plausible model for the mechanism of action of cytarabine. It is worth mentioning again that we do not know why inhibition of DNA synthesis is lethal to cells that are synthesizing DNA when the block is introduced. Although the means by which the S phase-specific drugs like cytarabine and fluorouracil inhibit DNA synthesis may be known, this does not constitute a complete understanding of the mechanism of the cytotoxic effect.

Cytarabine is given intravenously, by injection or by continuous infusion. There is no evidence that one method is better than the other. It is not active when taken orally. The drug is rapidly deaminated by cytidine deaminase in the liver and kidney.[79] The deaminated product, uracil arabinoside, is inactive and accounts for approximately 90 per cent of the drug eliminated in the urine. As the primary site of metabolism is the liver, the drug should be used at reduced dosage in patients with poor hepatic function.

Cytarabine exerts its primary toxic effects on the bone marrow (marrow depression, leukopenia, thrombocytopenia, and anemia with megaloblastosis) and the gastrointestinal tract (vomiting, diarrhea, and stomatitis).[80] The drug is primarily used for induction of remission in acute granulocytic and acute lymphocytic leukemias (Tables 10-2 and 10-3).

Antibiotics

Dactinomycin, Daunorubicin, and Mithramycin

Dactinomycin (actinomycin D), daunorubicin (daunomycin), and mithramycin are antibiotics that were isolated from different species of *Streptomyces* and found to have antitumor activity. Actinomycin D has proved a very useful tool in molecular biology. Its mechanism of action is understood in greater detail than that of daunorubicin or mithramycin, and it is used more widely clinically.

Dactinomycin
(actinomycin D)

Actinomycin D is composed of a phenoxazone ring system (the chromophore residue) and two identical cyclic polypeptides. In low concentrations the drug inhibits DNA-directed RNA synthesis.[81] At higher concentrations DNA synthesis is also inhibited. The receptor for actinomycin D is double-stranded DNA. The drug does not bind to RNA, and at concentrations that completely inhibit host cell RNA synthesis it does not inhibit the growth of RNA viruses like Mengovirus.[82] RNA viruses that replicate by producing a DNA that serves as a template for further RNA synthesis (e.g. Rous sarcoma virus) are inhibited by actinomycin D. Studies of the association of actinomycin D to synthetic

DNA duplexes demonstrate that deoxyguanosine is essential for binding to take place.[83] This is consonant with the observation that the transcription of ribosomal RNA, which is relatively rich in G-C pairs, is more sensitive to inhibition by actinomycin D than the rest of the RNA. The binding of actinomycin D to DNA is very tight. It is clear that actinomycin D intercalates between the base pairs in DNA. This has been demonstrated by spectroscopic, hydrodynamic, and kinetic studies[84] and by the observation that actinomycin D, like other known intercalating compounds, can unwind supercoiled, closed, circular DNA.[85]

The spectral changes that accompany the addition of deoxyguanosine to actinomycin in solution are similar to those that accompany the binding of the drug to DNA.[86] Thus it is possible to study the nature of the drug receptor interaction by X-ray diffraction analysis of co-crystallized complexes of actinomycin and deoxyguanosine.[87] These studies show that actinomycin D is a symmetrical molecule stabilized by two hydrogen bonds between the two valine residues in the cyclic pentapeptide side chains (see Figure 10-11).[88] The two cyclic polypeptide side chains lie in one axis with the planar chromophore region protruding on an axis almost perpendicular to them. In the complex of actinomycin D and deoxyguanosine (also illustrated in Figure 10-11), the chromophore lies between the two deoxyguanosine molecules. The guanine specificity for actinomycin binding is clearly determined by the two strong hydrogen bonds between the 2-amino-group of guanine and the carbonyl oxygen of the threonine residues in the polypeptide side chains.

In Figure 10-12, the actinomycin D and deoxyguanosine complex is shown from a different angle to demonstrate the spatial relationship between the chromophore ring system and the two guanine residues arranged as they would be oriented in opposite strands of the DNA double helix.[89] In this model the chromophore ring is intercalated between two G-C pairs, and the polypeptide units of actinomycin lie in the narrow groove of the DNA helix. One physical characteristic that distinguishes actinomycin D from its biologically inactive analogs is the very slow DNA-drug dissociation reaction. This tight binding is accounted for by the two intermolecular hydrogen bonds shown in Figure 10–11, two weaker

Actinomycin D

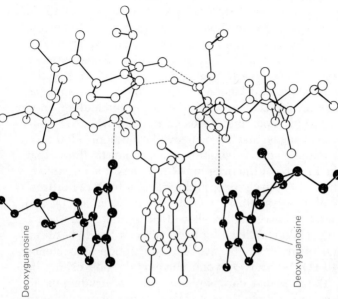

Actinomycin-deoxyguanosine complex

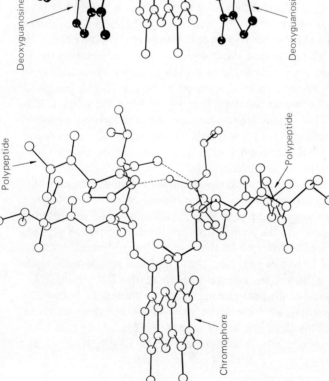

Figure 10-11 The structure of actinomycin D and an illustration of the actinomycin-deoxyguanosine complex. The twofold symmetry of the drug and the stabilizing hydrogen bonds (----) between the peptide side chains may be noted. In the actinomycin D-deoxyguanosine complex the two deoxy-guanosine molecules (•–•) stack on alternate sides of the chromophore ring. Strong hydrogen bonds (----) connect the 2-amino group of each guanosine with the carbonyl oxygen of the L-threonine residues in the polypeptide side chain. (Redrawn from Sobell *et al.*[88])

hydrogen bonds between the guanine N-3 and the N-H group on the threonines (shown in Figure 10-12 but not in Figure 10-11), numerous van der Waals contacts with both sugar-phosphate chains, and the planar interactions between the purine rings and the chromophore. This complex of the drug with the DNA template blocks the transcription of RNA by DNA-dependent RNA polymerase, which in turn is responsible for the cytotoxic effect.

Daunorubicin is an anthracine derivative that also interacts with DNA by intercalation[85] to inhibit RNA synthesis.[90] The nature of the interaction between daunorubicin and DNA and the effects of the drug on cell metabolism have not been worked out in the

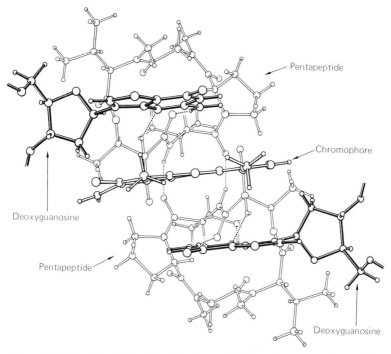

Pentapeptide

Chromophore

Deoxyguanosine

Pentapeptide

Deoxyguanosine

Figure 10-12 The relationship of actinomycin D to deoxyguanosine residues as they are oriented in opposite strands of the DNA double helix. Deoxyguanosine moieties are defined by the structures with the solid bonds; the actinomycin D by the structure with the open bonds. The region of actinomycin D defined by the bolder lines is the chromophore ring system protruding toward the observer. (Adapted from Sobell and Jain.[89])

same detail as have those of actinomycin D. In fact it is not entirely clear that the inhibition of nucleic acid synthesis is chiefly responsible for the cytotoxic effect.[91]

Mithramycin binds to DNA and inhibits RNA synthesis.[92] As with actinomycin D, guanine is required for the formation of the drug-DNA complex,[90] but mithramycin does not intercalate between the DNA bases.[85]

The oral absorption of actinomycin D is poor, and it must be administered intravenously. Daunorubicin and mithramycin are also given intravenously. Actinomycin D is an extremely irritating substance, and, as with some of the alkylating agents, local extravasation can produce a severe, prolonged reaction. It is therefore given by injection into the tubing of a rapidly flowing intravenous infusion. The administration of both actinomycin D and daunorubicin is often followed by nausea and vomiting. The drug concentration in the blood rapidly declines as it becomes tightly bound in the tissues.

Actinomycin D is a very toxic compound. It severely depresses the bone marrow. Ulcerations of the oral mucosa, proctitis and symptoms of gastrointestinal irritation, and alopecia occur commonly. When actinomycin D is given, erythematous reactions and necrosis can develop in skin areas previously exposed to radiation. Daunorubicin has a similar complex of toxic effects, and, in addition, it can produce a cardiotoxicity characterized by progressive tachycardia, hypotension, and dyspnea not associated with objective signs of congestive failure.[93] It is not clear whether or not this side effect is dose related, and the mechanism is unknown. Mithramycin can cause nausea, vomiting, malaise, fever, facial flushing and swelling, stomatitis, and glossitis soon after administration. The most severe of the later toxic manifestations (which include hepatic, renal, and bone-marrow damage) is bleeding. This can take the form of a severe and fatal hemorrhagic diathesis.[94] The hemorrhage probably results from a combination of liver dysfunction, thrombocytopenia and drug-induced qualitative changes in the platelets, direct injury to the vascular bed, and possibly an increase in fibrinolytic activity.[95]

Actinomycin D is useful in the treatment of trophoblastic tumors (choriocarcinoma) and is usually administered after resistance has developed to methotrexate. Actinomycin D and mithramycin are effective in some patients with testicular carcinomas. Actinomycin D is the most effective drug in the treatment of Wilms' tumor. Despite the biochemical similarity between actinomycin D and daunorubicin, their spectrum of antitumor activity is quite different. Daunorubicin, for example, possesses significant antileukemic activity, whereas actinomycin D does not. Mithramycin is employed against embryonal cell testicular tumors. It has the unique ability of lowering serum calcium levels in both normal people and patients with hypercalcemia secondary to metastatic neoplastic disease.[96] Though the mechanism of this effect is unknown, mithramycin may prove to be a useful drug in the treatment of Paget's disease[97] and the hypercalcemia of malignancy.[98]

The Vinca Alkaloids

Vincristine and Vinblastine

Several plant alkaloids have been found to block cell division in metaphase. These compounds include colchicine, podophyllotoxin, vincristine, and vinblastine. Of these, vincristine and vinblastine, both derived from the periwinkle (Vinca rosea), have proved to be the most valuable in treating neoplastic disease.

The mechanism of action of vincristine and vinblastine is not well understood in biochemical terms; however, some observations have been made that seem to define the cellular events affected by these drugs. At low concentrations vincristine and vinblastine arrest cell division in metaphase.[99] Studies on cells in culture indicate that vinblastine does not affect the phases of the cell cycle other than mitosis.[100] It has been demonstrated that vinblastine causes a reversible disruption of the mitotic spindle.[101] The spindle fibers are long strands, composed of bundles of microtubules connecting the two centrioles in the dividing cell; some spindle fibers connect the kinetochores of the chromosomes to the centrioles (Figure 10-13). The spindle fibers direct the appropriate segregation of the sister chromatids to opposite poles during anaphase. In telophase the microtubules disappear when the nuclear envelope forms.

	R
Vincristine	CHO
Vinblastine	CH_3

The observation that vinca alkaloids disrupt these microtubules has prompted a number of investigations on this process. When intact cells are exposed to low concentrations of vinblastine or vincristine, crystals of microtubular protein are formed and are readily visualized by electron microscopy.[102] The addition of vinblastine to high speed supernatants prepared from cell homogenates precipitates microtubular protein out of solution.[103] This precipitation probably does not result from a specific drug-receptor interaction, since other acidic structural proteins are also precipitated out of solution by vinblastine.[104] The association of colchicine with microtubular protein is apparently specific for its antimitotic activity,[105] but there is as yet no evidence that the binding of vinblastine or vincristine is specific (their sites of

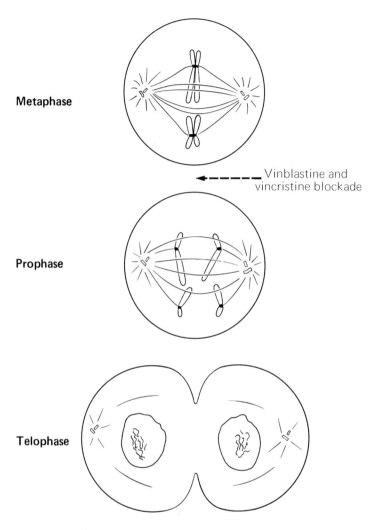

Metaphase

Vinblastine and
vincristine blockade

Prophase

Telophase

Figure 10-13 Diagrammatic representation of the mitotic spindle. Metaphase:
the sister chromatids of each chromosome are connected to the opposite poles
by spindle fibers (microtubules; prophase: the chromatids are separated; telophase: the spindle fibers dissolve with formation of the nuclear membrane. The
dashed arrow indicates that vinblastine and vincristine block mitosis at metaphase.

interaction differ from that of colchicine[106]). Nevertheless, it seems reasonable to predict that the microtubules are the cellular receptors involved in the antimitotic action of vinca alkaloid drugs. In addition to causing metaphase arrest the vinca alkaloids at higher concentrations inhibit the incorporation of uridine into RNA.[107,108] This is not a result of mitotic inhibition,[109] since, at these high levels, these drugs also cause dissolution of the nuclei, precipitation of intracellular material, and cell death.

Because of their unpredictable oral absorption, vincristine and vinblastine are administered intravenously. They are irritating substances, and extravasation during administration can cause cellulitis. Nausea and vomiting occasionally follow the administration of these drugs. The drugs are rapidly cleared from the blood as they are taken up by the tissues. Because the primary route of excretion is apparently in the bile, they must be employed with caution in patients with obstructive liver disease.

Despite their similarity in structure and mechanism of action, vincristine and vinblastine differ somewhat in their spectra of antitumor activity and the nature of their toxicity. Vincristine, for example, is very effective in inducing remission in acute leukemias while vinblastine is not. The reverse is true in Hodgkin's disease where vinblastine is more effective. Both drugs are used in the treatment of a variety of neoplasms (see Tables 10-2 and 10-3) and are often given in combination with other cytotoxic agents. As they produce metaphase arrest, it is possible that cell populations are partially synchronized by exposure to these drugs, and that a subsequent exposure to S phase-inhibiting agents might be enhanced.

Vinblastine and vincristine suppress the bone marrow and produce gastrointestinal disturbances and alopecia; they are both neurotoxic. Vinblastine is much more toxic to the marrow than vincristine, and vincristine is much more neurotoxic than vinblastine. Why vinblastine has a greater bone-marrow depressant effect is not known; however, this is the drug's major clinical toxicity. The chief limitation to vincristine therapy is a neurological toxicity characterized by parasthesias, muscle weakness, foot drop, loss of deep tendon reflexes in the lower extremities, neuritic pain, headache, vocal cord paralysis, ptosis, and diplopia. This neurotoxicity is usually reversed when the drug is withdrawn.

It is perhaps not surprising that the vinca alkaloids are neurotoxic; nerve cells constitute one of the richest sources of microtubular proteins. The neurotubule (microtubule) is a structural element of the neuron and may participate in the rapid movement of substances along the axon. In addition to neurotubules, neurons contain other fiber-like structures called neurofilaments. In human central and peripheral neurons exposed to vincristine disordered arrays of neurofibrillar structure ("neurofibrillary tangles") appear,[110] and microtubule-drug crystals form.[111] These changes are accompanied by axonal degeneration and myelin loss. Experiments in rabbits show that with vinblastine the changes are reversible on withdrawal of the drug, but with vincristine they seem to persist.[112] After systemic administration, the vinca alkaloids inhibit the incorporation of uridine into RNA by mouse brain.[113] The effect of vincristine is greater than vinblastine. It may be that vincristine, which is less charged than vinblastine, is more neurotoxic because it can pass through the blood-brain barrier somewhat more easily.

Miscellaneous Anticancer Drugs

Hydroxyurea

Hydroxyurea is an antitumor agent of simple structure that causes a relatively specific inhibition of DNA synthesis without inhibiting the incorporation of radioactive precursors into RNA or protein.[114] It kills cells that are synthesizing DNA at the time of exposure. Cells in other phases of growth survive, but they are prevented from entering the phase of DNA synthesis.[115] The drug does not affect the DNA polymerase reaction or the phosphoryla-

$$H_2N-\overset{\overset{\text{O}}{\|}}{C}-NH-OH$$

Hydroxyurea

tion of nucleotide precursors of DNA. It does cause a marked reduction in the soluble pool of deoxyribonucleotides without affecting the size of the ribonucleotide pools.[116] By an unknown mechanism, hydroxyurea inhibits the ribonucleotide reductase reaction (the conversion of ribonucleotides to deoxyribonucleotides).[117] The addition of deoxyribonucleosides to cells exposed to hydroxyurea can partially reverse the drug-induced inhibition of thymidine incorporation into DNA,[118] but this is not always the case.[114] At present the best evidence indicates that the biochemical locus of action of hydroxyurea is the ribonucleotide reductase reaction. The data, however, are not yet definitive, and there may be other effects that contribute to the cytotoxicity of this compound.

Hydroxyurea is well absorbed from the gastrointestinal tract. Peak plasma concentrations are achieved within 2 hours, and the drug is barely detectable in the serum after 24 hours. The route of excretion is renal, and about 80 per cent of the drug is eliminated in the urine in the first 12 hours.[119] The primary adverse reaction is bone-marrow depression. Less frequently, gastrointestinal symptoms, rashes, and alopecia develop. The principal indication for hydroxyurea is in the treatment of busulfan-resistant, chronic granulocytic leukemia.[120] Significant tumor response has also been reported for melanoma.

Procarbazine

Procarbazine, a methyl hydrazine derivative, is effective in inhibiting the growth of a number of experimental leukemias. The mechanism of action of this drug is unknown. Clearly one of its effects is to produce single-strand breaks in DNA. Though this has not been shown to cause the growth inhibitory effect of the drug, it may very well explain procarbazine's radiosensitization effect.

$$CH_3-NH-NH-CH_2- \bigcirc -CONH-CH \Big\langle {}^{CH_3}_{CH_3}$$

Procarbazine

Like some of the halogenated pyrimidines, procarbazine potenttiates the cytocidal effects of X-irradiation. It may do so by inhibiting the ability of the cells to repair the X-ray–induced DNA strand breakage.[121] Procarbazine is well absorbed after oral administration. The drug is excreted by the kidney as an oxidation product, N-isopropylterephthalamic acid.[122] The most common toxic effects are bonemarrow depression, nausea, vomiting, and anorexia. Procarbazine is an inhibitor of monoamine oxidase, and it potentiates the action of the phenothiazine group of tranquilizers. It appears to be incompatible with alcohol. When the two drugs are given together, intense flushing and malaise (as seen with alcohol and disulfiram) may follow. Like other hydrazines, procarbazine can produce a hemolytic anemia with hemoglobin denaturation and the formation of Heinz bodies in the erythrocytes. The drug is most often employed in the treatment of Hodgkin's disease that has become refractory to other agents.[123]

Pipobroman

Pipobroman is a derivative of piperazine that produces bonemarrow hypoplasia. Its mechanism of action is unknown. Pipobroman has a very limited application; it is almost solely restricted to the treatment of polycythemia vera,[124] though busulfan and chlorambucil are preferred agents. The toxic effects include bonemarrow depression with anemia and leukopenia. Pipobroman causes nausea, vomiting, abdominal cramping, diarrhea, and skin rashes.

Mitotane

Mitotane (o,p'-dichlorodiphenyldichloroethane) is an isomer of the insecticide DDD, which damages the cells of the adrenal cortex. The mechanism of this selective attack is unknown, but mitotane has been used with some success in the treatment of inoperable adrenal cortical carcinoma.[125] The drug is given orally, and it can produce nausea, vomiting, skin eruptions, diarrhea, mental depression, and muscle tremors.

L-Asparaginase

The literature on L-asparaginase was reviewed by Cooney and Handschumacher in 1970.[126] The use of this enzyme in the treatment of leukemia developed from the observation that guinea pig serum suppressed the growth of lymphosarcoma cells in mice.[127] It was subsequently demonstrated that the suppressive effect of the guinea pig serum was due to the presence of L-asparaginase, an enzyme that hydrolyzes L-asparagine to L-aspartic acid.[128] This enzyme has been shown to decrease the levels of L-asparagine in the blood.[129] Certain cancer cells have a nutritional requirement for L-asparagine, which results from a lower level of asparagine synthetase activity in the sensitive tumor cells than in other cell types. The sensitivity of experimental tumors to L-asparaginase is inversely correlated with the ability of the tumor cells to synthesize L-asparagine.[130] Resistant cells selected from sensitive-cell populations have an increased ability to synthesize asparagine.[131] Thus the application of this enzyme in cancer chemotherapy exploits a unique biochemical difference between certain neoplastic cells and normal cells to permit a selective therapeutic effect.

As expected, deprivation of L-asparagine inhibits the rate of protein synthesis early.[132] Nucleic acid synthesis is depressed later. The depression of protein synthesis is presumably a direct result of the limitation of availability of an essential substrate, L-asparagine. Deprivation of this amino acid, however, is followed by other biochemical changes in cells, like an increase in ribonuclease activity,[133] and the sequence of biochemical events responsible for the therapeutic effect has not been completely worked out.

Not all L-asparaginase preparations have effective antitumor activity. Two L-asparaginase enzymes are produced by *E. coli,* for example, and only one is active.[134] It is the principal source of the L-asparaginase used therapeutically. This enzyme has a molecular weight of approximately 140,000 daltons and is composed of several subunits.[135] It is administered intravenously and has a half-life in the plasma that is quite variable (reports range from eight to thirty hours[136]). The *E. coli* enzyme without antitumor activity is cleared from the plasma more rapidly than the active preparation.[137]

About 40 per cent of patients treated with L-asparaginase experience nausea, vomiting, and fever.[138] Acute hypersensitivity reactions, including respiratory distress, occur occasionally. The incidence of hypersensitivity reactions with repeated injection of L-asparaginase (a foreign protein) has not been as high as anticipated. Precipitating antibodies to the enzyme have been found in man.[139] Treatment with L-asparaginase can cause anorexia, impaired liver function, decreased serum albumin and cholesterol, azotemia, pancreatitis, bone-marrow depression, impaired renal function, and central nervous system dysfunction.

L-Asparaginase is used clinically to induce remission in acute leukemia. The best response rate has been achieved in acute lymphocytic leukemia.[139] The response rate for acute myelocytic leukemia is less than 20 per cent. The durations of unmaintained remissions are short, and maintenance therapy is continued with other agents.

Steroid Hormones

One way the rate of growth of specific cell populations in the body is controlled is by the growth-stimulating and growth-inhibiting action of hormones. The use of the glucocorticoids, the progestins, and the sex steroids in tumor therapy is a therapeutic application of the normal effects of these hormones on target cells. The steroid hormones are more selective than other anticancer drugs, because they act almost solely on those cells that, by virtue of their specific differentiation, contain receptors that are unique for these hormones.

It is fortunate that many tumors of target tissues retain their capacity to respond to the steroids. Androgens, which often have growth-inhibitory effects on cells that are stimulated to grow by the estrogens, have proved useful in the treatment of cancer of the breast. Similarly, the estrogens and progestins are growth inhibitory in carcinoma of the prostate, a target tissue for the androgens. The estrogens are also effective in treating carcinoma of the breast in late post-menopausal patients; however, they may stimulate the growth of breast tumors in pre-menopausal and early post-menopausal patients. The progestins produce temporary clinical remissions in about one-fourth of patients with carcinoma of the endometrium. The glucocorticoid steroids have an anti-anabolic effect on a variety of cell types such as lymphocytes and fibroblasts. This action is exploited therapeutically to induce remissions in acute lymphocytic leukemia. In addition to their therapeutic effects, the toxic effects of the steroids are for the most part an expression of target tissue response to prolonged high levels of these hormones.

References

1. R. Baserga: The relationship of the cell cycle to tumor growth and control of cell division: A review. *Cancer Res.* 25:581 (1965).

2. G. C. Mueller: The $G_1 \rightarrow S$ conversion: A target for cancer chemotherapy. *Cancer Res.* 29:2394 (1969).

3. C. W. Young and J. H. Burchenal: Cancer chemotherapy. *Ann. Rev. Pharmacol.* 11:369 (1971).

4. A. F. Hermens and G. W. Barendsen: Changes of cell proliferation characteristics in a rat rhabdomyosarcoma before and after X-irradiation. *Europ. J. Cancer* 5:173 (1969).

5. E. B. Krumbhaar and H. D. Krumbhaar: The blood and bone marrow in yellow cross gas (mustard gas) poisoning: changes produced in the bone marrow of fatal cases. *J. Med. Res.* 40:497 (1919).

6. A. Gilman: The initial clinical trial of nitrogen mustard. *Am. J. Surg.* 105:574 (1963).

7. D. R. Krieg: Ethyl methanesulfonate-induced reversion of bacteriophage T_4 rII mutants. *Genetics* 48:561 (1963).

8. M. Ochoa and E. Hirschberg: "Alkylating agents" in *Experimental Chemotherapy*, Vol. 5. ed. by R. J. Schnitzer and F. Hawking. New York: Academic Press, 1967, pp. 1–132.

9. H. B. Brewer, J. P. Comstock, and L. Aronow: Effects of nitrogen mustard on protein and nucleic acid synthesis in mouse fibroblasts growing *in vitro*. *Biochem. Pharmacol.* 8:281 (1961).

10. B. A. Booth, W. A. Creasey, and A. S. Sartorelli: Alterations in cellular metabolism associated with cell death induced by uracil mustard and 6-thioguanine. *Proc. Natl. Acad. Sci.* 52:1396 (1964).

11. P. D. Lawley and P. Brookes: Molecular mechanisms of the cytotoxic action of difunctional alkylating agents and of resistance to this action. *Nature* 206:480 (1965).

12. E. P. Geiduschek: Reversible DNA. *Proc. Natl. Acad. Sci. U.S.* 47:950 (1961).

13. K. W. Kohn, C. L. Spears, and P. Doty: Interstrand cross-linking of DNA by nitrogen mustard. *J. Mol. Biol.* 19:266 (1966).

14. P. D. Lawley and P. Brookes: Interstrand cross-linking of DNA by difunctional alkylating agents. *J. Mol. Biol.* 25:143 (1967).

15. P. D. Lawley, J. H. Lethbridge, P. A. Edwards, and K. V. Shooter: Inactivation of bacteriophage T$_7$ by mono- and difunctional sulfur mustards in relation to cross-linking and depurination of bacteriophage DNA. *J. Mol. Biol.* 39:181 (1969).

16 M. K. Wolpert and R. W. Ruddon: A study on the mechanism of resistance to nitrogen mustard (HN$_2$) in Ehrlich ascites tumor cells: Comparison of uptake of HN$_2$-^{14}C into sensitive and resistant cells. *Cancer Res.* 29:873 (1969).

17. R. B. Setlow and W. L. Carrier: The disappearance of thymine dimers from DNA: An error-correcting mechanism. *Proc. Natl. Acad. Sci. U.S.* 51:226 (1964).

18. A. R. Crathorn and J. J. Roberts: Mechanism of the cytotoxic action of alkylating agents in mammalian cells and evidence for the removal of alkylated groups from deoxyribonucleic acid. *Nature* 211:150 (1966).

19. B. D. Reid and I. G. Walker: The response of mammalian cells to alkylating agents. II. On the mechanism of the removal of sulfur-mustard-induced cross-links. *Biochim. Biophys. Acta* 179:179 (1969).

20. K. W. Kohn, N. H. Steigbigel, and C. L. Spears: Cross-linking and repair of DNA in sensitive and resistant strains of *E. coli* treated with nitrogen mustard. *Proc. Natl. Acad. Sci. U.S.* 53:1154 (1965).

21. G. P. Wheeler and B. J. Bowdon: Some effects of 1,3-bis (2-chloroethyl)-1 nitrosurea upon the synthesis of protein and nucleic acids *in vivo* and *in vitro*. *Cancer Res.* 25:1770 (1965).

22. G. P. Wheeler and S. Chumley: Alkylating activity of 1,3-bis (2-chloroethyl)-1-nitrosourea and related compounds. *J. Med. Chem.* 10:259 (1967).

23. G. P. Wheeler and J. A. Alexander: Studies with mustards. VI. Effects of alkylating agents upon nucleic acid synthesis in bilaterally grown sensitive and resistant tumors. *Cancer Res.* 24:1338 (1964).

24. H. G. Mandel: The physiologic disposition of some anticancer agents. *Pharm. Rev.* 11:743 (1959).

25. D. A. Karnofsky, I. Graef, and H. W. Smith: Studies on the mechanism of action of the nitrogen and sulfur mustards *in vivo*. *Am. J. Path.* 24:275 (1958).

26. F. M. Schabel, T. P. Johnston, G. S. McCaleb, J. A. Montgomery, W. R. Laster, and H. E. Skipper: Experimental evaluation of potential anticancer agents. VIII. Effects of certain nitrosoureas on intracerebral L1210 leukemia. *Cancer Res.* 23:725 (1963).

27. G. E. Foley, O. M. Friedman and B. P. Drolet: Studies on the mechanism of action of cytoxan: Evidence of activation *in vivo* and *in vitro*. *Cancer Res.* 21:57 (1961).

28. Choice of anti-cancer drugs in disseminated or non-resectable neoplastic disease. *Med. Letter Reference Handbook.* pp. 36–37 (1971).

29. T. C. Hall: Pharmacologic studies of cyclophosphamide (NSC-26271) and its congener phosphoramide mustard (NSC-69945). *Cancer Chemother. Rep.* 51:335 (1967).

30. F. S. Philips, S. S. Sternberg, A. P. Cronin, and P. M. Vidal: Cyclophosphamide and urinary bladder toxicity. *Cancer Res.* 21:1577 (1961).

31. V. T. DeVita, P. P. Carbone, A. H. Owens, G. L. Gold, M. J. Krant, and J. Edmonson: Clinical trials with 1,3-bis (2-chloroethyl)-1-nitrosourea, NSC-409962. *Cancer Res.* 25:1876 (1965).

32. J. R. Bertino (ed.) "Folate Antagonists as Chemotherapeutic Agents" *Ann. N.Y. Acad. Sci.* vol. 186 (1971).

33. M. T. Hakala and E. M. Suolinna: Specific protection of folate reductase against chemical and proteolytic inactivation. *Mol. Pharmacol.* 2:465 (1966).

34. W. C. Werkheiser: Specific binding of 4-amino folic acid analogues to folic acid reductase. *J. Biol. Chem.* 236:888 (1961).

35. S. Charache, P. T. Condit, and S. R. Humphreys: Studies on the folic acid vitamins. IV. The persistence of amethopterin in mammalian tissues. *Cancer* 13:236 (1960).

36. R. R. Rueckert and G. C. Mueller: Studies on unbalanced growth in tissue culture. I. Induction and consequences of thymidine deficiency. *Cancer Res.* 20:1584 (1960).

37. J. Borsa and G. F. Whitamore: Cell killing studies on the mode of action of methotrexate on L-cells *in vitro*. *Cancer Res.* 29:737 (1969).

38. J. Borsa and G. F. Whitamore: Studies relating to the mode of action of methotrexate. III. Inhibition of thymidylate synthetase in tissue culture cells and in cell-free systems. *Mol. Pharmacol.* 5:318 (1969).

39. A. Goldin, J. M. Venditti, I. Kline, and N. Mantel: Eradication of leukaemic cells (L 1210) by methotrexate and methotrexate plus citrovorum factor. *Nature* 212:1548 (1966).

40. R. L. Capizzi, R. C. De Conti, J. C. Marsh, and J. R. Bertino: Methotrexate therapy of head and neck cancer: Improvement in therapeutic index by the use of leucovorin "rescue." *Cancer Res.* 30:1782 (1970).

41. L. W. Law: Origin of the resistance of leukaemic cells to folic acid antagonists. *Nature* 169:628 (1952).

42. F. M. Sirotnak, G. J. Donati, and D. J. Hutchison: Genetic modification of the structure and amount of dihydrofolate reductase in amethopterin-resistant *Diplococcus pneumoniae*. *J. Biol. Chem.* 239:4298 (1964).

43. D. Kessel, T. C. Hall, and D. Roberts: Modes of uptake of methotrexate by normal and leukemic human leukocytes *in vitro* and their relation to drug response. *Cancer Res.* 28:564 (1968).

44. M. T. Hakala, S. F. Zakrzewski, and C. A. Nichol: Relation of folic acid reductase to amethopterin resistance in cultured mammalian cells. *J. Biol. Chem.* 236:952 (1961).

45. B. L. Hillcoat, V. Swett, and J. R. Bertino: Increase in dihydrofolate reductase activity in cultured mammalian cells after exposure to methotrexate. *Proc. Natl. Acad. Sci. U.S.* 58:1632 (1967).

46. E. S. Henderson. R. H. Adamson, and V. T. Oliverio: The metabolic fate of tritiated methotrexate. II. Absorption and excretion in man. *Cancer Res.* 25:1018 (1965).

47. D. G. Johns, J. W. Hollingsworth, A. R. Cashmore, I. H. Plenderleith, and J. R. Bertino: Methotrexate displacement in man. *J. Clin. Invest.* 43:621 (1964).

48. R. B. Rees, J. H. Bennett, H. I. Maibach, and H. L. Arnold: Methotrexate for psoriasis. *Arch. Dermatol.* 95:2 (1967).

49. M. A. Swanson and R. S. Schwartz: Immunosuppressive therapy. *New Eng. J. Med.* 277:163 (1967).

50. J. L. Way and R. E. Parks: Enzymatic synthesis of 5'-phosphate nucleotides of purine analogues. *J. Biol. Chem.* 231:467 (1958).

51. S. Tomizawa and L. Aronow: Studies on drug resistance in mammalian cells. II. 6-mercaptopurine resistance in mouse fibroblasts. *J. Pharm. Exptl. Ther.* 128:107 (1960).

52. R. W. Brockman: Resistance to purine antagonists in experimental leukemia systems. *Cancer Res.* 25:1596 (1965).

53. L. L. Bennett, R. W. Brockman, H. P. Schnebli, S. Chumley, G. J. Dixon, F. M. Schabel, E. A. Dulmadge, H. E. Skipper, J. A. Montgomery, and H. J. Thomas: Activity and mechanism of action of 6-methylthiopurine ribonucleoside in cancer cells resistant to 6-mercaptopurine. *Nature* 205:1276 (1965).

54. G. B. Elion and G. H. Hitchings: Metabolic basis for the actions of analogs of purines and pyrimidines. *Advances in Chemother.* 2:91 (1965).

55. J. S. Salser, D. J. Hutchison, and M. E. Balis: Studies on the mechanism of action of 6-mercaptopurine in cell-free preparations. *J. Biol. Chem.* 235:429 (1960).

56. A. Hampton: Reactions of ribonucleotide derivatives of purine analogues at the catalytic site of inosine 5'-phosphate dehydrogenase. *J. Biol. Chem.* 238:3068 (1963).

57. A. Hampton and A. Nomura: Iosine 5'-phosphate dehydrogenase. Site of inhibition by guanosine 5'-phosphate and of inactivation by 6-chloro- and 6-mercaptopurine ribonucleoside 5'-phosphates. *Biochemistry* 6:679 (1967).

58. R. J. McCollister, W. R. Gilbert, D. M. Ashton, and J. B. Wyngaarden: Pseudofeedback inhibition of purine synthesis by 6-mercaptopurine ribonucleotide and other purine analogues. *J. Biol. Chem.* 239:1560 (1964).

59. D. L. Hill and L. L. Bennett: Purification and properties of 5' phosphoribosyl pyrophosphate amidotransferase from adenocarcinoma 755 cells. *Biochemistry* 8:122 (1969).

60. R. P. Miech, R. York, and R. E. Parks: Adenosine triphosphate-guanosine 5'-phosphate phosphotransferase. II. Inhibition by 6-thioguanosine 5'-phosphate of the enzyme isolated from hog brain and sarcoma 180 ascites cells. *Mol. Pharmacol.* 5:30 (1969).

61. J. S. Salser and M. E. Balis: The mechanism of action of 6-mercaptopurine. II. Basis for specificity. *Cancer Res.* 25:544 (1965).

62. G. B. Elion: Actions of purine analogs: Enzyme specificity studies as a basis for interpretation and design. Cancer Res. 29:2448 (1969).

63. T. L. Loo, J. K. Luce, M. P. Sullivan, and E. Frei: Clinical pharmacologic observations on 6-mercaptopurine and 6-methylthiopurine ribonucleoside. Clin. Pharm. Ther. 9:180 (1968).

64. L. Hamilton and G. B. Elion: The fate of 6-mercaptopurine in man. Ann. N.Y. Acad. Sci. 60:304 (1954).

65. J. Shorey, S. Schenker, W. N. Suki and B. Combes: Hepatotoxicity of mercaptopurine. Arch. Int. Med. 122:54 (1968).

66. C. Heidelberger: Cancer chemotherapy with purine and pyrimidine analogues. Ann. Rev. Pharmacol. 7:101 (1967).

67. L. Cheong, M. A. Rich, and M. L. Edinoff: Mechanism of growth inhibition of H.Ep.#1 cells by 5-fluorodeoxycytidine and 5-fluorodeoxyuridine. Cancer Res. 20:1602 (1960).

68. K-U. Hartman and C. Heidelberger: Studies on fluorinated pyrimidines. XIII. Inhibition of thymidylate synthetase. J. Biol. Chem. 236:3006 (1961).

69. C. Heidelberger, G. Kaldor, K. L. Mukherjee, and P. B. Danneberg: Studies on fluorinated pyrimidines. XI. In vitro studies on tumor resistance. Cancer Res. 20:903 (1960).

70. K. L. Mukherjee and C. Heidelberger: Studies on fluorinated pyrimidines. IX. The degradation of 5-fluorouracil-6-C[14]. J. Biol. Chem. 235:433 (1960).

71. N. K. Chaudhuri, K. L. Mukherjee, and C. Heidelberger: Studies on fluorinated pyrimidines. VII. The degradative pathway. Biochem. Pharmacol. 1:328 (1958).

72. R. W. Handschumacher: Orotidylic acid decarboxylase: Inhibition studies with azauridine 5'-phosphate. J. Biol. Chem. 235:2917 (1960).

73. P. Calabresi and R. W. Turner: Beneficial effects of triacetylazauridine in psoriasis and mycosis fungoides: Ann. Int. Med. 64:352 (1966).

74. M. Y. Chu and G. A. Fisher: A proposed mechanism of action of 1-β-D-arabinofuranosylcytosine as an inhibitor of the growth of leukemic cells. Biochem. Pharmacol. 11:423 (1962).

75. E. C. Moore and S. S. Cohen: Effects of arabinonucleotides on ribonucleotide reduction by an enzyme system from rat tumor. J. Biol. Chem. 242:2116 (1967).

76. M. Y. Chu and G. A. Fisher: The incorporation of ^{3}H-cytosine arabinoside and its effect on murine leukemic cells (L5178 Y). Biochem. Pharmacol. 17:753 (1968).

77. F. L. Graham and G. F. Whitamore: Studies in mouse L-cells on the incorporation of 1-β-D-arabinofuranosylcytosine into DNA and on inhibition of DNA polymerase by 1-β-D-arabinofuranosylcytosine-5'-triphosphate. Cancer Res. 30:2636 (1970).

78. J. J. Furth and S. S. Cohen: Inhibition of mammalian DNA polymerase by the 5'-triphosphate of 1-β-D-arabinofuranosylcytosine and the

5'-triphosphate of 9-β-D-arabinofuranosyladenine. *Cancer Res.* 28:2061 (1968).

79. W. A. Creasy, R. J. Papac, M. E. Markiw, P. Calabresi, and A. D. Welch: Biochemical and pharmacological studies with 1-β-D-arabinofuranosylcytosine in man. *Biochem. Pharmacol.* 15:1417 (1966).

80. Cytarabine (Cytosar). *Clin. Pharm. Ther.* 11:155 (1970).

81. E. Reich, R. M. Franklin, A. J. Shatkin, and E. L. Tatum: Effect of actinomycin D on cellular nucleic acid synthesis and virus production. *Science* 134:556 (1961).

82. E. Reich, R. M. Franklin, A. J. Shatkin, and E. L. Tatum: Action of actinomycin D on animal cells and viruses. *Proc. Natl. Acad. Sci. U.S.* 48:1238 (1962).

83. I. H. Goldberg, M. Rabinowitz and E. Reich: Basis of actinomycin action. I. DNA binding and inhibition of RNA-polymerase synthetic reactions by actinomycin. *Proc. Natl. Acad. Sci. U.S.* 48:2094 (1962).

84. W. Müller and D. M. Crothers: Studies of the binding of actinomycin and related compounds to DNA. *J. Mol. Biol.* 35:251 (1968).

85. M. Waring: Variation of the supercoils in closed circular DNA by binding of antibiotics and drugs: Evidence for molecular models involving intercalation. *J. Mol. Biol.* 54:247 (1970).

86. W. Kersten: Interaction of actinomycin C with constituents of nucleic acids. *Biochim. Biophys. Acta* 47:610 (1961).

87. H. M. Sobell, S. C. Jain, T. D. Sakore, and C. E. Nordman: Stereochemistry of actinomycin-DNA binding. *Nature* 231:200 (1971).

88. H. M. Sobell, S. C. Jain, T. D. Sakore, G. Ponticello, and C. E. Nordman: Concerning the stereochemistry of actinomycin binding to DNA: An actinomycin-deoxyguanisine crystalline complex. *Cold Spring Harbor Symp.* Vol 36, in press (1971).

89. H. M. Sobel and S. C. Jain: The stereochemistry of actinomycin binding to DNA. II. Detailed molecular model of actinomycin-DNA complex and its implications. *J. Mol. Biol.* in press (1972).

90. D. C. Ward, E. Reich, and I. H. Goldberg: Base specificity in the interaction of polynucleotides with antibiotic drugs. *Science* 149:1259 (1965).

91. R. Silvestrini, A. DiMarco, and T. Dasdia: Interference of daunomycin with metabolic events of the cell cycle in synchronized cultures of rat fibroblasts. *Cancer Res.* 30:966 (1970).

92. G. Northrop, S. G. Taylor, and R. L. Northrop: Biochemical effects of mithramycin on cultured cells. *Cancer Res.* 29:1916 (1969).

93. G. Bonadonna and S. Monfardini: Cardiac Toxicity of daunorubicin. *Lancet* 1:837 (1969).

94. J. H. Brown and B. J. Kennedy: Mithramycin in the treatment of disseminated testicular neoplasms. *New Eng. J. Med.* 272:111 (1965).

95. R. W. Monto, R. W. Talley, M. J. Caldwell, W. C. Levin, and M. M. Guest: Observations on the mechanism of hemorrhagic toxicity in mithramycin (NSC 24559) therapy. *Cancer Res.* 29:697 (1969).

96. R. Parsons, M. Baum, and M. Self: Effect of mithramycin on calcium and hydroxyproline metabolism in patients with malignant disease. *Brit. Med. J.* 1:474 (1967).

97. W. G. Ryan, T. B. Schwartz, and C. P. Perlia: Effects of mithramycin on Paget's disease of bone. *Ann. Int. Med.* 70:549 (1969).

98. C. P. Perlia, N J. Gubisch, J. Wolter, D. Edelberg, M. M. Dederick, and S. G. Taylor: Mithramycin treatment of hypercalcemia. *Cancer* 25:389 (1970).

99. C. G. Palmer, D. Livengood, A. K. Warren, P. J. Simpson, and I. S. Johnson: The action of vincaleukoblastine on mitosis *in vitro. Exptl. Cell Res.* 20:198 (1960).

100. N. Bruchovsky, A. A. Owen, A. J. Becker, and J. E. Till: Effects of vinblastine on the proliferative capacity of L cells and their progress through the division cycle. *Cancer Res.* 25:1232 (1965).

101. S. E. Malawista, H. Sato, and K. G. Bensch: Vinblastine and griseofulvin reversibly disrupt the living mitotic spindle. *Science* 160:770 (1968).

102. K. G. Bensch and S. E. Malawista: Microtubular crystals in mammalian cells. *J. Cell. Biol.* 40:95 (1969).

103. J. B. Olmsted, K. Carlson, R. Klebe, F. Ruddle, and J. Rosenbaum: Isolation of microtubule protein from cultured mouse neuroblastoma cells. *Proc. Natl. Acad. Sci., U.S.* 65:129 (1970).

104. L. Wilson, J. Bryan, A. Ruby, and D. Mazia: Precipitation of proteins by vinblastine and calcium ions. *Proc. Natl. Acad. Sci. U.S.* 66:807 (1970).

105. L. Wilson and M. Friedkin: The biochemical events of mitosis. II. The *in vivo* and *in vitro* binding of colchicine in grasshopper embryos and its possible relation to inhibition of mitosis. *Biochemistry* 6:3126 (1967).

106. L. Wilson: Properties of colchicine binding protein from chick embryo brain. Interactions with vinca alkaloids and podophyllotoxin. *Biochemistry* 9:4999 (1970).

107. W. A. Creasey and M. E. Markiw: Biochemical effects of the vinca alkaloids. II. A comparison of the effects of colchicine, vinblastine and vincristine on the synthesis of ribonucleic acids in Ehrlich ascites carcinoma cells. *Biochim. Biophys. Acta* 87:601 (1964).

108. E. K. Wagner and B. Roizman: Effect of the vinca alkaloids on RNA synthesis in human cells *in vitro. Science* 162:569 (1968).

109. P. G. W. Plagemann: Vinblastine sulfate: Metaphase arrest, inhibition of RNA synthesis, and cytotoxicity in Novikoff rat hepatoma cells. *J. Nat. Canc. Inst.* 45:589 (1970).

110. M. L. Shelanski and H. Wisniewski: Neurofibrillary degeneration. *Arch. Neurol.* 20:199 (1969).

111. W. W. Schlaepfer: Vincristine-induced axonal alterations in rat peripheral nerve. *J. Neuropathol. and Exptl. Neurol.* 30:488 (1971).

112. F. J. Seil and P. W. Lampert: Neurofibrillary tangles induced by vincristine and vinblastine sulfate in central and peripheral neurons *in vitro*. *Exptl. Neurol.* 21:219 (1968).

113. B. M. Agustin and W. A. Creasey: Vinca alkaloids and the synthesis of RNA in mouse brain. *Nature* 215:965 (1967).

114. R. D. Pollak and H. S. Rosenkranz: Metabolic effects of hydroxyurea on BHK-21 cells transformed with polyoma virus. *Cancer Res.* 27:1214 (1967).

115. W. K. Sinclair: Hydroxyurea: Differential lethal effects on cultured mammalian cells during the cell cycle. *Science* 150:1729 (1965).

116. J. Neuhard: Studies on the acid-soluble nucleotide pool in *Escherichia coli*. IV. Effects of hydroxyurea. *Biochim. Biophys. Acta* 145:1 (1967).

117. M. K. Turner, R. Abrams, and I. Lieberman: Meso-α,β-diphenylsuccinate and hydroxyurea as inhibitors of deoxycytidylate synthesis in extracts of Ehrlich ascites and L cells. *J. Biol. Chem.* 241:5777 (1966).

118. C. W. Young, G. Schochetman, and D. A. Karnofsky: Hydroxyureainduced inhibition of deoxyribonucleotide synthesis: Studies in intact cells. *Cancer Res.* 27:526 (1967).

119. B. H. Bolton, L. A. Woods, D. T. Kaung, and R. L. Lawton: A simple method of colorimetric analysis for hydroxyurea (NSC-32065). *Cancer Chemother. Rep.* 46:1 (1965).

120. B. J. Kennedy and J. W. Yarbro: Metabolic and therapeutic effects of hydroxyurea in chronic myeloid leukemia. *J.A.M.A.* 195:1038 (1966).

121. H. Moroson and M. Furlan: Single-strand breaks in DNA of Ehrlich ascites tumor cells produced by methyl hydrazine. *Radiation Res.* 40:351 (1969).

122. V. T. Oliverio, C. Denham, V. T. DeVita, and M. G. Kelly: Some pharmacologic properties of a new antitumor agent, N-isopropyl-α (2-methylhydrazino)-p-toluamide hydrochloride (NSC-77213). *Cancer Chemother. Rep.* 42:1 (1964).

123. K. W. Brunner and C. W. Young: A methylhydrazine derivative in Hodgkin's disease and other malignant neoplasms. Therapeutic and toxic effects studied in 51 patients. *Ann. Intern. Med.* 63:69 (1965).

124. R. W. Monto, A. T. Pas, J. D. Battle, R. J. Rohn, J. Louis, and N. B. Louis: A-8103 in Polycythemia. *J.A.M.A.* 190:833 (1964).

125. A. M. Hutter and D. E. Kayhoe: Adrenal cortical carcinoma. *Am. J. Med.* 41:572 (1966).

126. D. A. Cooney and R. E. Handschumacher: L-Asparaginase and L-asparagine metabolism. *Ann. Rev. Pharmacol,* 10:421 (1970).

127. J. G. Kidd: Regression of transplanted lymphomas induced *in vivo* by means of normal guinea pig serum. I. Course of transplanted cancers of various kinds in mice and rats given guinea pig serum, horse serum, or rabbit serum. *J. Exp. Med.* 98:565 (1953).

128. J. D. Broome: Evidence that the L-asparaginase of guinea pig serum is responsible for its antilymphoma effects. I. Properties of the L-aspara-

ginase of guinea pig serum in relation to those of the antilymphoma substance. *J. Exp. Med.* 118:99 (1963).

129. D. A. Cooney and R. E. Handschumacher: Investigation of L-asparagine metabolism in animals and human subjects. *Proc. Am. Assoc. Canc. Res.* 9:15 (1968).

130. B. Horowitz, B. K. Madras, A. Meister, L. J. Old, E. A. Boyse, and E. Stockert: Asparagine synthetase activity of mouse leukemias. *Science* 160:533 (1968).

131. J. D. Broome: Studies on the mechanism of tumor inhibition by L-asparaginase. Effects of the enzyme on asparagine levels in the blood, normal tissues, and 6C3HED lymphomas of mice: Differences in asparagine formation and utilization in asparaginase sensitive and resistant lymphoma cells. *J. Exp. Med.* 127:1055 (1968).

132. L. T. Mashburn and G. S. Gordon: The effects of L-asparaginase on the amino acid incorporation of mouse lymphoid tumors. *Cancer Res.* 28:961 (1968).

133. L. T. Mashburn and L. M. Landin: Changes in ribonuclease activities in P1798 lymphosarcoma after asparaginase treatment. *Arch. Biochem. Biophys.* 125:721 (1968).

134. A. Campbell, L. T. Mashburn, E. A. Boyse, and L. J. Old: Two L-asparaginases from *Escherichia coli* B. Their separation, purification, and antitumor activity. *Biochemistry* 6:721 (1967).

135. H. A. Whelan and J. C. Wriston: Purification and properties of asparaginase from *E. coli* B. *Biochemistry* 8:2386 (1969).

136. R. L. Capizzi, J. R. Bertino, and R. E. Handschumacher: L-asparaginase. *Ann. Rev. Med.* 21:433 (1970).

137. E. A. Boyse, L. J. Old, H. A. Campbell, and L. T. Mashburn: Suppression of murine leukemias by L-asparaginase. Incidence of sensitivity among leukemias of various types: Comparative inhibitory activities of guinea pig serum L-asparaginase and *Escherichia coli* L-asparaginase. *J. Exp. Med.* 125:17 (1967).

138. C. M. Haskell, G. P. Canellos, B. G. Levanthal, P. P. Carbone, A. A. Serpick, and H. H. Hansen: L-asparaginase toxicity. *Cancer Res.* 29:974 (1969).

139. H. F. Oettgen, L. J. Old, E. A. Boyse, H. A. Campbell, F. S. Philips, B. D. Clarkson, L. Tallal, R. D. Leeper, M. K. Schwartz, and J. H. Kim: Inhibition of leukemias in man by L-asparaginase. *Cancer Res.* 27:2619 (1967).

Index

p4 > when need
9 > bacteriocidal

12 - contra indic of sulfa
13 - urinary tract disturb + sulf